Breast Cancer

Society Shapes an Epidemic

Anne S. Kasper, Ph.D.,
and Susan J. Ferguson, Ph.D.

St. Martin's Press
New York

ISBN 0-312-21710-2

Portions of chapter 9 in this volume are excerpted from *Living
Downstream: An Ecologist Looks at Cancer and the Environment* by
Sandra Steingraber, copyright © 1997 by Sandra Steingraber, Ph.D.,
reprinted by permission of Perseus Books Publishers, a member of
Perseus Books, L.L.C.

Library of Congress Cataloging-in-Publication Data available from the
Library of Congress

Printed in the United States of America

Design by Acme Art, Inc.

First edition: October 2000
10 9 8 7 6 5 4 3 2 1

Contents

PART ONE

Breast Cancer Diagnoses and Treatment—The Historical Context

PART TWO

Breast Cancer as a Social Problem

• The Economics of Breast Cancer

Preface and Acknowledgments

We, the editors, have compiled this volume, *Breast Cancer: Society Shapes an Epidemic,* so that our readers better understand the ways society shapes what we know about breast cancer. Although many books have been written about this disease, and breast cancer is featured regularly on television and radio, in newspapers, magazines, and in film, there is another story to tell—one that has not yet been told. We tell that story in this book. It is the story of the often difficult to discern, yet powerful ways that the social forces that we take for granted have deeply influenced and forged women's experiences of breast cancer. The chapters in this book critically examine these social forces and clarify how research science, the health care system, the economy, and the media, for example, make breast cancer more than just another disease to be treated. Our hope is that, in reading this book, you will find new ways to think about and understand the epidemic of breast cancer and the role society has played in creating this illness.

We also would like the reader to know that the nonalphabetical listing of the editors' last names does not imply first author status or senior authorship to either editor. Both editors contributed equally to the proposed and finished manuscript. This book has required an immense collaborative effort and the creative energies of both editors to complete. Each editor brought unique talents to this project that, when combined, resulted in an unconventional and incomparable journey of writing and scholarship. This journey has taken over four years to complete, but the resulting book contributes much to our social understanding of breast cancer.

We would like to express our deep appreciation to the contributing authors, each of whom brought gifts of impressive scholarship in diverse fields that resulted in chapters rich in analysis and insight. We would like to thank all of the contributors who responded to our call for more social research on breast cancer. We also want to acknowledge our debt to the many women of the Women's Health Movement, who inspired all of us to undertake this effort as part of the Movement's continuing work to enable women to take charge of their health and their lives. Women of the breast cancer advocacy movement also have inspired us with their enormous courage and resolve, as have the millions of women who have had or are living with breast cancer.

In addition, we would like to acknowledge the labor of several individuals who helped us complete this book. First and foremost, we would like to thank our editors at St. Martin's Press, Maura Burnett and Kristi Long, for their support and publishing insights. We especially appreciate the work done by our copyeditor, Roberta P. Scheer, and by the members of the production team at St. Martin's Press. At Grinnell College, we have received excellent administrative support from faculty secretaries: Faun Black, Vicki Bunnell, Patty Dale, Karen Groves, and Linda Price. Several Grinnell College students, who have worked as research assistants for Susan Ferguson, also have contributed to this book. Michelle Brunner, Alice Gates, Jennifer McNamee, Erin White, and Carla Talarico spent innumerable hours compiling bibliographies, tracking down sources in the library, copying articles, filing, reading chapter drafts, and organizing the literature on breast cancer. We pay a special tribute to Carla Talarico, who also served as an assistant editor on the compilation of the final manuscript. Carla's adept attention to details, superb editing skills, and queries to the authors enabled us to complete this manuscript in a timely fashion. We also are grateful for the generous research support from Grinnell College.

Susan Ferguson would like to acknowledge Joel Best, series editor at Aldine de Gruyter, who first encouraged her to do a book on breast cancer in 1996. Susan's academic interest in breast cancer began several years earlier in graduate school while reading Audre Lorde's *Cancer Journals* for a seminar on feminist theory. That academic interest soon became personal when a close friend was diagnosed with breast cancer. Following Angie's cancer treatments over the next couple of years refocused Susan's political and academic energies on women's health issues. Thank you Angie, for sharing your illness journey with me. Last, but not least, Susan would like to thank her editor at Mayfield Publishing Company, Serina Beauparlant, and her dear friends Laura Burrus, Deanna Shorb, and Gretchen Stiers for their advice and unwavering support on this project.

Anne Kasper extends her thanks to Alice J. Dan, Ph.D., Director of the Center for Research on Women and Gender at the University of Illinois at Chicago for her steadfast support. Additionally, she thanks Stephen Greenfield and his staff for their contributions at crucial steps in the preparation of the manuscript. Anne also offers her deepest appreciation to her husband, Tom Kasper, who has unfailingly encouraged and sustained her work in women's health for 30 years.

Foreword

As one of the "founding mothers" of the current breast cancer advocacy movement, I am fascinated with the question of why things happen at one point in time rather than another. Breast cancer has been around for a long time. What factors had to converge for it to become the issue of the day? This book, with its mission to take a look at the breast cancer movement from a social perspective, affords me the perfect opportunity to do some reflecting of my own.

Once you are diagnosed with breast cancer you become an outsider. You no longer belong to the world of the "temporarily immortal" but have joined the world of the "defectives." This world includes the disabled, chronically ill, mentally ill, homosexual, and everyone else who dwells on the tails of the bell curve. Although you can be treated for breast cancer you can never go back to the way you were before. Not only do you become a member of a new "club," but as with other marginalized groups, you become dependent on the insiders—the "well" majority—for care, answers, and more money for treatment and research. In order to be able to speak up and lobby for yourself with the ingroup, you must be able to publicly acknowledge your situation; in other words, to come out. How did a breast cancer diagnosis come to be a badge of honor rather than a point of shame? How did women move from private support groups to public advocacy efforts? When did companies realize that supporting breast cancer awareness would not taint them but rather enhance their position with their women customers? And what effect has empowering women with breast cancer had on the social institutions discussed so well in this book?

For me it started in Cambridge, Massachusetts, in the early 1990s with a patient named Susan Shapiro. Her mother had died of breast cancer and now her cancer had spread. She asked me where to find groups that were looking at breast cancer as a political issue. I knew of none. She put out a call to all women with cancer to meet in the fall and discuss the politics of cancer. And at that meeting she launched the Women's Community Cancer Project. She died a few months later, but the movement she helped bring about did not.

Other breast cancer advocacy groups were being formed by spontaneous combustion. In Oakland, California, another group, the Women's Cancer Resource Center, started, founded by a lesbian named Jackie Winnow. It too was a political group. There was a second group in the Bay Area, Breast Cancer Action, founded by Eleanor Pred, an older woman with breast cancer who modeled her work on AIDS activism.

In Washington, D.C., the Mary Helen Mautner Project for Lesbians with Cancer was formed by Susan Hester after Mautner, her partner, died of breast cancer. Its purpose was to provide support for lesbians with cancer, based on the model of the AIDS buddy programs.

These four groups emerged at around the same time. There were obvious differences: in two cases, the focus was lesbians, and in two, the focus was all women cancer patients. But all were based on the premise that there were political, not just personal, aspects of cancer that affected women.

All of these groups were aware of the work the AIDS movement had been doing. For the first time we were seeing people with a killer disease aggressively demanding more money for research, changes in insurance policies, and job protection. Women with breast cancer took note—particularly those women who had been part of the feminist movement and were geared, as the gay activists with AIDS were, to the idea of identifying oppression and confronting it politically.

At the time these groups were emerging I was finishing work on the first edition of *Dr. Susan Love's Breast Book*. As I went on my book tour, talking with women, I began to realize how deep women's anger was and how ready they were to do something. The key moment for me was in Salt Lake City in June 1990, when I gave a talk for 600 women. It was the middle of the afternoon, during the week, and the audience was mostly older women. It was a rather long talk, and at the end, I said, "we don't know the answers, and I don't know what we have to do to make President Bush wake up and do something about breast cancer. Maybe we should march topless to the White House." I was making a wisecrack, hoping to end a somber talk with a little lightness.

I got a great response, and afterwards women came up to me asking when the march was, how they could sign up for it, and what they could do to help organize it. I realized that throughout the country this issue touched all kinds of women, and that they were all fed up with the fact that this virtual epidemic was being ignored. I saw that it wasn't just in the big centers like San Francisco and Boston and Washington, D.C., where I'd expect to see political movements springing up. It was everywhere—everywhere women were ready to fight for attention to breast cancer.

I felt that we ought to have some sort of national organization to give these women the hook they needed to begin organizing. I went to Washington to give a talk to the Mautner Project. Before the talk, I went out to dinner with Susan Hester, the founder of the Project, and two of her friends. I was talking about the thoughts I had after the Salt Lake City speech. My idea was that maybe we should have a big march, and end it with the formation of a new national organization. Hester thought we needed to go about it the other way around: if we formed the organization, we could get its members to come to a big march.

When I left, I called Amy Langer, the president of NABCO, the National Association of Breast Cancer Organizations, a group that was dedicated to giving individuals and groups breast cancer information. I asked what she thought of the idea, and she liked it. I also contacted Nancy Brinker of the Komen Foundation.

The four of us—Susan, Amy, Nancy, and I—met for breakfast in Washington on December 11, 1990 during a breast cancer event and discussed it further. We all were enthusiastic, and the result was a planning meeting. We invited Sharon Greene, the executive director of Y-ME, a very large support group organization in Chicago. Then we got Ann McGuire from the Women's Community Cancer Project, and we invited Eleanor Pred from Breast Cancer Action and Kim Calder from Cancer Care and CANACT from New York.

We discussed whether any one of the existing groups wanted to take on the political piece and although everyone was very enthusiastic no one felt she could handle this aspect, so we decided to try to build a coalition of groups. The Komen Foundation dropped out and the other groups became the planning committee for the new coalition. We set up several task forces to figure out how we would go about it and what our goals would be. Amy Langer used NABCO's membership list and others threw in their lists for an invitation to an organizing meeting in May of 1991. Then we called an open meeting, to be held in Washington, and wrote to every women's group we knew.

We had no idea who would show up. On the day of the meeting the room was packed. There were representatives from all kinds of groups: the American Cancer Society and the American Jewish Congress were there. So was the Human Rights Campaign Fund, a large gay and lesbian group. There were members of breast cancer support groups from all around the country, such as Arm in Arm from Baltimore, the Linda Creed group from Philadelphia, SHARE from New York. Overall there were about 100 or so individuals representing 75 organizations. We were overwhelmed, and we started the National Breast Cancer Coalition on the spot. Out of that meeting came the first board of the Coalition.

And, as is so well documented in this book, the movement flourished. Advocates have become an expected presence on the National Cancer Institute's advisory boards and study sections. And a whole new group of women have cut their political teeth on lobbying for more breast cancer research dollars.

The breast cancer advocacy movement has been so successful in increasing awareness and funding that it has become a victim of its success. There are rival national groups (NABCO, Komen, NBCC, Y-ME) competing for local breast cancer survivor's loyalty and national corporations' public relations dollars. And advocacy has become institutionalized.

Which leads me to contemplate whether we can afford to cure breast cancer? I worry that there are too many companies, organizations, researchers, and universities depending on the breast cancer dollar. And then I remember polio and iron lungs and institutions that vanished with the onset of the vaccine. I see how the AIDS movement has changed now that we have effective therapy. Yes, we can afford to find out how to prevent this disease: we can find the cure. And we will. We will find it because of all of the millions of women around the world who have found their voice and determined that breast cancer is a political problem that must be eradicated!

Susan M. Love MD, MBA
Author *Dr Susan Love's Breast Book*
and *Dr Susan Love's Hormone Book*
Founder SusanLoveMD.com
Adjunct Professor of Surgery, UCLA School of Medicine

Living with Breast Cancer

Susan J. Ferguson, Ph.D., and Anne S. Kasper, Ph.D.

> Everyone who is born holds dual citizenship in the
> kingdom of the well and the kingdom of the sick.
> Although we all prefer to use only the good passport,
> sooner or later each of us is obliged, at least for a spell,
> to identify ourselves as citizens of that other place.
>
> —Susan Sontag, *Illness as Metaphor*

Breast cancer has affected the lives of millions of women as well as
their families, friends, and communities. More than 175,000
women were diagnosed with invasive breast cancer in 1999, and
approximately 44,000 died of the disease. These numbers are, quite
simply, staggering. How and why this disease has reached epidemic
proportions is the subject of this book. This book is not, however,
a guide to the latest treatments for the disease, nor is it a journal of
personal experiences with breast cancer. Instead, this book examines the social meanings of illness and the ways that society has
shaped what we know about breast cancer. The title, *Breast Cancer:
Society Shapes an Epidemic,* reflects this emphasis on understanding
how society has created and shaped our knowledge of breast cancer
as an illness. To say that breast cancer is socially constructed means

that cultural assumptions and biases influence our knowledge, perceptions, and experiences of breast cancer in this society. The chapters in the book explore this social construction of illness by presenting a critical assessment of scientific research, breast cancer policymaking, the media, environmental factors, the changing health care system, and their effects on breast cancer. The book also looks at breast cancer's historical roots as well as the contemporary breast cancer advocacy movement. Furthermore, it analyzes how society's troubling views of women in American culture have deeply influenced how women experience and understand breast cancer. In sum, this is a book that paints a critical picture of the ways that society has shaped what we know about breast cancer. The authors in this volume are concerned with this social construction of breast cancer, with viewing this illness through a social lens.

UNDERSTANDING BREAST CANCER
THROUGH A SOCIAL LENS

We most often think of breast cancer, and most diseases, in medical terms. We weigh its clinical signs and symptoms, how serious it is to our health and survival, what may have caused it, subsequent medical tests and treatments we may undergo, and the kinds of research that may be underway to understand it and, perhaps, find a cure. However, we rarely think about the ways that our culture has influenced what we know and do not know about breast cancer.

Whether or not we are aware of it, society and social institutions shape the occurrence of disease, the forces called upon to respond to disease, and the experience of illness. An editorial in the *American Journal of Public Health* reminds us that we have known this fact since Rudolf Virchow, the renowned nineteenth-century German pathologist, and others first wrote about social medicine. Quoting more contemporary authors, the editorial's authors explain the social construction of illness: "Societies in part create the disease they experience and, further, they materially shape the ways in which diseases are to be experienced." They add that, "the varieties of human affliction owe as much to the inventiveness of culture as they do to the vagaries of nature" (Link and Phelan 1996:471).

When we begin to look at breast cancer with a social lens rather than a medical one, we note that much changes. For example, instead of wanting to know the results of the latest clinical trial, we want to know why some forms of research are being undertaken while others are not, which scientists get funded and why, who is paying for breast cancer research, and who benefits from the findings. In other words, the vast public and private research enterprise can be viewed as a social institution, a powerful part of the culture that reaches into our lives in ways that are congruent with its own particular goals. The goals of the research establishment include finding answers to perplexing and pressing questions about disease, but the goals are also economic and political; these dimensions influence research priorities, means, and outcomes.

Utilizing a social lens also means examining the patient's experience of illness. For example, many of us assume that a woman's experience of breast cancer is determined by the disease itself. A breast malignancy may mean removing a woman's breast or part of it, causing the loss of a body part that has been transformed by disease. However, when a social perspective is applied, we begin to realize that this loss involves far more than a physical part of a woman's body. From her earliest years, a girl identifies with what it means to be female, and a myriad of messages suggest how she should view herself, and, perhaps more important, how society will view her. A complex array of meanings are attached to being female, not the least of which are the expectations that a woman should be physically attractive, sexually inviting, and maternal. No body part plays a more defining role in these expectations than the female breast. Freighted with these social expectations, many women who lose a breast often feel a loss of identity and self-worth, sometimes with enduring effects that can compromise their sense of well-being, their relationships, and their futures.

Applying a social lens to breast cancer also means looking at the social context of illness. The authors of *Women's Health: Complexities and Differences* offer one way to think about the social context of illness when addressing women's health needs, which involves moving away from the biomedical model of disease toward a social model of illness. They argue that women's health is *"embedded in communities,* not just in women's individual bodies" (Ruzek, Olesen, and Clarke 1997:13). These authors offer an inclusive model for addressing women's health that demands a recognition of the conditions of women's lives and work, such as race and ethnicity, education and income resources, housing and neighborhoods, social relationships and support, and other circumstances and experiences that shape their lives and health. They boldly state that, "American society must come to terms with this prerequisite to health, or all of the breast cancers 'caught early,' the chronic diseases avoided through positive health practices, and the benefits of new technologies will be undermined and overshadowed" (21).

Similarly, a social lens enables us to view changes in the social construction of breast cancer over time. For example, it was not long ago when breast cancer was treated as strictly a private matter. Breast cancer was not discussed publicly, and social norms ensured that it was generally ignored in research labs and medical conferences. Breast cancer was not a subject for policymakers and regulators, and it was confined to the occasional polite article in women's magazines. In fact, there was even a time in the early 1980s when Vincent DeVita, the director of the National Cancer Institute (NCI), in order to allocate maximum research dollars to other diseases, was willing to do away with breast cancer study sections.

However, the development of the breast cancer advocacy movement, large increases in research dollars, hearings in Congress, and vast amounts of attention in the media have changed this view of breast cancer. When we began this book in 1996, breast cancer was already sinking into the public's consciousness.

The impression today is that breast cancer is a growth industry, with Race for the Cure runs and walks in most major U.S. cities, the constant entry of new drugs and clinical trials to combat the disease, whole bookshelves devoted to the topic at local bookstores, and a cornucopia of tee-shirts, hats, pins, and pink ribbons. One cannot turn on the television or open a magazine without seeing advertisements promoting breast cancer awareness or certain types of breast cancer treatments. Moreover, many corporations are donating funds to breast cancer research, including American Express, Avon, Ford Motor Company, Gap, Hallmark Cards, Lee (jeans), and Yoplait (yogurt). It is important to realize that these corporations are directly benefiting from breast cancer awareness campaigns via their public relations, increased visibility, and profits. Even the U.S. Postal Service has jumped on the breast cancer bandwagon by issuing the first stamp ever to be used as a fund-raising vehicle for a social cause. The first breast cancer awareness stamp was issued in June 1996, and a second stamp, issued in July 1998, costs seven cents more than first class postage, with the extra funds donated to breast cancer research. The breast cancer stamps have been a public relations boon for the U.S. Postal Service, but it is not yet clear how much money has gone to breast cancer research. Much of the public discourse on breast cancer focuses on Breast Cancer Awareness Month every year, which not only benefits many corporations and organizations but now extends beyond the month of October to 12 months of publicity and self-promotions. In brief, this public discourse makes breast cancer one of the most definitive social issues today.

Thus, using a social lens to view breast cancer also enables us to examine the social forces, including corporate public relations, pharmaceutical companies, and nonprofit organizations, that have shaped the public discourse surrounding breast cancer. One of the most powerful forces in shaping the growing public awareness of breast cancer is the media. Increasingly, women's breast cancer narratives and art work appear in the mainstream press and are often treated as media events in and of themselves. One of the most famous incidents occurred in August 1993, when the *New York Times Magazine* ran a cover photo of a mastectomy self-portrait by photographer Matuschka. The cover photo showed Matuschka's mastectomy-scarred chest with the headline "You Can't Look Away Anymore." The public outcry concerning this cover initiated discussions about the lack of visibility of women's breast cancer experiences and treatments.

Since that 1993 cover photo, breast cancer is no longer an invisible or silent illness. The stories of women with breast cancer appear frequently in the press, especially those of well known women. For example, the *New York Times Magazine* ran excerpts from Peggy Orenstein's cancer diary in June 1997. Orenstein, a respected author and researcher, was 35 years old when her breast cancer was diagnosed. When Linda McCartney died from breast cancer in April 1998, newspapers around the world reported the story. In June 1998, the media followed a team of women living with breast cancer who climbed Mt. McKinley, the highest peak in North America. The film *Climb Every Step* was made of their journey. The group was primarily sponsored by the Breast Cancer Fund, and while no woman in the team made the summit, the climb and surrounding media blitz raised awareness and funds for breast cancer research (MacPherson 1999). In late 1999, the media focused on the attempts to rescue Dr. Jerri Nielson, a physician for a crew of researchers at the inaccessible Amundsen-Scott South Pole Station. Nielson diagnosed her own breast cancer in mid-July 1999 and proceeded to treat herself with chemotherapy because she could not be evacuated during several months of severe weather. Nielson was finally evacuated for emergency treatment of her breast cancer in October 1999.

The reality of breast cancer lies behind all these media reports and public relations campaigns. It lies with the many not-so-famous women who represent the 1.5 million American women who will be diagnosed with breast cancer in the next decade and the half-million women whose lives will be lost. The reality also lies with the millions of women currently living with breast cancer. There is no question that these epidemic numbers warrant enormous concern for and attention to breast cancer.

How did this social change in the awareness and activism around breast cancer take place? Why is breast cancer the "popular" health issue, replacing HIV/AIDS as the number one health concern? How has breast cancer come to be constructed as a major social problem in our society? Moreover, how has breast cancer had an impact on social institutions, including the family, politics, law, medicine, and the arts?

WHY WE WROTE THIS BOOK

This book explores many of these social issues surrounding breast cancer. While breast cancer is no longer simply an individual woman's worst fear, it is unclear how and why breast cancer has become a social problem, one that captures the attention of the public on television, in movies, magazines, and even the *Wall Street Journal*. A review of the breast cancer literature reveals that no one has yet, comprehensively, addressed the powerful and controversial social forces that construct our individual and collective responses to this illness. We believe that this book is the next logical step in our understanding of how and why breast cancer has a profound effect on the lives of all American women.

We have written this book in the spirit of the contemporary feminist Women's Health Movement and with the belief that the more we understand about women's health and the contested ground and inequalities of women's lives, the better for us all. We owe deep appreciation to the many women who have written books about their experiences with breast cancer, such as Rose Kushner's *Breast Cancer: A Personal History and Investigative Report* (1975) and Audre Lorde's *Cancer Journals* (1980). Many brave and insightful books have been written since the 1980s. The daring with which these writers, past and present, have challenged society's refusal to pay attention to breast cancer and the enormous suffering that results has given us much inspiration.

Our goals in writing the book are several. First, we hope to better understand breast cancer as a social phenomenon, even as a social problem. We have asked the question, How do social forces, such as gender and political power, shape how we understand and experience breast cancer? Second, we hope to bring attention and clarity to the social concepts and structures that frame breast cancer. If we are fortunate, this book will prompt more research into the social causes of breast cancer and provide added strength and arguments for the breast cancer advocacy movement. Finally, we also hope that the critical analysis found in all of the chapters will prompt readers to think in new ways about social institutions and social forces that many of us take for granted. Whether we think of the economy, the health care system, or poverty, for example, these entities are not immutable. Rather, like all social phenomena, they are in constant flux and open to question and change. Questioning the status quo of breast cancer will help all of us better understand this social problem.

WHAT IS KNOWN ABOUT BREAST CANCER

One way of understanding breast cancer as a social problem is to examine the current data. When we look at breast cancer data, we find that breast cancer incidence and mortality vary greatly around the world. Western industrialized countries tend to have higher rates of breast cancer than Asian countries and many countries in the developing world. In 1995, the United States had the fifteenth highest rate of breast cancer mortality among 46 countries. Ireland, Denmark, and the Netherlands had the three highest rates, while China and Albania had the lowest rates of breast cancer deaths (American Cancer Society [ACS] 1998). Why countries have varying rates of breast cancer remains unclear, although some evidence points to differences in diet, industrial processes, and longevity as contributing factors.

In the United States, breast cancer is the most common type of cancer found among women, and it is the second leading cause of cancer deaths among American women. For many years, breast cancer was the primary cause of cancer deaths among women in the United States; now lung cancer is the primary cause. Still, the U.S. Department of Health and Human Services estimated that, in 1999, there were approximately 175,000 new cases of breast cancer, and about 43,300 women were expected to die from breast cancer (HHS 1999). These high rates of breast cancer occurrence and mortality vary across states and geographical regions. For example, between 1990 and 1994, the eastern states of Massachusetts, New Jersey, and Connecticut had higher incidence rates of breast cancer than other states. Moreover, Washington, D.C., New Hampshire, and New Jersey had some of the highest mortality rates from breast cancer (ACS 1999). However, these incidence and mortality rates also vary by age, race-ethnicity, socioeconomic status, and sexual orientation.

مليح

AGE DIFFERENCES

The incidence of and mortality from breast cancer increase with age, with the odds of a woman developing breast cancer significantly increasing as she ages. For example, up to age 39, a woman has a 1 in 227 chance of developing breast cancer. From age 40 to 59, a woman's chance of developing the disease is 1 in 25, and from age 60 to 79, a woman's chance is 1 in 15. From age 80 on, a woman's chance of developing breast cancer is 1 in 8 (ACS 1998). This last statistic, without the age criterion mentioned, is the one most often heard in media reports about breast cancer, and it has frightened many women. The accurate reading of this statistic means that the 1 in 8 chance of developing breast cancer applies to women over a lifetime of 80 years. These age-associated risks of breast cancer are important, and we know that cancer, in general, is a disease of aging.

Yet, research shows that the use of breast cancer screening tests, specifically periodic mammography and physical breast examination by a physician, decline with age, especially for women over the age of 65 (Burg, Lane, and Polednak 1990). The reasons for this decline are not entirely clear, although it may be due in part to the inability of older women to pay out-of-pocket for health care. Moreover, until recently, Medicare paid for mammograms every other year only, rather than annually.

RACIAL-ETHNIC DIFFERENCES

The incidence and mortality from breast cancer also differ among racial-ethnic groups of women. For example breast cancer rates for African American women are lower than for white women but higher than for Latinas. However, five-year survival rates are lower and death rates are higher for African American women than for either white women or Latinas with breast cancer. Some of the reasons for these statistics are that African American women have higher rates of poverty, are more likely to be diagnosed later, and are often undertreated when compared to their white and Latina counterparts (National Women's Health Network 1996).

Breast cancer incidence and mortality for Latinas is lower than that for either white or African American women. However, the incidence of breast cancer among Latinas is increasing faster than among other groups of women. Moreover, Latinas who are diagnosed with breast cancer are less likely to reach the five-year survival marker than white women. Latinas represent a diverse population, including women who are from Cuba, Puerto Rico, Mexico, and other Central and South American countries. These different subpopulations have different incidence and mortality rates, and more research is warranted on these understudied populations. A few of the reasons for their poorer statistics is that Latinas are the least likely group to be insured of all major racial-ethnic groups, they often face language barriers in getting health care, and they report not being encouraged by health care providers to seek regular breast cancer screening (National Women's Health Network 1996a).

Incidence rates also vary widely for Asian American women with breast cancer, from low rates for both Korean and Vietnamese women to the highest rates among Native Hawaiian women. Moreover, mortality rates for Asian American women are the lowest among racial-ethnic groups in the United States. However, it is important to note that when Asian women migrate to the United States, their risk of breast cancer increases sixfold as compared to women in their native countries. This increase has been at least partially explained by the women's exposure to Western lifestyles, particularly diet and nutritional factors. Asian women also are the least likely of any racial-ethnic group to have an annual gynecological exam or to ever have had a mammogram. Mistrust of Western medicine, cultural beliefs and practices, and certain socioeconomic factors may explain these low rates of health care services among Asian American women (National Women's Health Network 1996b).

In general, Native American women also have lower breast cancer incidence rates than most other groups of women, including white and African American women. However, incidence rates for Native American women vary by region, with the lowest rates in states such as Arizona and New Mexico, and higher in Alaska. Breast cancer mortality rates for most Native American women are lower than for white, African American, and Latina women, reflecting the lower incidence rates among Native American women. However, the five-year breast cancer survival rate for American Indian women is lower than that of all other ethnic and racial groups in the United States. This lower survival rate may be due to lack of access to health care services. Although the Indian Health Service provides free health care to Native Americans, many are unable to use it. For example, the National Women's Health Network reported in 1996 that no Indian Health Service facilities exist in California, which has the second largest population of Native Americans in the United States.

These differences in the incidence, survival, and mortality rates from breast cancer among racial-ethnic groups of women raise numerous questions about the causation, diagnosis, and treatment of breast cancer in diverse communities. Some of these differences have been attributed to differences in access to medical care and diagnosis at a later stage of disease. Racial differences in breast cancer also are attributed to socioeconomic and cultural factors, such as poverty, inadequate housing, discrimination, language barriers, and nutritional and exercise patterns. Other economic factors, such as having health insurance or the ability to pay for health care, also affect breast cancer diagnosis and treatment outcomes.

SEXUALITY DIFFERENCES

To date, there have been few studies that have investigated breast cancer incidence and mortality rate differences between heterosexual women and lesbians. In 1993, a study by Suzanne Haynes found that lesbians had a two to three times greater risk of developing breast cancer than heterosexual women. Haynes theorized this result based on data from the National Lesbian Health Care Survey, where she found that lesbians tended to have higher body-mass indexes (ratio of weight to height), higher alcohol consumption, and higher rates of late childbearing or no childbearing (Galst 1999). This early study has been challenged on a number of levels, including the limitations of having a sample that was not randomly drawn from the lesbian population and questions concerning how the calculations were done to estimate risk. However, Stephanie Roberts and a team of researchers (1998) studied breast cancer risk factors among lesbians and heterosexual women who received care at Lyon-Martin Women's Health Services in San Francisco between 1995 and 1997. They found that among their sample of 1,019 low-income lesbians and heterosexual women, lesbians do tend to have higher body-mass indexes and fewer pregnancies than heterosexual women, but they do not consume more alcohol. Based on the former two variables, Roberts et al. conclude that lesbians may have a greater risk of developing breast cancer than do heterosexual women. Other researchers argue that lesbians are at greater risk because they see doctors less frequently for routine gynecological exams, whereas heterosexual women see doctors more often for birth control and prenatal care, and therefore, have their breasts checked more frequently. Researchers also have found that lesbians report facing discrimination when they seek medical care, leading many lesbians to delay or refuse regular health care services. The less frequent contact lesbians have with health care providers, the less likely they are to have breast cancer detected at earlier stages. Overall, more research is needed to thoroughly examine this relationship between sexual orientation and breast cancer.

OVERVIEW OF THE BOOK

The book addresses a number of powerful and controversial social issues surrounding breast cancer. It does so in order to provide the reader with an understanding of the complex forces that combine to construct our individual and collective responses to this illness, and why breast cancer has a profound effect on the lives of all American women.

Part One begins by setting the historical context of breast cancer diagnoses and treatment. Chapter One, "Inventing a Curable Disease: Historical Perspectives on Breast Cancer," by Barron H. Lerner, M.D., Ph.D., provides a history of breast cancer, including when breast cancer was first discovered and diagnosed by physicians. This chapter looks at the medical construction of breast cancer, including how breast cancer has been defined differently over time. Particularly interesting is how breast cancer, which initially was defined as an "incurable disease" until the end of the nineteenth century, became constructed as a "curable" disease. Lerner argues that historical analysis is a particularly effective approach for demonstrating how medicine is a social process. For example, late nineteenth-century Johns Hopkins University surgeon William Halsted advanced a new model of breast cancer as a slow growing disease that long remained localized to the breast and nearby tissues. Halsted and his followers argued that an extremely extensive operation, radical mastectomy, could cure breast cancers that were discovered early enough. Yet, this attempt to transform breast cancer into a curable disease reflected such social factors as the growing authority and professionalization of surgery and the rise of the modern hospital where surgeons could perform operations that were both technologically sophisticated and potentially lucrative. Ultimately, the disappearance of the radical mastectomy after 1985 had as much to do with the rise of feminism and patients' rights as with scientific evidence that the operation was unnecessary. As with radical mastectomy, Lerner argues that current debates over breast cancer diagnosis and treatment are socially constructed and unlikely to be resolved by clinical research alone.

In Chapter Two, entitled "Deformities and Diseased: The Medicalization of Women's Breasts," Susan J. Ferguson, Ph.D., discusses medicalization, a process through which natural human experiences come to be seen as conditions requiring treatment. In this chapter, Ferguson argues that women's breasts have been medicalized by members of the medical establishment, including plastic and reconstructive surgeons, the American Medical Association (AMA), the manufacturers of breast implants, and the U.S. Food and Drug Administration (FDA). Specifically, these groups promote the medicalization of women's breasts by defining women with small breasts as "deformed" or "diseased." Moreover, the medical establishment promotes breast reconstruction after mastectomy as an integral part of breast cancer treatment, medicalizing what is otherwise an elective and cosmetic procedure. In a fascinating historical account of the often bizarre and dangerous materials used as breast implants over time, Ferguson reveals the sometimes life-threatening physical, emotional, and financial costs women pay for these procedures. She also details the failure of the medical establishment to investigate the safety of these devices and their implantation in women's bodies, as well as its failure to inform women of the potential risks of these surgeries. The chapter concludes with several suggestions to redress the medicalization of women's breasts and the social control that is its result.

Divided into three sections, Part Two of this book focuses on breast cancer as a social problem. The first section emphasizes the economics of breast cancer, the second looks at women's experiences of breast cancer, and the third section addresses the politics of breast cancer.

The first chapter in the section on the economics of breast cancer is "Breast Cancer and the Evolving Health Care System," by Ellen R. Shaffer, M.P.H. Shaffer addresses whether the current health care system is meeting, and if it can meet, the health care needs of women with breast cancer. She argues that reform of the U.S. health care system is a breast cancer issue because the fragmented organization and profit-driven financing of the current system obstruct access to high quality care for women with breast cancer. Too often, Shaffer demonstrates, diagnosis is delayed or inaccurate, treatment does not conform to recommendations based on the latest medical evidence, and women are unable to participate in making medical decisions about their own health care. Moreover, the rise of corporate medicine has compounded existing inequalities based on gender, social class, race, and insurance status. While many early detection programs have proliferated, breast cancer policy and advocacy have yet to focus on and overcome system-based barriers to quality and access to the full range of care, not just detection. Shaffer concludes the chapter by showing how active patients and model health care providers can point the way to patient-responsive, coordinated, evidence-based, and equitable care for breast cancer patients.

The second chapter in this section is "Profits from Pain: The Political Economy of Breast Cancer," by Jane S. Zones, Ph.D. Zones argues that one of the reasons so many resources are invested in detection, diagnosis, and treatment of breast cancer is because they are profitable, whereas investments in prevention will not bring large financial returns. Zones argues that increasing resources directed at detecting and treating breast cancer have encouraged the development of innovative products and procedures and that the prominence of breast cancer has become a means of creating wealth. Commercial enterprises have sought to increase their market share by producing new commodities and services, making exaggerated claims of benefit or minimizing risk, creating demand, and limiting competition. New breast cancer drugs, high-dose chemotherapy, genetic testing, and screening mammography illustrate these economic strategies. Moreover, Zones argues, interlacing corporate interests and public relations present a formidable challenge to women's best interests regarding breast cancer. Zones concludes that the financial interests in breast cancer have limited and distorted the information that is available to affected women and their advocates.

The second section of Part Two focuses on women, their bodies, and the illness experience. Chapter Five, "Women's Experiences of Breast Cancer," by Marcy E. Rosenbaum, Ph.D., and Gun M. Roos, Ph.D., explores how women perceive and experience breast cancer. The authors argue that women's experiences of breast cancer are inextricably woven with their social worlds. That is, the women struggle with the incongruence between societal expectations for women with breast cancer and their personal experiences of the illness. The chapter includes the voices of women with breast cancer and how they grapple with pervasive and constraining social meanings about breasts and breast cancer that surround this illness. The authors demonstrate that breast cancer is not just a personal process but, rather, an experience filtered through the meanings constructed by the social contexts in which women live. Women respond to these meanings in a variety of ways that include acceptance, rejection, and the struggle to balance between competing meanings. The persistent and often onerous social meanings available to women serve to mute expression of the myriad ways women can and do respond to breast cancer. The authors conclude by describing an expansion of social models that are needed to enable women to make more meaningful sense of their breast cancer experiences.

In Chapter Six, "Barriers and Burdens: Poor Women Face Breast Cancer," Anne S. Kasper, Ph.D., explores what it means to be poor and have breast cancer and why the experience of breast cancer is different for poor women. She reports on a study she conducted with 24 poor, urban women with breast cancer in order to understand why economically disadvantaged women are diagnosed with later stage breast cancer and are less likely to survive the disease than other women. Kasper argues that the barriers and burdens of poverty set the stage for the inappropriate and inferior cancer treatment received by the majority of the 24 women. Using descriptions of the women's life circumstances and breast cancer experiences, the chapter illustrates how difficult it was for the women to find appropriate and timely treatment for their illness. The women encountered a range of obstacles to medical services, faced significant treatment delays, and received substandard quality of care. Some of the women were unable to get a mammogram or see a doctor when they knew it was necessary, others were denied treatment for lack of funds, and one woman was left untreated a year after being diagnosed. Several women were forced to pay out of their own pockets, some went into debt either to pay for care or simply to survive while they were sick, and others were harassed by collection agencies for payments they could not meet. This chapter demonstrates how social inequality shapes women's access to care and the consequences for their health and survival.

The third section of Part Two focuses on the politics of breast cancer. In "Breast Cancer Policymaking," Carol S. Weisman,

Ph.D., discusses the intersecting roles played by federal agencies (the National Cancer Institute, the U.S. Food and Drug Administration, and the National Institutes of Health), the American Cancer Society, Congress, industry, and women's health advocates in influencing the policies, funding, and health services to address breast cancer. Weisman describes breast cancer policymaking as the decisions made by society to allocate resources to research, programs, and services to prevent and treat breast cancer. Although the definition of breast cancer as a social problem that requires public policy responses can be dated to the 1970s, the 1990s witnessed an unprecedented surge of breast cancer policymaking. This chapter considers the political opportunities that made this policy surge possible, the dynamics, the multiple stakeholders who participate in breast cancer policymaking, and some implications and unintended consequences of single-issue or disease-specific policymaking for women's health. Weisman illustrates her arguments with a case study of the controversial issue concerning the effectiveness of screening mammography for women in their forties.

Chapter Eight, "Controversies in Breast Cancer Research," by Sue V. Rosser, Ph.D., provides a feminist critique of breast cancer research and science. Rosser argues that the ways scientific work is structured influences our knowledge about the biology and the causes of the disease. Rosser argues that a male-dominated, hierarchical model has created blinders and biases in the biomedical model of scientific research. Rosser further argues that the current trends and controversies in breast cancer research serve as examples of the many problems that women's health in general and breast cancer specifically have suffered. As the incidence of breast cancer has increased during the last 30 years, biases in research have translated into problems with prevention, screening, determining risk, detection, and treatment of the disease. The chapter examines how conflicting policies and messages surrounding mammography screening, bone marrow transplant procedures for advanced breast cancer, the anticancer drug tamoxifen, and breast implants result from biases in scientific research and policy.

In the last chapter in this section on the politics of breast cancer, "The Environmental Link to Breast Cancer," Sandra Steingraber, Ph.D., analyzes why there is no comprehensive and coordinated investigation into how environmental factors may be a cause of breast cancer. She argues that early detection cannot account for all the increase in the incidence of breast cancer. Rather, Steingraber points to the exponential rise in the production and use of toxic chemicals that occurred at the end of World War II. The chapter includes a review of much of the evidence that implicates a myriad of agents, such as pesticides, herbicides, hormone-disrupting chemicals, hazardous wastes, polluted water sources, workplace carcinogens, and radiation, as possible causes of breast cancer. The author also critically reviews the current argument that the science does not support in-depth research into these environmental factors. Steingraber concludes that a primary obstacle to an environmental investigation into breast cancer is that it would place in question the foundations of an industrial, capitalist, and growth-based global economy.

Part Three of this volume focuses on breast cancer and social change. In Chapter Ten, "Breast Cancer in Popular Women's Magazines from 1913 to 1996," Jennifer R. Fosket, Angela Karran, and Christine LaFia, Ph.D., analyze stories about breast cancer in women's magazines from 1913, when the first article appeared in the Ladies' Home Journal, to 1996. Their research reveals how women's knowledge of breast cancer is created, reproduced, and sustained over time by the media. The chapter demonstrates that the media and popular culture serve to transmit and shape notions of women's identity, sexuality, femininity, motherhood, and responses to breast cancer. The authors argue that representations of breast cancer in popular culture convey profound social and ideological messages and expectations to women with breast cancer. For example, women are depicted in magazine articles as being personally responsible for preventing, detecting, and surviving their breast cancer. By focusing on the behaviors of individual women, media messages succeed in propagating a blame-the-victim ideology. Furthermore, these media messages shift the focus away from the important social, economic, and political causes and consequences of breast cancer.

"Sister Support: Women Create a Breast Cancer Movement," by Barbara A. Brenner, J.D., describes how thousands of informal, community-based breast cancer support groups arose to address women's unmet needs for social support and then coalesced into an organized political movement for breast cancer advocacy. Brenner recounts how this process began in the mid-1970s, during the early years of the contemporary Women's Health Movement, when women came together for support following a breast cancer diagnosis. By the early 1990s, there was more than one national breast cancer organization, and efforts to increase research funding had met with considerable success. Today, women with breast cancer participate in some of the decision-making processes for research funding. However, at the same time, grass-roots activists have raised questions about the nature and direction of breast cancer research. In addition, they have pointed to the failure of the breast cancer movement to reflect the experiences of the full diversity of women at risk and diagnosed with breast cancer. Brenner demonstrates that these and other controversial issues, such as funding sources, alliances with industry and medicine, the growth of grass-roots feminist activism, and environmental causes of breast cancer, are bringing into focus differences among breast cancer organizations that will determine the future direction and impact of the breast cancer movement.

The concluding chapter, "Eliminating Breast Cancer from Our Future," written by the editors, looks toward the issues that are ahead for breast cancer as an illness and as a social problem. The editors map a future for breast cancer that is based on the chapter analyses of the social forces currently influencing breast cancer, and answer this challenging question: What changes can be anticipated given the research, analyses, and controversies presented in this book? The editors also present directions for research, policy, advocacy, and health services that would be in the best interests of all women, and particularly women with breast cancer.

We expect that you will find the chapters in this book stimulating, and even troubling, but in a way that might promote positive social action. We also hope this book enables you to see and comprehend breast cancer in ways that may not have occurred to you before. Or, perhaps you will see connections that were just outside your view but now become visible and important to your understanding of breast cancer. We hope you will share your newly acquired insights and knowledge with other women and men. Perhaps our most earnest aspiration is that you will feel empowered to play a role, however small or large, in critically examining and changing the ways that society and social institutions have shaped our understanding of and experiences with breast cancer.

REFERENCES

American Cancer Society (ACS). 1998. "American Cancer Society—Cancer Facts and Figures 1998: Graphical Data." At http://www.cancer.org/statistics/cff98/graphicaldata.html (August 31, 1999).

———. 1999. "1990-1994 Cancer Incidence and Mortality Rates." At http://www2.cancer.org/epi/dsp_incidence.cfm (November 23, 1999).

Burg, Mary Ann, Dorothy S. Lane, and Anthony P. Polednak. 1990. "Group Differences in the Use of Breast Cancer Screening Tests." *Journal of Aging and Health* 2(4):514-30.

Department of Health and Human Services (HHS). May 25, 1999. "HHS Fact Sheet: Advancing the Science, Improving the Treatments for Breast Cancer." At http://www.hhs.gov (August 31, 1999).

Galst, Liz. 1999. "Lesbians and Cancer Risk." *MAMM Magazine* (December/January). At http://www.hrc.org/issues/lesbians/mamm.html.

Kushner, Rose. 1975. *Breast Cancer: A Personal History and Investigative Report*. New York: Harcourt Brace Jovanovich.

Link, Bruce G., and Jo C. Phelan. 1996. "Editorial: Understanding Sociodemographic Differences in Health—The Role of Fundamental Social Causes." *American Journal of Public Health* 86:471-72.

Lorde, Audre. 1980. *The Cancer Journals*. Argyle, N.Y.: Spinsters Ink.

MacPherson, Myra. 1999. "The Climb of Their Lives." *Health* 13(3):92.

National Women's Health Network. 1996. *Breast Cancer and African American Women.* Washington, D.C.: National Women's Health Network.

————. 1996a. *Breast Cancer and Latinas.* Washington, D.C.: National Women's Health Network.

————. 1996b. *Breast Cancer and Asian American Women.* Washington, D.C.: National Women's Health Network.

————. 1996c. *Breast Cancer and Native American Women.* Washington, D.C.: National Women's Health Network.

Roberts, Stephanie A., Suzanne L. Dibble, Jennifer L. Scanlon, Steven M. Paul, and Heather Davids. 1998. "Differences in Risk Factors for Breast Cancer: Lesbian and Heterosexual Women." *Journal of the Gay and Lesbian Medical Association* 2(3):93-103.

Ruzek, Sheryl B., Virginia L. Olesen, and Adele E. Clarke. 1997. *Women's Health. Complexities and Differences.* Columbus: Ohio State University Press.

Sontag, Susan. 1977. *Illness as Metaphor.* New York: Vintage Books.

PART ONE

BREAST CANCER DIAGNOSES AND TREATMENT— THE HISTORICAL CONTEXT

CHAPTER ONE

Inventing a Curable Disease: Historical Perspectives on Breast Cancer

Barron H. Lerner, M.D., Ph.D.

Perhaps the most contentious issue in the history of cancer therapy is the radical mastectomy. During the first half of the twentieth century, this operation came to exemplify what "scientific surgery" could achieve in the treatment of both breast and other cancers. Yet, by the 1970s, feminist critics assailed radical mastectomy as a needlessly disfiguring operation that male surgeons were unwilling to abandon. As such, it exemplified a central theme in the critique of twentieth-century medicine: the powerless patient as a victim of the well-meaning but imperious physician.

Yet, the history of breast cancer hardly begins or ends with radical mastectomy. For thousands of years, physicians defined and treated the disease in complex ways. Revisiting this history demonstrates how diseases, such as breast cancer, cannot be understood apart from the surrounding sociocultural setting. While biological findings are of great importance, so, too, are the ways in which such data are constructed.

Take the work of William Halsted, the renowned turn-of-last-century Johns Hopkins University surgeon, whose theories served as the foundation for the major theme of this chapter: the transformation of breast cancer from a lethal to a supposedly curable disease. Believing that breast cancer was initially a localized disease that spread in a gradual and orderly manner from the breast into nearby tissues, Halsted devised and popularized an extensive surgical procedure—the radical mastectomy—that removed as much potentially cancerous tissue as possible. Halsted's disciples diligently emphasized how their chief's operation could permanently cure breast cancers that were detected early enough in their growth.

Such a construct was built on research that supported early, aggressive treatment of breast cancer. Yet, the interpretation of such data was inextricably linked to the social milieu in which the disease was investigated and debated. As we shall see, the paradigm of early detection and radical mastectomy triumphed because it was congruent with a series of cultural, economic, political, and gender considerations, such as the growing dominance of a biomedical model of disease, the agenda of the American Cancer Society (ACS), the professionalization of surgery, the rise of the hospital, the association of cancer treatment with powerful military metaphors, and the idea that females should subjugate all concerns of appearance and sexuality to ostensibly improve their chances of permanent cure from cancer.

However, even the notion of "cured" breast cancer was not driven by statistical data alone. That is, what constituted a "cure" did not exist independently but had to be constructed and then disseminated to clinicians and the public. Indeed, in the late 1940s, a small group of statisticians and iconoclastic physicians would explicitly question the standard definition of cure. Depending on how data were presented, these critics claimed, studies that purportedly demonstrated the curability of breast cancer by radical mastectomy might themselves be misleading. Over the next decades, definitive statistical proof emerged showing that radical mastectomy did not increase the chance of permanent cure from breast cancer. As of the year 2000, the operation is almost never used, having been replaced by less extensive surgical procedures, often in conjunction with radiotherapy or chemotherapy.

Yet, radical mastectomy fell into disrepute not only as a result of research studies but also due to changing notions of gender and power. Both using and expanding upon concepts of feminism and patients' rights that arose in the 1970s, women with breast cancer began to demand less mutilating operations as well as full participation in medical decision making. As much as the changing data, it was this challenge to medical authority that finally ended the monopoly of radical mastectomy.

Although the debates over radical mastectomy have subsided, controversies about the early detection of breast cancer and the value of various therapeutic interventions continue to rage. History reminds us that such disputes are unlikely to be settled by science alone.

THE HISTORICAL CONSTRUCTION OF DISEASE

Several scholars have used history to demonstrate how disease is socially constructed (Jordanova 1995; Wright and Treacher 1982). While not discounting the existence of pathological entities that contribute to illness, these authors emphasize how society shapes biological findings into discrete entities we consider to be diseases. As Charles Rosenberg has written, "A disease does not exist until society decides that it does—by perceiving, naming and responding to it" (1989:1-2). This analysis applies most obviously to conditions in which biological mechanisms remain unclear and issues of patient behavior are central. Thus, alcoholism became a disease in the 1940s when post-Prohibition researchers and activists changed their focus from banning liquor to helping those who drank excessively. Conversely, the classification of homosexuality as a mental illness was discarded in 1973 as a result of political pressure from gay activists (Bayer 1987).

Such a model may seem less convincing for diseases that appear more "real," such as a myocardial infarction or pneumonia. After all, cardiac patients experiencing intense chest pain can most assuredly claim that they have objective disease. Yet, even in such cases, social factors can influence how such experiences are labeled and interpreted. As Robert Aronowitz (1998) has shown, the diagnosis of angina pectoris in the early 1900s meant something quite different to doctors and patients than does myocardial ischemia in today's era of invasive cardiac technology. Consumption in the nineteenth century was understood as a wasting illness that resulted from heredity and exposure to decaying waste. After the discovery of the causative bacterium in 1882, however, consumption gradually became known as pulmonary tuberculosis, a communicable disease amenable to preventive public health efforts (Rothman 1994).

In order to clarify how meanings of disease may change over time, Rosenberg has proposed an alternative model to social construction: that of *framing* disease. That is, the same biological phenomenon—whether pus in the lungs, the blockage of a blood vessel around the heart, or the deterioration of kidney function— is framed differently as a result of the changing social surroundings in which the phenomenon is interpreted (Rosenberg 1989). Whether one uses the language of construction or framing, the history of breast cancer well demonstrates how conceptualizations of disease are intimately influenced by those who define and describe such entities.

EARLIEST CONSTRUCTS OF BREAST CANCER

Descriptions of what was likely breast cancer can be found as far back as the Edwin Smith Surgical Papyrus, which dates from the Egyptian Pyramid Age (3000-2500 B.C.E.). Hippocrates, the Greek physician credited with placing medicine on a rational basis, also wrote of "hard tumors within the breast" in the fifth century B.C.E. (Lewison 1955:5). It was Galen, a second-century A.D. Greek physician living in Rome, who first situated breast cancer within a broader explanatory framework of disease. Galen, following the humoral theory, believed that cancer, like all diseases, resulted from an imbalance of the body's four humors—blood, phlegm, black bile, and yellow bile. Breast cancer, he claimed, was caused by an excess of black bile, which could best be treated by bleeding, purgation, and a special diet. Thus, Galen was among the first to conceptualize breast cancer as merely a localized manifestation of a systemic disease affecting the whole body (Martensen 1994). Yet, even Galen insisted that the breast should be cut off "when the tumor is situated on the surface of the body" (de Moulin 1983:9).

Citing such evidence, some historians have characterized the history of breast cancer as an ongoing debate as to whether the disease was a systemic phenomenon or a localized process amenable to aggressive surgery. The latter theory achieved increasing prominence beginning in the late 1800s, building on the laboratory investigations of German scientists such as Rudolf Virchow, who believed that cancer arose from isolated collections of cells that had become diseased, and Richard von Volkmann, who claimed that cancer initially spread along local lymphatic tissues rather than via the blood (Baum 1986; de Moulin 1983).

Such findings encouraged late nineteenth-century surgeons, such as England's Charles Moore, to treat breast cancer by surgically removing the breast, the surrounding skin and fat, and the axillary (underarm) lymph nodes to which the cancer first spread. Von Volkmann also excised the tissue overlying the two chest wall muscles for more advanced cases. Yet, some physicians retained their skepticism about the value of surgery. "[W]e may," wrote Sir James Paget in 1853, "dismiss all hope that the operation will be a final remedy for the disease." To be sure, breast cancers at this time were usually far advanced, often involving more than a quarter of the breast. Accordingly, many physicians concluded that an aggressive operation "only accelerates [the disease's] progress and fatal termination" (Lewison 1955:15, 13).

Not until the work of William Halsted in the 1890s did extensive surgery become standard treatment. Halsted, whose training in Germany had familiarized him with Virchow's teachings, consolidated the work of earlier surgeons into a coherent theory of breast cancer as a localized disease that spread centrifugally in a slow, ordered manner. Halsted believed that a careful, meticulous operation that removed the breast, axillary nodes, and chest wall muscles using "an exceedingly wide berth" potentially removed all cancerous cells and could thus produce a "cure of cancer of the breast" (1894-95:297). Halsted's data (1898) seemed to support his claims. In 1898, for example, he reported that 40 of 76 cases (53 percent) were alive after three years—a considerable achievement for a disease with such a grim prognosis. Given such statistics, it is not surprising that the Halsted radical mastectomy became the treatment of choice for breast cancer by the early 1900s.

WHAT IS MEANT BY "CURE"?

Despite the popularity of the radical mastectomy, what Halsted meant by the term "cure" was far from straightforward. He and his contemporaries were well aware that the procedure did nothing for distant breast cancer that had already silently spread beyond the operative site to the liver, bones, or lungs. In such cases, which were the majority in Halsted's era, the goal of radical mastectomy was to remove the tumor thoroughly enough to prevent localized recurrence and, in so doing, potentially provide women with three or more years of disease-free existence. Although such women were considered "cured," as many as three-quarters of them would eventually die when the previously silent areas of breast cancer began to grow (Meyer 1967).

Sensing this ambiguity, several commentators attempted to clarify the ability of surgery to cure cancer. One such author was the British physician Charles Childe, whose book *Control of a Scourge* equated cure from cancer with "freedom from recurrence" or "lasting relief" in which a patient ultimately died "without ever having experienced any sign or symptom whatsoever of a return of the disease" (1907:2). Childe's redefinition stemmed from his belief that breast and other cancers were curable if rapidly discovered and removed. Building on Halsted's ideas, Childe emphasized that cancers only remained localized—and thus potentially curable—temporarily. "A period exists in every cancer," he wrote, "when it is local, when it is operable, when it is curable." The goal of treatment, therefore, was "to catch the case early enough." It was not the disease that was incurable, Childe concluded, but "the delay that makes it so" (111, 142, 144). This philosophy produced a seeming paradox in which the largest operations were used for the smallest breast cancers. Whereas surgeons advocated radical mastectomy for cancers that had not evidently spread beyond the breast, women with obviously systemic disease often received smaller operations designed to ease symptoms but not to cure.

Numerous studies over the next several decades appeared to validate this approach, demonstrating that radical mastectomy was most effective for cancers confined to the breast (termed Stage I disease). For example, Robert Greenough and Grantley Taylor, using the newly adopted criterion of five-year survival, reported that 62 percent of women with Stage I breast cancer treated between 1921 and 1923 had lived at least five years. In contrast, only 21 percent of women survived this long if the cancer had already spread to the axillary nodes (Stage II) or beyond (Stages III and IV) prior to surgery (Greenough and Taylor 1934). As physicians were now equating five-year survival with "cure," these statistics supported the curability of early, localized cases of breast cancer.

Yet, this new notion of breast cancer as surgically curable arose not merely as a result of such data. As the death rate from infectious diseases declined in the early 1900s, mortality from cancer was rising. As of 1930, cancer was the second leading cause of death in the United States; by 1946, breast cancer killed more women than any other cancer (U.S. Public Health Service 1949:14). As early as 1910, many Western nations, including the United States, Canada, and England, began public health campaigns to control cancer. Because it seemed to be such a promising strategy for lowering cancer mortality, the combination of early detection and radical mastectomy was eagerly promoted by health officials and physicians.

This emphasis on early surgical intervention was most pronounced in the United States, where a voluntary organization, the American Society for the Control of Cancer (ASCC), was founded in 1913. Building on the promotional techniques of tuberculosis crusaders, ASCC members fervently urged Americans to overcome the fatalism and fear that surrounded the "dread disease" and to heed the "danger signals" of incipient cancers. Thus, "any lump, especially in the breast" needed to undergo immediate removal and evaluation (Patterson 1987; Ross 1987:23). Having so strongly tied its own fortunes to early surgical intervention, the ASCC (later the American Cancer Society [ACS]) would remain among the staunchest devotees of this strategy.

Also contributing to American enthusiasm for early, radical surgery was the triumph of a biomedical model of disease—that is, an emphasis on the physiological disturbances that occurred when someone became sick. To some degree, earlier physicians had viewed illnesses as individualized experiences that affected each patient differently. By the early 1900s, however, physicians and medical educators had begun to stress the role of laboratory investigation in identifying specific biological entities that could be treated similarly among all patients (Maulitz 1979). Halsted's radical mastectomy, which drew on both animal experimentation and his studies of breast cancer pathology, well embodied this more reductionist approach to disease.

It was no surprise that the growing authority of the radical mastectomy coincided with the professionalization of surgery in the early twentieth century. This development could be traced directly back to Halsted, who had not only sought to make surgery "scientific," but developed the country's first system for training surgical residents. The perennial reverence for Halsted, whose gentle surgical technique was analogized to that of a "Venetian or Florentine intaglio cutter or a master worker in mosaic," helped to legitimate the notion that careful, properly performed radical surgery could cure otherwise lethal breast cancers (Bland 1981; Lewison 1955:25; Martensen 1998). In this manner, as Christopher Lawrence (1992) has argued, an operation, such as radical mastectomy, was justified in part because it was the type of intervention that surgeons themselves had decided must be valuable. Also promoting the use of aggressive surgery in this era was the rise of the modern hospital, where surgeons performed operations that were both technologically sophisticated and potentially lucrative (Rosenberg 1987).

The great desire of the American Cancer Society (ACS), surgeons, and other physicians to champion early detection manifested itself in the language such groups used. In 1936, for example, the ACS formed the Women's Field Army to promote the early detection and treatment of breast, uterine, and other women's cancers. Borrowing and expanding upon battle metaphors used in venereal disease and tuberculosis control, women in the Army called for "trench warfare with a vengeance against a ruthless killer" (Black 1995:273). Physicians used similar terminology, arguing that "victory" over breast cancer required "a carefully planned military campaign" and an "increase [in] the caliber of our weapons" (Haagensen 1956:587; McDivitt 1971:269). The language of battle demonstrated the great investment that activists and physicians had made in early detection; in turn, such unambiguous military terminology validated the need to intervene early and decisively.

Building on the success of the Pap smear, which allowed doctors to identify and treat potentially cancerous lesions of the cervix, the ACS by the late 1940s accelerated its efforts to find even smaller, presumably more curable, breast cancers. Rather than simply asking women to report lumps promptly, anticancer propaganda now urged women to examine their breasts at home and advised clinicians to examine breasts during routine office visits (Haagensen 1950). As usual, discovered lumps, if cancerous, would be treated with radical mastectomy.

Yet, several factors mitigated against widespread adoption of breast examination. Some women, for example, claimed that monthly self-examination caused unnecessary worry. Conversely, others feared the outcome of successful detection of an early cancer: radical surgical removal of one or both breasts. In addition, Leslie Reagan has argued that, during the 1930s and through the early 1950s, "sexualized and dangerous meanings" necessarily accompanied the display of private female parts to male physicians (1997:1781). Although educational literature attempted to downplay this issue, such concerns discouraged some women from participating in early detection efforts.

Despite these drawbacks, the ACS persevered, using breast cancer as a test case for its credo that early detection and radical surgery saved lives from cancer. Society members fervently hoped that breast cancer's easily accessible location on the body and its reputation as the most dreaded of tumors would inspire women to search for small, curable cancers. Many women approached this task eagerly. "[D]on't let fear prevent an early diagnosis," urged breast cancer patient Genevieve Zeiss in a 1957 *Ladies' Home Journal* article (54). Because rates of breast cancer were high among both the wealthy and the poor (Dorn and Cutler 1958:104), such entreaties applied equally to private and clinic patients. Similarly, prompt radical surgery was seen as advantageous both for older women, who had higher rates of breast cancer, and for younger women, who often had more aggressive tumors.

Yet, if social class or age bias did not foster the aggressive use of radical mastectomy, other cultural and gender considerations played major roles. The message that women needed to find and report breast lumps fit well with public health strategies in Western countries, which increasingly sought to change individual behaviors rather than improve environmental conditions (Starr 1982:180-97). Cultural notions of personal responsibility for one's health resonated particularly strongly in America; breast cancer was no exception. As one health official noted, "The key to breast cancer control lies in the hands of women themselves" (Kaiser 1950:1203). Both popular and medical articles consistently offered the same moral: "Responsible" women who complied with early detection and radical mastectomy would be rewarded with a cure; those who delayed were "guilty" of "negligence" and thus more likely to die (Miller and Pendergrass 1954:424, 422). The gendering of these messages was clear. Given the traditional cultural assumption that females were responsible for the health of their families, women who disregarded educational messages put their loved ones at risk as well (Reagan 1997).

Radical mastectomy achieved great popularity in America because it made sense both medically and socially. By the 1950s, however, a group of critics began to question the value of both early detection and radical surgery. As in the past, what constituted a "cure" was not so straightforward.

CHALLENGES TO EARLY DETECTION AND RADICAL MASTECTOMY

Although radical mastectomy had become the treatment of choice for breast cancer, occasionally commentators criticized its dramatic effects on a woman's appearance. One early opponent, English surgeon Geoffrey Keynes, argued that the operation was needlessly disfiguring because it left many women with sunken chest walls and weak, swollen arms. By the 1920s, Keynes (1937) was removing only the tumor or the breast and then inserting radium needles into the nearby tissue. It was not until the 1950s, however, that critics offered a more persistent challenge to Halsted.

Most of these later commentators supported an alternative explanation of cancer growth known as biological predeterminism. This theory, first proposed by Los Angeles breast surgeon Ian MacDonald in 1951, argued that the major factors that determined the outcome of breast cancer cases were the biological aggressiveness of the tumor and the patient's response to the tumor. In other words, fulminant cancers generally killed women while more slow-growing ones did not (MacDonald 1951).

There was an important corollary to the predeterminists' emphasis on the variable biological activity of breast cancer: It challenged universally accepted assumptions about the need to discover tumors promptly. Although most predeterminists supported early detection and its ability to find smaller lesions, their emphasis on the cancer's intrinsic virulence indicated the ultimate limitations of such a strategy. "[E]arliness or lateness of treatment," estimated Wallace Park and James Lees, "will raise or lower the overall curability rate by a maximum of 5 to 10 percent" (1951:144).

How did Park and Lees generate such a low figure? For one thing, they, like many other predeterminists, had formal training in biometrics. Rather than simply terming as "cured" all patients who had survived five years after radical mastectomy, these biometricians used sophisticated statistical techniques to argue that high cure rates were more apparent than real. First, argued Park and Lees, patients continued to die from breast cancer more than five years after their operation. Second, despite decades of aggressive advocacy of early detection and radical mastectomy, mortality from breast cancer in the United States—roughly 25 per 100,000 women—had not budged since 1930. Rates in Canada and England also were unchanged (Kraus and Oppenheim 1965; Shimkin 1963). If so many more women were being cured, asked the predeterminists, why wasn't the death rate falling? One possible explanation was that physicians were inaccurately designating as "cures" the surgical removal of the roughly 20 percent of slow-growing breast cancers that would never have killed the patient in the first place. "Curing nonlethal lesions," wrote Canadian biometrician Neil McKinnon in 1955, "does not reduce mortality" (p. 620).

This last argument would become more compelling with the growing use of mammography after 1970. With its ability to detect tiny cancers that neither women nor physicians could feel, mammography represented a major advance in early detection. As of the 1990s, roughly 10 to 20 percent of tumors found on mammograms were noninvasive *in situ* lesions (Cady et al. 1996). Although only some of these lesions would ultimately become cancerous, most physicians termed them carcinoma *in situ* or Stage 0 cancer and treated them with mastectomy. Certain doctors even wrote that early detection and surgical removal of these precancers, which by definition had not yet spread, generated a 100 percent cure rate (Hutter et al. 1969). What these operations were curing, however, was far from clear.

As they challenged the impact of early detection on cure rates, the biological predeterminists also questioned whether radical mastectomy was the best operation for achieving a cure. There was general agreement that Halsted's procedure could cure breast cancers that remained localized for a long period. Yet, New York pathologists Maurice Black and Francis Speer argued in 1953, many so-called early breast cancers were virulent and thus had already metastasized throughout the body. In such cases, radical mastectomy was too little: If the cancer had already spread beyond the reach of the surgeon's scalpel, a localized operation in the region of the breast, no matter how radical, could not produce a cure.

At the same time, the predeterminists, questioning the old adage of larger operations for smaller cancers, argued that radical mastectomy was too much. Since those cases most likely to be cured were localized to the breast and perhaps a small number of axillary nodes, why was removal of so much additional tissue required? By the 1950s, a small number of surgeons, often working in conjunction with

radiotherapists, had begun to perform less extensive surgical procedures for presumably localized breast cancers. These operations
included removal of the tumor alone (lumpectomy), part of the breast
(partial mastectomy), or only the breast (simple or total mastectomy). Many proponents of these conservative procedures resided in
Canada or Europe, where radical mastectomy had not produced as
fierce an allegiance as it had in the United States. Among the
advocates of less radical surgery was Robert McWhirter, a Scottish
physician who employed simple mastectomy and local irradiation.
An American who promoted conservative surgery as curative was
Cleveland surgeon George Crile, Jr., who stopped performing radical
mastectomies in 1955 (Crile 1961; McWhirter 1948).

By the 1970s, the medical literature had begun to generate some
definitive data about early detection and radical mastectomy. As the
more moderate of the predeterminists had argued, prompt tumor
discovery had both benefits and limitations. For example, the famous
Health Insurance Plan (HIP) study of the 1960s revealed that breast
examination and mammography lowered breast cancer mortality
among women age 50 to 74 by 30 percent but had little impact on
women in their forties (Shapiro 1979). Given the intense cultural
support for improving the curability of breast cancer, however,
dispassionate evaluation of such data was nearly impossible. As one
surgeon stated in 1969, biological predeterminism needed to be
"annihilated" (Cutler and Connelly 1969:772).

In the case of radical mastectomy, research was much more
conclusive. By the late 1970s, dozens of studies had found that it
was no more curative than more conservative procedures; the
extensive surgery limited local recurrence of the cancer but did not
prolong survival (McPherson and Fox 1977). The most authoritative studies were conducted by Bernard Fisher, a University of
Pittsburgh surgeon who, as chairman of the federally funded
National Surgical Adjuvant Breast and Bowel Project (NSABP),
organized a series of randomized controlled trials comparing
treatment alternatives. Randomized trials, first used in the 1940s,

eliminated many of the methodological problems of earlier research. Fisher's studies, NSABP-04 and NSABP-06, were especially important because they appeared to provide statistical proof of the old predeterminist claims that breast cancer became systemic early in its course and that radical mastectomy was thus needlessly extensive (Fisher 1992).

Yet, even as research questioned radical mastectomy, American surgeons were slow to abandon the procedure. As Canadians and Europeans switched to more conservative operations, the number of radical mastectomies performed in the United States fell from 51,000 to only 46,000 between 1965 and 1974 (Montini and Ruzek 1989). On the one hand, the persistence of radical surgery stemmed from skepticism about the data of Crile, McWhirter, and others; the final results of Fisher's trials would not be published until 1985 (Fisher 1992). At the same time, the continued use of radical mastectomy reflected the reluctance of surgeons throughout the country to abandon a familiar, reliable treatment for one that seemed riskier. Performing the more complete operation, surgeons believed, would save more women's lives while saving themselves from possible lawsuits. When the decline of radical mastectomy finally began in the late 1970s, much of the impetus would come from outside of the medical profession.

REVOLT AGAINST RADICAL MASTECTOMY

Throughout the twentieth century, patients influenced how their breast cancers were treated. For example, the earliest data on breast-conserving surgery and radiotherapy came from the hundreds of women who had declined radical mastectomy (Daland 1927). "It may seem strange to you," a 62-year-old woman told her surgeon in 1958, "but I have a horror of losing my breast" (Cope 1970:7). Nevertheless, as with other diseases, the treatment of breast cancer up until the 1970s largely involved the dissemination of recommendations from the physician to mostly compliant patients (Katz 1984). Prior to the rise of bioethics and patient autonomy, few questioned the authority of physicians to determine appropriate therapy. Thus, upon learning from her surgeon husband that she needed a radical mastectomy, Marion Flexner wrote "I tried hard not to disappoint him" (Flexner 1947:57).

Given their lack of power both as patients and as females in a male dominated society, women had been particularly obligated to follow the advice of their physicians. Historically, male doctors had used this dual source of authority to incorporate beliefs about appropriate female behavior into their medical recommendations. For instance, in the early 1900s, doctors' opinions about proper family size and patients' economic circumstances became conflated with the medical indications for tubal ligation and hysterectomy (Lerner 1994). Similarly gendered assumptions about women and their bodies permeated the breast cancer literature. In 1951, for example, one surgeon argued that breast cancer patients should have their second breast removed prophylactically; except for "possible sexual enhancement," George Pack wrote, breasts in women unlikely to ever breast feed were "useless" (1951:931). Another physician, Irving Ariel, warned that avoidance of radical mastectomy due to "feminine whims" might result in a "dead woman with a somewhat more pleasant-appearing chest wall" (1978:62).

After 1970, however, the feminist, consumerist, and patients' rights movements directly contested the ability of the medical profession to control treatment decisions. Many of the first challenges to the authority of breast surgeons actually came from courageous whistle blowers within the medical profession. Foremost among them was Crile, a provocateur who prided himself on questioning routine procedures that had "acquired an odor of sanctity by sheer longevity" ("Focus on George Crile, Jr., M.D." 1964). By the early 1970s, Crile (1973), William Nolen (1971), and other daring surgeons had gone public, writing articles in women's magazines, such as *Vogue* and *Ms.*, that denounced radical mastectomy as mutilating and implored breast cancer patients to demand a complete list of treatment options. Of particular note was a confrontational article written by Boston surgeon Oliver Cope in 1970. In the eyes of his conservative Boston colleagues, Cope had committed two sins—first, advocating partial mastectomy and radiation and, second, publishing his work in, of all places, the *Radcliffe Quarterly.* "Women should know there are alternatives," he wrote: "They don't need to be railroaded into having their breast removed" (1970:9).

Such sentiments achieved great resonance among feminists, who sought "equality and individual self-determination in every aspect of life" (Ruzek 1978:34). The Women's Health Movement, a loosely based network of activists, women health care providers, and grassroots organizations, argued that such qualities were particularly lacking in the medical system. Doctors, these women argued, were "condescending, paternalistic, judgmental, and non-informative" (Ruzek 1978:32). To the authors of *Our Bodies, Ourselves,* the influential health manual published by the Boston Women's Health Collective in 1973, breast cancer was one of many areas in which women patients remained uninformed and victimized.

To be sure, not all women questioned medical authority and demanded less radical surgery. Those who did so most vocally tended to be upper-middle-class white women with a strong feminist bent. Yet, the overall trend toward empowerment was unmistakable. By the late 1970s, many breast cancer survivors had written books or articles in women's magazines stressing autonomy and self-determination. The subtitle of Rosamond Campion's *The Invisible Worm* (1972), for example, was "a woman's right to choose an alternate to radical surgery." Other women—including Betty Ford and Happy Rockefeller—either described or published personal accounts of their breast cancer, detailing how their struggles with diagnosis, treatment alternatives, and possible breast reconstruction permeated their daily lives ("Breast Cancer: Fear and Facts" 1974).

These narratives encouraged readers to view breast cancer not as a monolithic disease but as an illness that varied from woman to woman (Bayh and Kotz 1979; Lorde 1980; Rollin 1976). Most notable among these authors was Rose Kushner (1975), a Maryland journalist diagnosed with breast cancer in 1974 who relentlessly fought both the Halsted radical and the "one-step" procedure in which women found to have positive biopsies during surgery received immediate mastectomies while still under anesthesia.

While some surgeons welcomed a more activist patient role, others responded to women's attempts to influence treatment decisions with anger or amazement. "Women," wrote one doctor, "are marching on clinics and private offices waving copies of *McCall's*, *Good Housekeeping, Ms., Playgirl*, or the supplement of their local newspaper" (Holleb 1975:145). Campion wrote that a surgeon had called her a "very silly and stubborn woman" for challenging the operation he believed would save her life (1972: 33). Yet, spurred by patients with breast cancer and other diseases, the traditional paternalistic structure of medicine was slowly changing. As a result of the Women's Health Movement, feminist activism, the rise of bioethics, and, in the case of breast cancer, laws passed by state legislatures, greater degrees of informed consent and patient autonomy gradually became components of the medical encounter (Montini and Ruzek 1989; Rothman 1991). Indeed, as more women "refused to consent to radical mastectomies" and searched for surgeons "willing to perform more conservative and less disfiguring operations" (Maisel 1971:152), offering procedures other than radical mastectomy had become a necessary business decision.

If social factors such as feminism and consumerism had thus induced physicians to revisit the clinical indications for radical mastectomy, the medical literature also supported such a strategy. By 1978, early results of NSABP-04 were available, showing no difference in five-year survival among women treated with radical mastectomy versus total mastectomy with or without radiotherapy. In 1979, a National Institutes of Health (NIH) consensus conference proclaimed the death of the Halsted paradigm: Potential cures of breast cancer required not radical mastectomy but lesser surgery, often combined with radiotherapy or systemic chemotherapy to kill cancer cells that had spread throughout the body ("Treatment of Primary Breast Cancer" 1979). As early as 1975 Fisher wrote that breast cancer was no longer "purely a surgical problem" (p. 142). Only 5,000 radical mastectomies were performed in America in 1983, down from 46,000 in 1974 (Montini and Ruzek 1989).

The fact that 5,000 radical mastectomies were still being done as late as 1983, however, indicates that traditional beliefs about breast cancer remained entrenched. So, too, did the fact that the operation that largely replaced radical mastectomy for the treatment of localized cancers was not one of the very conservative procedures, such as lumpectomy or partial mastectomy, proven effective in controlled trials. Rather, women most often received a modified radical mastectomy, which preserved the chest wall muscles but still entailed breast removal and lymph node dissection. In a sense, the modified procedure, still the most common operation for invasive breast cancer, is no more "medically indicated" than was the radical mastectomy. Rather, it has remained in favor among physicians and patients because it best addresses the persistent cultural ambiguity about how aggressively to treat localized breast cancer. On the one hand, the modified radical preserves enough tissue to minimize anatomic deformity and permit breast reconstruction; on the other hand, it is extensive enough to satisfy the persistent belief that the safest strategy is to remove as many potentially cancerous cells as possible.

CONCLUSION

Historical analysis is a particularly effective approach for demonstrating how diseases such as breast cancer are socially constructed. Although historical debates about breast cancer have involved detailed analyses of clinical studies, the ways that such data have been framed have greatly influenced their acceptance or rejection by clinicians and patients. Thus, studies supporting early detection and radical mastectomy received particularly favorable attention in the United States because they were consistent with social forces avidly promoting a cure for breast cancer: the triumph of a biomedical model of disease, the professionalization of surgery, the rise of the technologically sophisticated hospital, and the strong cultural predisposition that more intervention, even if ultimately unsuccessful, is a less risky strategy (Feinstein 1985). Yet, as critics of this strategy pointed out, even an ostensibly scientific term such as cure was itself socially constructed. Simply surviving five years after a radical mastectomy did not necessarily prove that a woman was cured, that the surgery itself had prolonged her life, or that such an extensive operation had been necessary in the first place.

Similarly, the decline of radical mastectomy reflected both the results of increasingly rigorous clinical trials and the social context in which such trials were interpreted. By the 1970s, it was no longer acceptable to defend radical mastectomy because it was a revered operation that dated back to Halsted. Newly empowered women patients, biostatisticians, oncologists, radiotherapists, and many surgeons themselves had grown increasingly dissatisfied with a procedure that suddenly seemed outdated and mutilating as opposed to curative.

This historical account demonstrates that breast cancer continues to be socially constructed. For one thing, commentators still routinely use military metaphors, debating whether the recent encouraging decline in breast cancer mortality proves that we are finally "winning the war" on the disease (Lerner 1998). Advocates of such terminology argue that it increases funding for research and empowers individual women who are "fighting" breast cancer. Yet, this choice of language reminds us of the vested interests of certain organizations and individuals in proving that early detection does or does not work. Thus, rather than reasonably evaluating the ability of various early detection strategies to improve cure rates, we continue to dispute the merits of early detection itself (Kolata 1997). As such, women and clinicians may be left without helpful guideposts as they discuss screening options such as mammography.

A similar divisiveness characterizes debates over breast cancer treatment. While radical mastectomy is almost never used today, other aggressive, potentially curative interventions—such as high-dose chemotherapy (HDC) and bone marrow transplant—have taken its place (Altman 1996). As in the past, however, there are numerous social factors that may encourage us to see such treatments as curative, including the marketing of chemotherapeutic agents, the ascendancy of oncologists in treating breast cancer, the profitability of high technology procedures, and, most importantly, the enduring zeal with which American society approaches the possibility of cure.

At least one factor has changed dramatically since the early twentieth century. Ever since feminist and consumer activists challenged medical decision making in the 1970s, patients have taken a central role in choosing among screening and treatment strategies. Indeed, well-informed patients are now as likely as physicians to select an aggressive therapeutic strategy, such as bone marrow transplant. Concurrently, it has been breast cancer survivors and other women, taking a lesson from those infected with HIV, who have catapulted breast cancer into the media spotlight in the United States. As chapter 11 of this book discusses, breast cancer advocacy has become a central focus for many women's organizations and foundations. Federal funding for breast cancer research increased from $75 to a projected $550 million from 1991 to 1997 (Belkin 1996).

Yet, such developments have generated criticism. For example, some commentators have claimed that advances in breast cancer screening and treatment have mostly benefited middle- and upper-class women. Poor women and women of color, they point out, have persistently lower rates of breast cancer screening and shorter survival after diagnosis (chapter 6 of this volume, Lyman et al.

1997). Both domestic and foreign critics have argued that money raised by America's war on breast cancer has been spent poorly. That is, because research has overemphasized expensive technologies for detecting and curing the disease, there has been insufficient scrutiny of the potential causes of breast cancer, such as poor dietary habits or environmental exposures (Proctor 1995).

Such controversies remind us that medicine is a *social* process. Our knowledge about the biology of breast cancer will continue to be influenced by the ways in which terms such as early detection, cure, and war on cancer, are understood. A better appreciation of how breast cancer is socially constructed may help physicians and patients reach more rational clinical decisions and enable policymakers to develop more equitable, cost-effective screening and treatment recommendations.

NOTES

AUTHOR'S NOTE: The author would like to thank Susan Ferguson, Anne Kasper, and David Rothman for their comments, Jennifer Roemer for research assistance, and Susan Lauer for technical assistance. Dr. Lerner receives funding from the Burroughs Wellcome Fund and the Angelica Berrie Gold Foundation. He is a Robert Wood Johnson Foundation Generalist Physician Faculty Scholar (Project # 031491).

REFERENCES

Altman, Roberta. 1996. *Waking Up, Fighting Back: The Politics of Breast Cancer.* Boston: Little, Brown.

Ariel, Irving M. 1978. "The Treatment of Breast Cancer by Radical and Super Radical Mastectomy." *Resident & Staff Physician* (September) 57-62.

Aronowitz, Robert A. 1998. *Making Sense of Illness: Studies in Twentieth Century Medical Thought.* Cambridge: Cambridge University Press.

Baum, Michael. 1986. "The History of Breast Cancer." Pp. 95-105 in *Breast Disease,* ed. John F. Forbes. Edinburgh: Churchill Livingstone.

Bayer, Ronald. 1987. *Homosexuality and American Psychiatry: The Politics of Diagnosis.* Princeton: Princeton University Press.

Bayh, Marvella, and Mary Lynn Kotz. 1979. *Marvella: A Personal Journey.* New York: Harcourt Brace Jovanovich.

Belkin, Lisa. 1996. "How Breast Cancer Became This Year's Hot Charity." *New York Times Magazine* (December 22) 40.

Black, Margaret. 1995. "What Did Popular Women's Magazines from 1929 to 1949 Say About Breast Cancer?" *Cancer Nursing* 18:270-77.

Black, Maurice M., and Francis D. Speer. 1953. "Biologic Variability of Breast Carcinoma in Relation to Diagnosis and Therapy." *New York State Journal of Medicine* 53:1560-63.

Bland, Cornelia S. 1981. "The Halsted Mastectomy: Present Illness and Past History." *Western Journal of Medicine* 134:549-55.

"Breast Cancer: Fear and Facts." 1974. *Time* (November 4) 107-10.

Cady, Blake, Michael D. Stone, John G. Schuler, Ravi R. Thakur, Molly A. Warner, and Philip T. Lavin. 1996. "The New Era in Breast Cancer: Invasion, Size, and Nodal Involvement Dramatically Decreasing as a Result of Mammographic Screening." *Archives of Surgery* 131:301-08.

Campion, Rosamond. 1972. *The Invisible Worm: A Woman's Right to Choose an Alternate to Radical Surgery.* New York: Macmillan.

Childe, Charles P. 1907. *The Control of a Scourge.* New York: E. P. Dutton.

Cope, Oliver. 1970. "Breast Cancer: Has the Time Come for A Less Mutilating Treatment?" *Radcliffe Quarterly* (June) 6-11.

Crile, George Jr. 1961. "Simplified Treatment of Cancer of the Breast: Early Results of a Clinical Study." *Annals of Surgery* 153:745-61.

———. 1973. "Breast Cancer: A Patient's Bill of Rights." *Ms.* (September) 66.

Cutler, Sidney J., and Roger R. Connelly. 1969. "Mammary Cancer Trends." *Cancer* 23:767-74.

Daland, Ernest M. 1927. "Untreated Cases of Breast Cancer." *Surgery, Gynecology and Obstetrics* 44:264-68.

de Moulin, Daniel. 1983. *A Short History of Breast Cancer.* Boston: Martinus Nijhoff.

Dorn, Harold F., and Sidney J. Cutler. 1958. *Morbidity from Cancer in the United States.* Public Health Monograph No. 56. Washington, D.C.: U.S. Department of Health, Education and Welfare.

Feinstein, Alvan R. 1985. "The 'Chagrin Factor' and Qualitative Decision Analysis." *Archives of Internal Medicine* 145:1257-59.

Fisher, Bernard. 1975. "What We Have Learned and Are Learning from Cooperative Clinical Trials." Pp. 141-44 in *Early Breast Cancer: Detection and Treatment,* ed. H. Stephen Gallagher. New York: John Wiley.

———. 1992. "The Evolution of Paradigms for the Management of Breast Cancer: A Personal Perspective." *Cancer Research* 52:2371-83.

Flexner, Marion W. 1947. "Cancer—I've Had It." *Ladies' Home Journal* (May) 57.

"Focus on George Crile, Jr., M.D." 1964. *Roche Medical Image.* February.

Greenough, Robert B., and Grantley W. Taylor. 1934. "Cancer of the Breast: End-Results." *New England Journal of Medicine* 210:831-35.

Haagensen, Cushman D. 1950. *Carcinoma of the Breast.* New York: American Cancer Society.

———. 1956. *Diseases of the Breast.* 1st ed. Philadelphia: W. B. Saunders.

Halsted, William S. 1898. "A Clinical and Histological Study of Certain Adenocarcinomata of the Breast." *Transactions of the American Surgical Association* 16:144-81.

———. 1894-95. "The Results of Operations for the Cure of Cancer of the Breast Performed at the Johns Hopkins Hospital from June 1889 to January 1894." *Johns Hopkins Hospital Reports* 4:297-350.

Holleb, Arthur I. 1975. "Response to Demands for Patient Participation in Treatment Selection: A Panel Discussion." Pp. 145-50 in *Early Breast Cancer: Detection and Treatment,* ed. H. Stephen Gallagher. New York: John Wiley.

Hutter, Robert V. P., Ruth E. Snyder, John C. Lucas, Frank W. Foote Jr., and Joseph H. Farrow. 1969. "Clinical and Pathologic Correlation with Mammographic Findings in Lobular Carcinoma in Situ." *Cancer* 23:826-39.

Jordanova, Ludmilla. 1995. "The Social Construction of Medical Knowledge." *Social History of Medicine* 8:361-81.

Kaiser, Raymond F. 1950. "Why Cancer 'Control.'" *Public Health Reports* 65:1203-08.

Katz, Jay. 1984. *The Silent World of Doctor and Patient.* New York: Free Press.

Keynes, Geoffrey. 1937. "The Place of Radium in the Treatment of Cancer of the Breast." *Annals of Surgery* 106:619-30.

Kolata, Gina. 1997. "Stand on Mammograms Greeted by Outrage." *New York Times* (January 28) C1, C8.

Krúm, Arthur S., and Abraham Oppenheim. 1965. "Trend of Mortality from Cancer of the Breast." *Journal of the American Medical Association* 194:201-02.

Kushner, Rose. 1975. *Breast Cancer: A Personal History and an Investigative Report.* New York: Harcourt Brace Jovanovich.

Lawrence, Christopher. 1992. "Democratic, Divine and Heroic: The History and Historiography of Surgery." Pp. 1-47 in *Medical Theory, Surgical Practice,* ed. Christopher Lawrence. London: Routledge.

Lerner, Barron H. 1994. "Constructing Medical Indications: The Sterilization of Women with Heart Disease or Tuberculosis." *Journal of the History of Medicine and Allied Sciences* 49:362-79.

———. 1998. "Fighting the War on Breast Cancer: Debates over Early Detection, 1945 to the Present." *Annals of Internal Medicine* 129:74-78.

Lewison, Edward F. 1955. *Breast Cancer and Its Diagnosis and Treatment.* Baltimore: Williams & Wilkins.

Lorde, Audre. 1980. *The Cancer Journals.* San Francisco: Spinsters.

Lyman, Gary H., Nicole M. Kuderer, Stephen L. Lyman, Charles E. Cox, Douglas D. Reintgen, and Paul P. Baekey. 1997. "Importance of Race on Breast Cancer Survival." *Annals of Surgical Oncology* 4:80-87.

MacDonald, Ian. 1951. "Biological Predetermination in Human Cancer." *Surgery, Gynecology and Obstetrics* 92:443-52.

Maisel, Albert Q. 1971. "Controversy Over Breast Cancer." *Reader's Digest* (December) 151-56.

Martensen, Robert F. 1998. "When the 'Truly Conservative' Went 'Radical': The Genesis, Development, and Persistence of the Radical Mastectomy as a Curative Treatment for Breast Cancer." Presented at the New York Academy of Medicine, June 1, New York, N.Y.

Martensen, Robert L. 1994. "Cancer: Medical History and the Framing of a Disease." *Journal of the American Medical Association* 271:1901.

Maulitz, Russell C. 1979. "'Physician Versus Bacteriologist': The Ideology of Science in Clinical Medicine." Pp. 91-107 in *The Therapeutic Revolution: Essays in the Social History of Medicine,* ed. Morris J. Vogel and Charles E. Rosenberg. Philadelphia: University of Pennsylvania Press.

McDivitt, Robert W. 1971. "Detection and Management of 'Early Breast Cancer.'" *Johns Hopkins Medical Journal* 129:269-73.

McKinnon, Neil E. 1955. "Limitations in Diagnosis and Treatment of Breast and Other Cancers." *Canadian Medical Association Journal* 73:614-25.

McPherson, Kim and Maurice S. Fox. 1977. "Treatment of Breast Cancer." Pp. 308-22 in *Costs, Risks, and Benefits of Surgery,* ed. John P. Bunker, Benjamin A. Barnes, and Frederick Mosteller. New York: Oxford University Press.

McWhirter, Robert. 1948. "The Value of Simple Mastectomy and Radiotherapy in the Treatment of Cancer of the Breast." *British Journal of Radiology* 21:599-610.

Meyer, Kenneth K. 1967. "The 'Cure' of Cancer of the Breast." Pp. 3-9 in *Current Concepts in Breast Cancer*, ed. Albert Segaloff, Kenneth K. Meyer, and Selma DeBakey. Baltimore: Williams & Wilkins.

Miller, Marlyn W., and Eugene P. Pendergrass. 1954. "Some Observations Concerned with Carcinoma of the Breast, Part V." *Pennsylvania Medical Journal* 57:421-25.

Montini, Theresa and Sheryl Ruzek. 1989. "Overturning Orthodoxy: The Emergence of Breast Cancer Treatment Policy." *Research in the Sociology of Health Care* 8:3-32.

Nolen, William A. 1971. "The Operation Women Fear Most." *McCall's* (April) 52.

Pack, George T. 1951. "Argument for Bilateral Mastectomy." *Surgery* 29:929-31.

Park, Wallace W., and James C. Lees. 1951. "The Absolute Curability of Cancer of the Breast." *Surgery, Gynecology and Obstetrics* 93:129-52.

Patterson, James T. 1987. *The Dread Disease: Cancer and Modern American Culture.* Cambridge: Harvard University Press.

Proctor, Robert N. 1995. *Cancer Wars: How Politics Shapes What We Know and Don't Know about Cancer.* New York: Basic Books.

Reagan, Leslie J. 1997. "Engendering the Dread Disease: Women, Men, and Cancer." *American Journal of Public Health* 87:1779-87.

Rollin, Betty. 1976. *First You Cry.* New York: J. B. Lippincott.

Rosenberg, Charles E. 1987 *The Care of Strangers: The Rise of America's Hospital System.* New York: Basic Books.

———. 1989. "Disease in History: Frames and Framers." *Milbank Quarterly* 67 (Suppl. 1):1-15.

Ross, Walter S. 1987. *Crusade: The Official History of the American Cancer Society.* New York: Arbor House.

Rothman, David J. 1991. *Strangers at the Bedside: How Law and Bioethics Transformed Medical Decision Making.* New York: Basic Books.

Rothman, Sheila M. 1994. *Living in the Shadow of Death: Tuberculosis and the Social Experience of Medical Illness in American History.* New York: Basic Books.

Ruzek, Sheryl Burt. 1978. *The Women's Health Movement: Feminist Alternatives to Medical Control.* New York: Praeger.

Shapiro, Sam. 1979. "Evidence on Screening for Breast Cancer from a Randomized Trial." Pp. 19-36 in *Control of Breast Cancer Through Mass Screening*, ed. Philip Strax. Littleton, Mass.: PSG Publishing.

Shimkin, Michael B. 1963. "Cancer of the Breast." *Journal of the American Medical Association* 183:358-61.

Starr, Paul. 1982. *The Social Transformation of American Medicine.* New York: Basic Books.

"Treatment of Primary Breast Cancer." 1979. *New England Journal of Medicine* 301:340.

U.S. Public Health Service. 1949. *Vital Statistics of the United States, 1947, Part I.* Washington, D.C.: GPO.

Wright, Peter, and Andrew Treacher. 1982. "Introduction." Pp. 1-22 in *The Problem of Medical Knowledge: Examining the Social Construction of Medicine*, ed. Peter Wright and Andrew Treacher. Edinburgh: Edinburgh University Press.

Zeiss, Genevieve. 1957. "A New Life After Breast Cancer." *Ladies' Home Journal* (October) 52.

CHAPTER TWO

Deformities and Diseased: The Medicalization of Women's Breasts

Susan J. Ferguson, Ph.D.

> We may not have a cure for every disease, alas, but
> there's no reason we can't have a disease for every cure.
> —Barbara Ehrenreich, 1992

For more than 30 years, medical sociologists have argued that the institution of medicine is an agent of social control. In his classic essay, Irving Kenneth Zola argues that as more of human experience becomes medicalized—that is, as natural human experiences and processes come to be seen as conditions that require medical attention—physicians enjoy increased control over people's lives (1971). Sociologists Diana Scully and Catherine Kohler Riessman further discuss how doctors historically have exercised social control over women by medicalizing women's experiences, such as childbirth, premenstrual syndrome, and menopause.

In addition to women's experiences concerning reproduction, women's bodies and weight have been medicalized. As Riessman argues, "Weight . . . illustrates in a most graphic form how power relations are maintained through medical social control, how women internalize their oppression by desiring to be thin and turning to doctors for help" (1992:205). Although many specialists, including general surgeons, nutritionists, and endocrinologists treat weight problems and obesity, this task frequently falls to the plastic surgeon (Riessman 1992). In 1990, liposuction, which consists of "sucking fat cells out from underneath [the] skin with a vacuum device," was the most frequently performed elective plastic surgery among women (Morgan 1991:28). Eight years later, in 1998, liposuction was still the most frequently performed elective plastic surgery on women. In fact, liposuction procedures have increased 57 percent since 1996, from 109,353 procedures to 172,079 in 1998, and have increased 264 percent since 1992. Of the 172,079 liposuction procedures in 1998, only 11 percent were performed on men, while 89 percent were performed on women (ASPRS 1999).

While other examples of the medicalization of women's lives, such as reproduction, sexuality, menstruation, and weight, have been well researched, few sociologists have addressed the medicalization of women's breasts.[1] The overwhelming number of U.S. women who have undergone breast augmentation and reconstruction suggests an area in need of study. Every year until 1992, when the U. S. Food and Drug Administration (FDA) first restricted access to breast implants, approximately 150,000 women received breast implants (Parker 1995). From 1992 until 1996, the number of women who received breast implants decreased dramatically (Bruning 1995). However, since 1996, breast surgery has increased substantially, with 202,061 women receiving breast implants in 1998. Breast augmentation alone has increased 51 percent, from 87,704 procedures in 1996 to 132,378 procedures in 1998, and it has increased 302 percent since the FDA restrictions of 1992 (ASPRS 1999). Thus, it is estimated that more than two million U.S. women and three million women worldwide currently have or have had breast implants (Parker 1995; Regush 1992; Shapiro 1999). Approximately 20 percent of these women sought breast implants for reconstructive purposes following cancer or other surgery, but only 10 percent of all women who undergo mastectomies opt for reconstructive surgery of any kind (Johnson 1992; Mellican 1995). The majority of women (roughly 80 percent) sought breast implants for augmentation or enlargement (Coco 1994; Panarites 1993; Wolfe 1991).

Some might argue that these data do not constitute evidence for the medicalization of women's breasts because women elect to have cosmetic surgery, and because breast augmentation and reconstruction are not medically necessary. However, the medical establishment—including plastic and reconstructive surgeons, the American Medical Association (AMA), the manufacturers of breast implants, and the FDA—contributes to women's decisions to have breast surgery through the process of medicalization. Specifically, in the present examination of breast augmentation and reconstruction, it becomes clear that women with a different number of breasts or different sized breasts are considered deviant. Moreover, small breasts have been labeled as "diseased" by members of the medical establishment (Coco 1994:111). Mammaplasty, or breast augmentation and reconstruction, has been used to cure women of this "disease" and to promote conformity to societal norms of beauty and femininity. Thus, breast reconstruction and augmentation are used as forms of social control over women. These procedures are problematic for women because they are expensive, time consuming, and associated with chronic and disabling health problems (Davis 1991). Moreover, they often involve hospitalization, the risk of infection, and additional surgery and anesthesia.

Importantly, it must be acknowledged that women have not been acquiescent victims in the medicalization of their breasts. As Peter Conrad argues, "[i]t is clear that patients are not necessarily passive and can be active participants in the process of medicalization" (1996:148). I agree with Conrad's argument that many women willingly participate in this process, and some women even find mammaplasty empowering. For example, one woman writes about her decision to have silicone breast implants as self-affirming: "I got [silicone implants] for me and I feel great." Similarly, a woman who underwent a mastectomy writes about her choice of breast implants, "I did not have to grieve the loss of my breasts" (Coco 1994:122-23). Other women say they choose breast implants to improve their body image or to raise their self-esteem. While recognizing the importance of these women's perceptions and actions, this chapter focuses on understanding the specific structural constraints under which women choose breast augmentation and reconstruction. Thus, it emphasizes the institutional agents of medicalization and social control rather than women's individual agency.

This chapter begins by examining the history of breast augmentation and reconstruction, and the multiple health problems associated with these procedures. Next, the social construction of women's health is examined, with an emphasis on how women's breasts have been medicalized. This examination focuses particularly on the roles of the American Society of Plastic and Reconstructive Surgeons (ASPRS), the AMA, and the companies that manufacture breast implants in reinforcing the ideology that women's breasts are diseased. In addition, this chapter demonstrates how each of these institutions profits from the medicalization of women's breasts and the continued practice of breast augmentation and reconstruction. Thus, this chapter primarily concentrates on these members of the medical establishment; however, the role of the FDA in reinforcing the ideology that women's breasts are diseased also is briefly considered. Finally, suggestions for social change are presented, which include ideological, structural, and individual level solutions.

HISTORY OF BREAST AUGMENTATION AND RECONSTRUCTION

The history of breast augmentation and reconstructive surgery is the cornerstone of this chapter's argument that women's breasts have been medicalized, and that physicians have exercised social control over women through breast augmentation and reconstruction. Importantly, the history of breast augmentation and reconstruction demonstrates U.S. society's obsession with breast size and shape. This account also demonstrates the lengths to which medical professionals went to construct and to reinforce the ideology that women's breasts are "deformed" and "diseased." Similarly, the literature shows the extreme risks that women were willing to take [in attempts to conform to a societal beauty standard.]Throughout history, women have sustained serious, and even fatal, health problems associated with these procedures. The history of breast augmentation and reconstruction and the various problems associated with these procedures provides the historical and social contexts through which the more recent controversy over the safety of breast implants can be examined.

THE EARLY ATTEMPTS AT BREAST AUGMENTATION

In 1947, *Newsweek* recalled that the first surgical correction of the female breast was performed in Europe in the seventeenth century when a barber removed both breasts from a woman who suffered pain and embarrassment because of their extreme weight. The purpose of most breast surgery between that time and the early twentieth century was either to remove a tumor or to reduce the size of large breasts for health reasons. It was not until the 1890s that the problem of so-called breast deformity—that is, breasts whose size or shape differed substantially from the "correct breast shape"—was taken seriously by the surgical profession in both Europe and the United States; even then, conservative doctors were reluctant to admit a need for cosmetic or vanity reconstruction ("Light on Breast Surgery" 1947:60; Haiken 1997).

Although breast implants have been available in the United States for only the last 45 years, doctors have been injecting substances into women's breasts to enlarge them since the late nineteenth century. The first substance known to be injected into women's breasts was paraffin or wax. Robert Gersuny of Vienna pioneered the use of paraffin injections for breast augmentation in the 1890s, and it remained a popular procedure until World War I (Haiken 1997:235). In 1912, doctors began to receive complaints associated with the injections, including hard lumps, inflammation, and cancer. Complications were sometimes so severe that doctors performed mastectomies to correct the problems caused by the paraffin. Despite the seriousness of these complications, "doctors, and even *entrepreneurial laypeople* [emphasis added], continued doing wax injections" (Guthrie with Podolsky 1994:3) for the purposes of breast augmentation or reconstruction through the 1950s and 1960s (Bridges and Vasey 1993:2640).

These initial attempts to alter the size and shape of women's breasts represent an unfortunate pattern. Throughout the twentieth century, doctors have continued to inject and implant substances into women's breasts in the absence of data on their safety. Plastic surgeons Randolph Guthrie and Doug Podolsky, in their historical text on breast implants, state, "[f]or more than a century, breast enlargement and restoration methods have been devised not through standardized scientific methods but on an apparently whimsical trial-and-error basis" (1994: 3). Indeed, historical and popular sources report that the materials used to enlarge women's breasts included small glass balls, plastic wool, animal fat, ox cartilage, and ivory ("Light on Breast Surgery" 1947; "Hope for the Flat-Chested" 1967). This odd variety of materials—none demonstrated to be safe or appropriate for implantation into humans— reveals physicians' desire to create and reinforce normative breast size and shape, or what the editors of an investigative report on breast implants in Ms. magazine referred to as "the patriarchy's ideal breasts" ("Beauty and the Breast" 1996:45).

Historical documents suggest that at least some of these procedures were performed on otherwise healthy women who suffered from a "breast deformity"—breasts considered too small or poorly shaped. As the ideal beauty image for women changed throughout this century, so did the trends in breast surgery. Carol Tavris, a social psychologist, writes, "[c]urvy, full-breasted women [were] in fashion in the early 1900s, 1950s, and increasingly, today." Tavris asserts that cultural trends in beauty, femininity, and breast size may have fueled many of the earliest attempts at breast augmentation surgery. Importantly, Tavris also points out that "with the dawn of the 1990s, media images of women began to celebrate a hybrid form that is all but impossible for most women: big-breasted but narrow-hipped" (1992:30, 32-33). The increase in breast augmentation during the 1990s suggests that women are trying to approximate this virtually unattainable ideal figure.

After the initial attempts at using paraffin injections for breast augmentation, Elizabeth Haiken observes in her history of cosmetic surgery, doctors tried a variety of new techniques. She states: "In the 1920s and 1930s, some surgeons experimented with a technique known as autologous fat transplantation, in which fatty tissue was transferred surgically from the abdomen and buttocks to the breast, but they found that the body tended to reabsorb fat quickly, sometimes in unshapely ways, and that lumps that resulted from this process made the early detection of cancer difficult" (Haiken 1997:236). Moreover, because this surgery resulted in visible scarring, surgeons in the 1940s experimented with transplants that included most of the skin. These tissue grafts also had problematic results, and doctors began looking at other types of implant material.

In the mid-1950s, surgeons began implanting natural sea sponges into women's breasts. When women's immune systems rejected the natural sponges, doctors then tried using synthetic sponges made from polyvinyl alcohol, including a product called Ivalon. The synthetic sponges eventually failed, too: Fibrous scar tissue would form around the sponge and enter into all of the holes of the sponge. In 1957, *Time* reported that the "main objection among the surgeons to this type of operation is that Ivalon does not stay spongy, but shrinks 20 percent and becomes as hard as a baseball" ("Building up Bosoms" 1957:59). In 1955, doctors tried to correct this problem by placing the synthetic sponges in a polyethylene sac; and by 1960, it was estimated that "approximately 16,600 polyvinyl or polyethylene implants were in place, performed by 184 of the 294 existing plastic surgeons at that time" (Glatt, Afifi, and Noone 1999:200). However, doctors eventually abandoned this method because of an abnormally high infection rate associated with materials in the polyethylene sac. Despite the high failure rate, doctors continued to try different types of synthetic sponges, including Polistan, introduced in 1959, Etheron, introduced in 1960, and Hydron, introduced in 1961 (Haiken 1997:243).

Synthetic sponges were utilized for breast augmentation throughout the 1950s and 1960s, including "one that looked like a ball of bubble wrap" (Guthrie with Podolsky 1994:6). A compressible implant filled with air, this implant initially appeared to be successful. Soon, however, doctors became aware of problems with the air-filled implants: Guthrie and Podolsky report that when the implants were squeezed or when the women experienced a change in air pressure such as that experienced in an airplane, the cells inside were known to break, causing a loud pop (p. 6). Other complications included high rates of infection and extrusion, which occurs when the implant wears against and eventually breaks through the skin of the breast.

THE USE OF SILICONE IN BREAST AUGMENTATION

In the last 35 years, the most popular method of breast augmentation and reconstruction has been the silicone-gel-filled implant (Johnson 1992). Since the 1940s, silicone has been used in medical devices such as artificial joints, cardiac pacemakers, artificial heart valves, penile and testicular implants, intravenous tubing, catheters, and lenses used in the eyes. A synthetic plastic, silicone exists in three physical forms: silicone liquid or oil, silicone gel, and a hard, rubberlike material known as an elastomer (Bruning 1995; Hatcher, Brooks, and Love 1993). When first developed, silicone was thought to be an "ideal synthetic soft tissue" (Bridges and Vasey 1993:2639). In the late 1940s, plastic surgeons began using injections of liquid silicone to fill out body parts, including the face, lips, and breasts (Bridges and Vasey 1993:2639; Bruning 1995:6; Vasey and Feldstein 1993:16).

Several sources suggest that silicone injections for the purpose of breast augmentation originated in Japan during World War II. Known as the Sakurai formula (named after the Japanese physician who first performed the procedure), this procedure was developed for and used on Japanese prostitutes, who noticed that American servicemen preferred larger-breasted women (Panarites 1993; Swartz 1995). Investigative journalist John Byrne reports that this situation was discovered when "a transformer coolant made of silicone was suddenly disappearing from the docks of Yokohama Harbor in Japan . . . Large doses of the doctored industrial fluid were [being] injected directly into [the prostitutes'] breasts" (1996: 46). Haiken states that "Japanese cosmetologists pioneered the use of silicone to enlarge the breasts of Japanese prostitutes during the war, after such solutions as goats' milk and paraffin were found wanting" (1997: 246). The complex power relations in this example are striking: Japanese prostitutes had their bodies altered via a potentially life-threatening procedure so that they would appeal to American servicemen. Thus, the history of breast implants reveals not only sexist but also racist and imperialistic motivations. Moreover, this history reveals the ways that a woman's ability to choose breast augmentation and reconstruction is constrained by her specific historical, sociocultural, and economic situation.

Silicone injections for breast augmentation first became popular in the United States during the 1950s (Troutwine 1993). As the Japanese had experimented during World War II, U.S. physicians, like Harvey D. Kagan, also had been performing experimental breast procedures on U.S. women since the mid-1940s. Moreover, Kagan had been using a *nonsterile industrial version* of liquid silicone manufactured by Dow Corning called Dow Corn ing 200 Fluid (Byrne 1996:46). (Liquid silicone was initially created during World War II when the U.S. government jointly commissioned Corning Glass and Dow Chemical to find a substitute for rubber, which was in short supply [Burkholz 1994:77].) Byrne reports that the

> [a]ccidental injection of silicone into the bloodstream could result, albeit infrequently, in blindness and even death. Many women suffered from gangrene, pneumonia, massive infection, and collapsed lungs. In some cases, silicone migrated to other parts of the body, accumulating in large lumps. Sometimes, the lumps could be surgically removed. In other cases, however, surgeons found it impossible to excise them without undue disfigurement. Sometimes, to avoid gangrene or the migration of infections to the brain and lungs, surgeons had to perform mastectomies. (p. 46)

The complications from these injections were so serious and potentially life threatening that Nevada and California passed emergency legislation making silicone injections a felony and a misdemeanor, respectively (Byrne 1996). Haiken states: "In 1964, concerned about such reports, Dow Corning voluntarily listed liquid silicone with the Food and Drug Administration as a drug rather than an implant material; the FDA reclassified liquid silicone as a new drug in early 1965, in an attempt to restrict its use" (1997: 247). The FDA finally banned direct injection of silicone into women's breasts in 1965 (Panarites 1993).

Significantly, this history establishes an early record of medical knowledge and intervention concerning the problems associated with the insertion of silicone into the body. Tragically, instead of limiting the medical use of silicone, doctors and medical researchers already had developed implants with sacs that they hoped would contain the silicone. In fact, the first breast implant was called Silastic, and it was invented by plastic surgeons Thomas D. Cronin and Frank Gerow in collaboration with Dow Corning. The silicone rubber envelope filled with liquid silicone was first implanted in March 1962 (Haiken 1997:256).

The story of Timmie Jean Lindsey, the first U.S. woman to receive silicone-gel breast implants, also demonstrates physicians' ability to influence women to have breast augmentation surgery. As Lindsey told reporters, in 1961 she went to a charity hospital to have her tattoos removed. She was the recently divorced mother of six children, and she wanted to remove the tattoos because, she said, they were reminders "of all the wrong turns she'd taken in her life." The doctors who removed Lindsey's tattoos then offered to enlarge her breasts with silicone-gel-filled implants. Lindsey agreed to the procedure and reported seeing dramatic results: Six weeks after the operation, she felt that men had begun to notice her more. As a result, she felt more attractive and enjoyed increased self-esteem (*Frontline* 1996; Swartz 1995). Amazingly, more than 30 years later, Lindsey still has the original implants in her body, and she has reported only minor health problems.

HEALTH PROBLEMS
ASSOCIATED WITH SILICONE BREAST IMPLANTS

Other women have not been so lucky. Multiple health problems have been linked to implants and specifically to silicone-gel-filled implants; still, doctors have continued to augment and reconstruct women's breasts with silicone. One of the reasons why silicone was thought to be an ideal synthetic soft tissue was that researchers believed that silicone was biologically inert; that is, it was assumed that silicone would not deteriorate or cause reactions in the body (Bridges and Vasey 1993; Guthrie with Podolsky 1994). Later studies would reveal that the opposite was true: Silicone *does* break down when injected or implanted into the body, causing both local and systemic, immediate and long-term reactions.

Some of the health problems associated with breast implants include capsular contracture, or the painful hardening of scar tissue around the breast implant; chronic chest pain; calcium deposits; hematoma, or the accumulation of blood under the skin; infection; skin necrosis or decay; changes in nipple or breast sensation; and extrusion (Davis 1991; FDA 1994, 1999; Miller 1993; Panarites 1993; Parker 1995; Segal 1992). Thus, in addition to the risks of anesthesia and surgery in general, breast implants have numerous surgical risks that result from placing a foreign object in the body.

The Public Citizen Health Research Group, a nonprofit consumer advocacy organization, reported that a total of 1.4 million complications had occurred in women with breast implants by 1988. Specifically, Public Citizen estimated that 155,500 women had reported ruptured implants or infections; 123,300 women had reported capsular contracture; and 310,000 women had reported "uncomfortably firm breasts" (Johnson 1992:2). These data were so alarming that Public Citizen petitioned the FDA to ban silicone breast implants. However, in December 1988, an FDA advisory panel voted against the ban (Haiken 1997). The FDA would not officially restrict the use of silicone implants by imposing a general moratorium until three years later, in January 1992.

The FDA currently identifies all of these risks on their web page of information on breast implants. An additional risk is the subsequent surgery, often needed by women with breast implants. The current (1999) FDA informational bulletin states:

> Surgery may be needed to treat a serious problem with the implant, or to remove a ruptured implant and, if desired, replace it. A recent study found that 24 percent of women with breast implants experience adverse events resulting in surgery during the first five years after implantation (silicone and saline implants were combined). The likelihood of needing additional surgery was greater for reconstruction than for augmentation . . . Additional surgeries may result in (additional) loss of breast tissue.

One study of supplemental surgical risks of breast implantation states, "our patient observations suggest a limit to the number of chest wall operations a woman can sustain before deformity or restriction of movement occurs. A device-specific reimplantation rate of 41.6 percent is simply unacceptable" (Shanklin and Smalley 1998:2474). These researchers imply that breast implants are defective devices because they have a nearly 42 percent failure rate that requires replacing them.

Moreover, the FDA bulletin explicitly states that repeat surgeries are required because of the limited temporal quality of implants: "Breast implants *are not lifetime devices* and cannot be expected to last forever. Some implants deflate (or rupture) in the first few months after being implanted and some deflate after several years; yet others are intact 10 or more years after surgery" (FDA 1999). In their 1998 study, Rod Rohrich and his colleagues conclude that implant failure increased markedly with age and that a significant number of implants will fail after eight to ten years. The average length of time before an implant ruptures was 13.4 years (p. 2306).

In addition to these localized and more immediate reactions, women also have reported the following chronic problems associated with silicone-gel-filled implants: swelling and/or joint pain or arthritis-like pain; swelling of the hands and feet; numbness; unusual hair loss; loss of energy; unexplained and unusual fatigue; increased vulnerability to colds, viruses, and flu; symptoms similar to those of connective tissue disorders, such as lupus, scleroderma, or rheumatoid arthritis; tightness, redness, or swelling of the skin; and swollen glands or lymph nodes (FDA 1994, 1999; Marcusson and Bjarnason 1999). Herbert Burkholz points out that research on the health problems associated with breast implants goes back almost three decades. He states: "According to studies at the University of Texas dating back to the 1970s, the human immune system reacts to silicone in breast implants by making antibodies against it. The antibodies then attack the silicone and whatever tissues are associated with it, with arthritis, scleroderma, and lupus as some of the consequences. Joint pain, rashes, and flu symptoms also result" (1994: 78). Thus, research done in the 1970s also shows an early medical awareness of chronic health problems associated with breast implants. Based on these studies, more doctors should have been alert to the risks of using these devices.

BREAST IMPLANTS AND CANCER

Some researchers also have suggested that breast implants are associated with increased incidence of cancer, due to either the silicone gel or the polyurethane foam coverings on some implants (Davis 1991; FDA 1994; Miller 1993; Panarites 1993; Parker 1995; Segal 1992). In fact, the polyurethane foam that constitutes the envelope surrounding the liquid silicone contains TDA (the chemical 2,4-toluene diamine), which is a known carcinogen in animals (Panarites 1993). While many researchers also are questioning the carcinogenicity of silicone gel, most agree that breast implants pose serious and potentially life-threatening problems for women, as they may interfere with the ability to detect tumors or other changes in mammograms (Johnson 1992; Wolfe 1991). The FDA reports that breast implants may interfere with mammograms because they "delay or hinder the early detection of breast cancer by hiding suspicious lesions" (1999). This interference is problematic because breast cancer is often detected much later in women who have breast implants, and this delay can be fatal. Burkholz observes:

> Studies show that on average, by the time that cancer is discovered in a woman with implants, the tumors are five to six times the volume of tumors found in women without implants. Further studies show that 45 percent of women with implants had cancer that had already spread to the lymph nodes at the time of diagnosis. The figure for women without implants whose cancer had been discovered by mammography was only 6 percent. (1994: 80)

Moreover, the FDA warns that "a radiologist may find it difficult to distinguish calcium deposits in the scar tissue around the implant from a breast tumor when he or she is interpreting the mammogram" (FDA 1999). When this situation occurs, the FDA recommends a tissue biopsy. Finally, mammography with breast implants is problematic because it requires severe breast compression, which could result in implant rupture. To reduce the risk of implant rupture, a trained technician needs to push the implant back and gently pull the breast tissue into view. Needless to say, numerous factors, including the size and location of the implant, the amount of breast tissue, and the degree of capsular contracture all affect how well the breast tissue can be imaged during mammography (FDA 1999).

In addition, four recent medical studies also question the potentially harmful effects of silicone breast implants on breast-feeding infants (Berlin 1994; Flick 1994; Levine and Ilowite 1994; Liau, Ito, and Koren 1994). There is some evidence that silicone may be transmitted through breast milk causing abnormal esophageal motility (difficulty in swallowing food) in infants (Levine and Ilowite 1994). The medical concern is great enough that European physicians recommend that mothers with breast implants refrain from breast feeding their infants. Given this research and the confirmed data on the incidence of silicone leakage or rupture of breast implants, why has similar concern not been expressed among U.S. physicians?

AUTOIMMUNE DISORDERS
AND CONNECTIVE TISSUE DISEASES

Since the 1980s, physicians and medical researchers primarily have debated the question of whether silicone implants cause autoimmune disorders and connective tissue diseases, two of the most serious systemic reactions associated with the silicone implants. So far, medical research has been inconclusive. While some studies suggest a linkage between silicone implants and autoimmune disorders, others suggest that the current scientific evidence does not indicate causation. Some studies (one conducted by the Mayo Clinic, the other by Harvard University and Brigham and Women's Hospital) find that silicone-gel-filled breast implants are *not* associated with increased risks for autoimmune dysfunction and connective tissue diseases (Gabriel et al. 1994; Washburn 1996). Even though the results of these studies have been published in scientific journals, critics argue that, like previous experiments, the results from these studies are flawed. Specifically, critics suggest that because connective tissue diseases are so rare in the general population, the samples in these studies were not large enough to assess whether women with breast implants really experienced increased risk for connective tissue disorders. Further, critics argue that the researchers did not consider the long latency period often associated between the exposure to silicone (as a result of rupture or silicone bleed) and the onset of symptoms.[2] Finally, critics suggest that these studies considered only traditional or classical examples of connective tissue disease; atypical symptoms were not accounted for (Washburn 1996). Some researchers suggest that the multiple symptoms reported by thousands of women (approximately 400,000) may indicate a new type of disease that has yet to be recognized and classified by the medical community.

In addition, there may be a conflict of interest in the way some of this research on the safety of breast implants was conducted, depending on which interest groups funded the studies. For example, Marcia Angell, physician and executive editor of the *New England Journal of Medicine,* acknowledges that the Mayo Clinic study "was partially funded by the American Society of Plastic and Reconstructive Surgeons' Educational Foundation, which in turn received funds from Dow Corning and other breast implant manufacturers" (1996:143). Both the ASPRS and Dow Corning have a vested interest in finding no fault with these implants. Scientists on both sides of the debate agree that more studies (and better-designed, independent studies) are needed to discover the true effects of silicone on the human body (Angell 1994, 1996; Bridges 1994; Gabriel et al. 1994).

THE COSTS OF BREAST SURGERY

Regardless of the specific findings on autoimmune disorders, enough women are reporting significant health problems to raise questions concerning why physicians would condone or promote the use of silicone implants for breast augmentation and reconstruction. While the intent of plastic surgeons and breast implant manufacturers was not to create more health problems in women, it cannot be denied that, until recent litigation, both groups have profited enormously from not only the initial breast implant procedure but also the often necessary follow-up surgeries. In fact, a report in *American Demographics* by Marc Spiegler shows that the breast implant business has never been better, especially since the FDA moratorium on silicone implants. He argues that "[p]lastic surgeons have been reaping the benefits of the silicone scare in both directions. The number of breast-implant-removal procedures soared 47 percent between 1992 and 1994, from 25,700 to 37,900" (1996: 13). According to the ASPRS, in 1996 there were only 3,013 breast implants removed, but in 1998 this number jumped back up to 32,262 removals, a 971 percent increase between 1996 and 1998 (ASPRS 1999).

How can the increase in breast implant removals be explained? The primary reason is that many women are afraid of retaining the implants for fear of disease. Another reason is that many women were advised by their lawyers to have the silicone implants removed to make a stronger legal case for claiming damages. In addition, many of the women who have had silicone breast implants removed replace them with other types of implants. Spiegler states that "[i]n 1994, 68 percent of women who had implants removed opted to replace them right away, up from 60 percent in 1992. This means that at least two-thirds of implant procedures are currently done for repeat customers" (1996: 13). Similarly, of the 32,262 implants removed in 1998, 83 percent were replaced with new implants (ASPRS 1999).

The effects of medical social control also can be observed when considering the enormous amounts of time, energy, and money expended by women who have undergone breast implant procedures. Even without the major consequent health problems, this surgery is time consuming and physically painful. Moreover, this elective surgery places an enormous financial burden on women, and costs are typically not covered by health insurance unless as part of breast cancer care. In 1992, the average surgeon's fee for breast augmentation or reconstruction with an implant ranged from $2,340 to $2,754 (Bruning 1995), and the average cost to a patient undergoing implant surgery in 1992 was $4,500 (Johnson 1992). In 1998, surgeons' fees for breast augmentation ranged between $3,077 and $3,292; for breast reconstruction, surgeons' fees ranged from $2,971 to $9,435, depending upon the type of procedure used. Note that these fees do *not* include anesthesia, operating room facilities, or other related expenses (ASPRS 1999).

Moreover, initial surgeries represent only part of the cost of breast augmentation and reconstruction because many women have to have the implants removed or replaced. Since the average life span of an implant is approximately ten years, many women may undergo replacement surgery multiple times during their lives (Miller 1993; Wartik 1993). A recent study published in the *Annals of Plastic Surgery* reported that only 30 percent of implants that were 6 to 15 years old had remained intact (Washburn 1996). Explantation, or removal of implants, is even more expensive than implantation: One source reports that in 1992 explantation surgery could cost more than $5,000 (Wartik 1993), and even more if the implant ruptured and leaked silicone throughout the chest cavity, requiring more extensive surgery.

Just as most insurance companies cover the costs of breast implantation only for reconstruction purposes after cancer, not for augmentation (DLR Research Note 1994), not all insurance companies cover the cost of explantation. Of those that do, they only do so when it is deemed medically necessary. Thus, individual women and their families are carrying the primary financial burdens of breast implants and many of their consequent health problems.

THE MEDICALIZATION OF WOMEN'S BREASTS

This history of breast augmentation and reconstruction and the multiple health risks associated with these procedures illustrates U.S. society's obsession with the perfect breast. Further, this history suggests ways that physicians have exercised social control over women, by keeping women in doctors' offices and on surgeons' tables for procedures that are not medically necessary. Given this history and the fact that breasts are not essential to maintaining good health, why have doctors tried for so long to perfect a method of breast augmentation and reconstruction? Similarly, why have women continued to pursue these options even when more information became available concerning the dangers involved with breast implants? (Data show that in 1998, 132,378 U.S. women had breast augmentation surgery [ASPRS 1999]—most with saline implants—which have not yet been proven to be safe [Bruning 1995; Spiegler 1996].) The answer to these questions lies in the social construction of women's health, and, specifically, in the medicalization of women's breasts. As breast cancer warrior Audre Lorde writes, in a society "where the superficial is supreme, the idea that a woman can be beautiful and one-breasted is considered depraved, or at best, bizarre, a threat to 'morale'" (1980: 65). Women with small breasts are similarly constructed as deviant: They supposedly lack the capacity for sexual pleasure, femininity, and maternity. The next section explores the process by which women with small breasts or a different number of breasts came to be seen as deformed or diseased. The American Society for Plastic and Reconstructive Surgeons (ASPRS), the manufacturers of breast implants, the American Medical Association (AMA), and the U.S. Food and Drug Administration (FDA) all played roles in the medicalization of women's breasts.

THE ROLE OF PHYSICIANS AND THE ASPRS

Physicians and, especially, plastic surgeons have been prominent actors in the medicalization of women's breasts. Physicians have primarily contributed to the belief that women who undergo breast cancer surgery are "deformed" by including reconstructive surgery in the definition of breast cancer treatment. Citing current medical literature on breast cancer and reconstruction, sociologist Anne Kasper quotes one study that says, "*not* electing reconstruction may add to the cost of medical and psychiatric follow-up, and will mean repeated purchases of external prostheses by the patient" (1995:199). This statement is highly problematic: It neither addresses the real risks involved with reconstruction nor challenges the ideology that women with a different number of breasts are considered "deformed" or "diseased." Instead, this statement reflects the belief that women who undergo mastectomy are in need of further medical treatment. By suggesting that reconstruction is a natural part of breast cancer treatment, physicians contribute to the belief that women with one or no breasts are unnatural.

While individual physicians clearly have contributed to the belief that small breasts are "deformities" or "diseased," and that women who undergo breast cancer surgery should also undergo reconstructive surgery, the American Society for Plastic and Reconstructive Surgeons (ASPRS) also has played a critical role in the process of medicalizing women's breasts. In fact, the ASPRS was one of the first medical groups to identify the condition "micromastia," or abnormal smallness of the breasts. In 1957 *Time* magazine reported that at its annual meeting, "the American Society of Plastic and Reconstructive Surgery was divided over the desirability of a drastic remedy [for micromastia]: surgery to pad out the breasts, using either body fat or a sponge-like synthetic" ("Building Up Bosoms" 1957:59). The fact that the ASPRS recognized "micromastia" as a problem in need of a remedy as early as 1957 supports the argument that the American Society for Plastic and Reconstructive Surgeons, which currently represents 90 percent of all plastic surgeons in the United States, contributes to the social construction of women's breasts as diseased.

In other historical documents, women's health specifically was constructed in terms of their breast size. Women with small breasts were said to suffer from extreme "neuroses" or "psychological disturbances" as a result of their breast size ("Light on Breast Surgery" 1947:60). For example, the ASPRS issued the following statement during a 1983 practice enhancement campaign: "There is substantial and enlarging medical knowledge to the effect that these deformities [small breasts] are really a disease which result in the patient's feelings of inadequacy, lack of self-confidence, distortion of body image, and a total lack of well-being due to a lack of perceived femininity" (Coco 1994:111). This statement illustrates well the social construction of illness by taking a natural, normal condition like women's breast size and making it a deviant condition in need of medical treatment. This example also is strikingly similar to other attempts to medicalize women's normal body functioning, such as premenstrual syndrome and menopause: Physicians successfully linked these natural human experiences with mental illness or psychological dysfunction—conditions that historically have been treated as deviant (Conrad and Schneider 1985). Thus, the ASPRS was successful in constructing women's small breasts as a double pathology: Small breasts, themselves, were considered to be a disease, and the psychological effects small breasts could have on a woman's self-esteem were seen to cause a trauma so severe that they also were labeled a disease.

In addition to defining small breasts as diseased, the ASPRS contributed to the process of medicalization by petitioning the FDA in 1982 to deregulate breast implants, as they considered implants to be "medically necessary" devices (Troutwine 1993:48-49). Jane Zones reports that the ASPRS petition failed: "The FDA General and Plastic Surgical Devices Advisory Panel, after several hearings, voted in January 1983 to recommend to the FDA Commissioner that the implants continue to be classified as Class III devices in the absence of convincing evidence of long-term safety" (1992: 226). Thus, the ASPRS further contributed to the medicalization of women's breasts by attempting to get the government to recognize, at least initially, that breast implants were a form of medical treatment.

The position of the ASPRS also is problematic because physicians have profited enormously from the medicalization of women's breasts (Zones 1992). Writer Mimi Swartz argues that the market for cosmetic surgery increased during the 1970s and 1980s because, at $4,000 a surgery, a "boob job" was seen as relatively inexpensive for middle-class women. Moreover, Swartz says, "the doctors and hospitals loved it almost as much as the patients: The surgery was not covered by insurance, so there were no reimbursements to wait for. Augmentation mammaplasty was strictly COD" (1995: 92). By 1992, women were spending $450 million a year on breast augmentation (Regush 1992). The profits have continued to grow in spite of the FDA restrictions and the media scare of the early 1990s. In 1998, when breast implant surgery cost approximately $6,000, women were spending close to $800 million a year on breast augmentation alone.[3]

In addition, the ASPRS eventually lobbied for and received insurance reimbursements for breast augmentation after they constructed another illness called "hypoplasia," for extreme flat-chestedness (Swartz 1995:92). Thus, the ASPRS maximized the profits of its members on breast augmentation surgery by expanding the market from middle-class women, who could afford to pay for the surgery out-of-pocket, to larger numbers of women, who could be medically diagnosed as suffering from the "diseases" of micromastia or hypoplasia, thereby qualifying for insurance reimbursement.

This situation is further complicated by the fact that, while all breast augmentation and reconstruction procedures carry the risk of injury, illness, and even death, very few women were informed of these risks by individual plastic surgeons or the ASPRS (Panarites 1993; Parker 1995). In fact, the following evidence suggests that the ASPRS and other medical societies attempted to hide this information. In 1992, the ASPRS put pressure on the FDA to dilute warnings about the safety of silicone breast implants on a form designed to ensure that women give informed consent to the procedures. The ASPRS asked the FDA to change the following statement, "Although there is no evidence that silicone used in breast implants causes cancer in humans, the possibility has not been ruled out," to "There is no evidence that silicone used in breast implants causes cancer in humans" (Troutwine 1993:49-50). This change in language represents an attempt on the part of the ASPRS to minimize the potential health risks associated with breast implants and to reduce public suspicion about their safety.

Physicians also failed to inform individual women about the risks of breast implants. Author Susan Zimmermann's research shows that plastic surgeons gave their patients breast implant brochures in the 1970s and 1980s that misinformed women of the specific health risks related to the procedure and falsely stated that the implants were lifetime devices (1998: 98-100). Moreover, breast implant packages come with a manufacturer's warning that includes a long list of problems including: "infection; extrusion of implant/ interruption in wound healing; blood clots; hematoma (accumulation of blood under the skin); calcification (hardening); fluid accumulation; skin necrosis (decay); change in nipple sensation; and other" (Goldrich 1988:22). Since, presumably, women are under anesthesia when the surgeons open the breast implant packages, women often do not get a chance to read the package inserts. These examples demonstrate the failure of the ASPRS and individual plastic surgeons to provide safety information to women about to undergo breast augmentation surgery.

THE MANUFACTURERS OF BREAST IMPLANTS

While the ASPRS played an instrumental role in the processes of medicalization and social control, this organization did not act alone in targeting women for breast augmentation procedures. Gayle Troutwine argues that breast implant manufacturers aggressively marketed implants to ASPRS doctors by promoting their "beauty-enhancing" qualities and by offering warranties and replacement implants if an implant failed. Troutwine further argues that not one of the advertisements that appeared in the *Journal of Plastic and Reconstructive Surgery* expressed any concern for women's health or for the common problems associated with implants, such as encapsulation or rupture. Instead, the advertisements focused on large breasts as fulfilling women's "natural" needs, or the ads appealed to the sexual desires of male surgeons. Breast augmentation surgery was such a profitable business that breast implant manufacturers soon began to directly target women consumers in addition to ASPRS surgeons. Troutwine writes: "By the mid-1980s, emboldened by desire for more profits, some manufacturers placed ads in magazines like *Cosmopolitan*. These ads hawked the same message: Large breasts are desirable, and silicone-gel-filled (and sometimes polyurethane-covered) implants can fulfill this desire risk-free" (1993: 48).

Today, advertisements for breast augmentation can be found in many newspapers and magazines. An advertisement suggesting that breast augmentation could improve a woman's self-esteem was even recently aired on television during a daytime soap opera (ABC 9/1/99). The advertising is working, and it is reaching a younger audience. Breast augmentation surgery for teenagers, girls under the age of 19, has increased dramatically. In some cases, breast implants are at the top of gift lists for teenage girls (Warren 1999:A2). Thus, the importance of breast implant manufacturers in this process of medicalization cannot be underestimated: Implant manufacturers like Dow Corning,[4] Bristol-Myers Squibb, and 3M have promoted and profited from women's dissatisfaction with their breast size or shape.

THE AMERICAN MEDICAL ASSOCIATION

Similar to the position taken by the ASPRS, the American Medical Association (AMA) also was critical of the FDA's attempts to publish complete information on the health risks associated with breast implants. In 1991 James Todd, then president of the AMA, stated that the FDA warnings "may raise unnecessary concerns to a woman whose decision has been made in all probability" (Troutwine 1993:50). Moreover, after the 1992 FDA moratorium on silicone breast implants, the AMA's Council on Scientific Affairs published their recommendations for the continued use of silicone breast implants in specific situations in the *Journal of the American Medical Association (JAMA)*. In effect, while supporting an establishment of a national registry of all breast implant patients and the FDA's request that women be fully warned about the risks and benefits of breast implant surgery, the AMA also supported the continued availability of silicone implants and surgical procedures for breast implantation. The recommendations state, "[t]hat the AMA, based on current scientific knowledge, supports the continued practice of breast augmentation or reconstruction with currently marketed implants when indicated." Moreover, the AMA voted to "urge the FDA and its commissioner, David A. Kessler, to adopt, endorse, and promulgate the recommendation of its advisory panel, thus allowing silicone-gel-filled breast implants to remain on the market pending further studies" (Council on Scientific Affairs 1993:2602). Thus, the ASPRS, the manufacturers of breast implants, and the AMA all have contributed to the medicalization and marketing of women's breasts.

THE FDA'S PARTICIPATION IN MEDICALIZATION AND SOCIAL CONTROL

The ASPRS and the AMA are not the only organizations that have participated in the medicalization of women's breasts: The FDA also had a role in the social control of women. Specifically, prior to 1992, the FDA participated in these processes by failing to adequately regulate breast implants (Troutwine 1993) and by asserting that breast implants must be kept available because of a public health concern for women who had undergone mastectomies.

The FDA's failure to regulate breast implants began in 1976, when Congress passed the Safe Medical Devices Amendment. This legislation gave the FDA power to regulate medical devices that might pose a health risk. The amendment contained a grandfather clause, a provision that freed from regulation any medical devices already in use when the amendment was created. Thus, since breast implants were considered to be medical devices, they were not subject to FDA regulation (FDA 1994, 1999). However, the law directed that the FDA eventually would require scientific evidence of safety and effectiveness of many of these pre-1976 devices (FDA 1999:1). Even though reports associating silicone breast implants with autoimmune disease emerged in the early 1980s, the FDA was slow in researching breast implant safety. Finally, in 1988, the FDA gave breast implant manufacturers 30 months to produce evidence on product safety. By 1991, only four companies had complied, so the FDA asked for more data (Sharp 1999:1506). The FDA did not take definitive actions to regulate breast implants until January 1992, when FDA Commissioner David Kessler called for a moratorium on silicone breast implants (Miller 1993). The lack of regulation on the part of the FDA communicated that women's health problems, especially those that occur as a result of cosmetic surgery, were not important enough to monitor.

After declaring the moratorium on silicone breast implants, the FDA created a public health panic by not providing women who already had implants with clear and accurate information about what to do. Instead, the FDA attempted to navigate a problematic middle ground when it advised women *not* to have explantation because the surgical risk may be higher: The "FDA believes . . . that information currently available is insufficient to warrant the surgical removal of the implants since any surgical procedure carries a certain amount of risk" (Johnson 1992:CRS-4). Thus, the FDA's 1992 decision to place a moratorium on the use of silicone-gel-filled breast implants presented women who had already undergone implant surgery with a complicated choice: Women could leave the implants in, risking rupture, painful hardening of breasts, and other complications, or they could choose to have the implants removed but potentially face complications from that surgery. Thus, the FDA effectively placed women in a Catch-22 situation.

The position of the FDA that reconstructive surgery following mastectomy is "an integral part of the cancer treatment" also clearly contributed to the medicalization of women's breasts (Panarites 1993:191). Specifically, this statement suggests that women who are missing one or both breasts are in need of medical treatment; in other words, women's bodies are considered "deformed" or "diseased" if they have a different number of breasts. Other statements by the FDA similarly suggest that the FDA's inaction was, in part, motivated by this notion. For instance, in 1991, while the FDA was waiting for implant manufacturers to supply safety data, they did not attempt to halt the use of implants: On the contrary, the FDA ensured that implants would still be made available, "citing a compelling public health need, especially for reconstruction patients" (Segal 1992:8-9). Moreover, in April 1992, the FDA modified the moratorium on breast implants and allowed silicone-gel-filled implants back on the market in controlled clinical studies "for reconstruction after mastectomy, correction of congenital deformities, or replacement for ruptured silicione implants for augmentation" (FDA 1999).

Ironically, the FDA's apparent concern for women's health did not focus on carcinogens in the environment or problems with high-fat diets that may be contributing to high rates of breast cancer in the United States (see chapter 9 of this volume). Instead, the FDA chose to focus on the psychological trauma experienced by women recovering from the loss of one or both breasts. Certainly the latter issue is important to address, but the FDA and the medical establishment should refocus their attention and energy on the causes of breast cancer instead of on its treatment. Thus, similar to the ASPRS, which asserted that small breasts are "deformities" or "diseased," the FDA also contributed to the medicalization of women's breasts by reinforcing the idea that women who have a breast removed via mastectomy are deformed.

In addition to the FDA's participation in the medicalization of women's breasts, their history of inaction also constitutes social control. The FDA recognizes that their role is not to prove the safety of implants; David Kessler, who assumed the post of FDA commissioner in 1990, asserts that "the burden of proving safety rests with the manufacturer" (Johnson 1992:CRS-5). However, we must ask why the FDA continued to allow breast implants to be used in the absence of clear information on their safety. Specifically, if the FDA received approximately 5,000 complaints related to the safety of breast implants between 1983 and 1992 (Johnson 1992:1), what prevented the FDA from acting sooner? The record shows that the FDA was aware of and concerned about the safety of silicone breast implants long before the 1992 moratorium. In 1965, for example, the FDA reportedly recognized that silicone injections violated its rule on untested procedures; acting on this concern, the FDA "seized silicone supplies in the office of several California doctors" ("Escalation" 1965:113). Moreover, after the FDA was petitioned to ban silicone implants by the Public Citizen Health Advisory Group in 1988, they failed to act until three more years had passed and thousands more women had had breast augmentation surgery. Thus, many scholars, health advocates, and investigative journalists agree that the FDA dropped the ball by not investigating and acting on the health problems associated with silicone breast implants sooner (Burkholz 1994; Miller 1993; Panarites 1993; Troutwine 1993). By allowing implant manufacturers and physicians to market breast implants for so long, the FDA also facilitated those groups' social control of women.

Since 1992, the FDA has called for safety and effectiveness data for saline-filled implants and has cleared several manufacturers to market them. In 1994, the FDA approved a pilot study on breast implants filled with a purified form of soybean oil (FDA 1999:2). Research on silicone implants also continues, including a 1998 study to assess the rupture rate of breast implants in a sample of 1,200 women. Also in 1998, the Department of Health and Human Services (DHHS) asked the National Academy of Sciences, Institute of Medicine:

> . . . to conduct an independent, unbiased review of all past and ongoing scientific research regarding the safety of silicone breast implants. A committee of experts in relevant scientific and clinical areas will evaluate past and ongoing studies of the relationship, if any, between implants and systemic disease; assess the biologic and immunologic effects of silicone and other chemical components of breast implant[s]; and assess the impact of breast implants, if any, on the offspring of women with implants or the accuracy of mammograms. (FDA 1999:3)

That more research is needed is evident from the available data: From 1985 until September 10, 1998, the FDA received 127,500 adverse reaction reports for silicone-gel-filled breast implants. During the same time period, there have been 49,661 adverse reaction reports for saline-filled implants. Included in these adverse reports for both types of breast implants are 118 reports of death allegedly related to breast implants (FDA 1999). The public debate about the safety of silicone breast implants also is unabated, with different groups submitting citizen's petitions to the FDA requesting that the FDA either ease restrictions on silicone implants or revoke their availability. As of October 1997, the FDA refused to comply with either request, citing "insufficient information to change the current regulatory policy on silicone gel implants" (FDA 1999:2).

CONCLUSION

> To "choose" a procedure that may harden the breasts, result in loss of sensation, and introduce a range of serious health problems isn't a choice, it's a scripted response. And it's worthy of the Stepford wives.
>
> —Laura Shapiro et al., 1992

A close examination of the history of breast augmentation and reconstruction, in addition to the recent scandal surrounding silicone breast implants, reveals that women's breasts have been medicalized in a number of ways. By defining women's breasts as diseased, the medical establishment has exercised social control over women, as evidenced by the accounts of women suffering from painful, debilitating diseases as a result of mammaplasty (Troutwine 1993; Washburn 1996). The enormous amounts of time, energy, and money associated with breast augmentation and reconstruction constitute evidence of social control. In addition to the physical and emotional distress of breast augmentation and reconstruction, these procedures also are financially burdensome. When one considers that breast implants may need to be removed or replaced many times throughout a woman's life, and that these procedures are often not covered by insurance, the costs to women increase enormously. While the controversy over the safety of breast implants is still being debated, women continue to express their pain and frustration: "I never thought I could feel so limited," writes one woman who underwent silicone breast implant surgery and suffered a number of health complications. Another woman writes, "I have osteoporosis from taking steroids to treat my lupus and cognitive problems [associated with her silicone breast implants]. I stopped working in 1995 because of loss of function. I've lost my health, never to regain it" (Washburn 1996:55, 48).

Clearly, American women have suffered needlessly because of the policies of plastic surgeons, the manufacturers of breast implants, the AMA, and the FDA. Several ideological, structural, and individual level solutions can counter this medicalization and social control of women. First, women's breasts should be demedicalized and viewed as natural, healthy tissue regardless of their size, shape, and number. Breast augmentation and reconstruction no longer should be considered a medical imperative for women who have small breasts or for women who undergo breast cancer surgery. Because the cosmetic surgery and breast implant industries are largely profit driven, the first step in the process of demedicalization involves removing the profit incentive for physicians, breast implant manufacturers, and lawyers. Ideally, this change would accompany larger changes in the U.S. health care system; these changes might include redistributing health care to a larger population and shifting the emphasis from high-cost, elective procedures performed by specialists to prevention, health education, and primary care.

In the absence of these larger changes, changes in the medical education of physicians would facilitate the demedicalization of women's breasts. Diana Scully's work on gynecologists' training (1980) effectively demonstrates that medical education is a process of socialization into the medical establishment; medical education becomes a powerful tool for shaping physicians' approaches to health, illness, and medical care.

Finally, the lobbying power of medical societies, like the ASPRS and the AMA, should be decreased. Their disregard for the safety record of breast implants suggests that these groups are acting not in the interest of women's health but in the interest of increasing profit and maintaining their power.

In addition to demedicalizing women's breasts, women should have more control over the processes of breast augmentation and reconstruction. Currently 233,586 women per year undergo breast augmentation or reconstructive surgery (ASPRS 1999); until the demand for this surgery decreases, women should be made fully aware of the risks involved with these procedures.

Regulations also should be placed on the advertising practices of plastic surgeons and breast implant manufacturers since advertising clearly contributes to the perception that women need breast augmentation and reconstruction. This step is particularly important because advertising, which plays a major role in the cosmetic surgery industry, increasingly targets younger women. Specifically, advertisements should reflect the potential health complications from breast augmentation and reconstruction. Moreover, individual plastic surgeons should be required to inform patients of the long-term financial costs of breast implants. The FDA could facilitate this process by increasing its efforts to educate women about breast implants and ensuring that cancer patients receive information about alternatives to reconstructive surgery. The current information found on the FDA's web page is an excellent start at educating women about the multiple risks involved with breast implants. Further, the FDA needs to do its job as a regulatory agency by requiring thorough scientific testing of the safety of all medical devices. More specifically, the FDA should develop new regulatory procedures aimed at evaluating medical devices with the stricter standards used on pharmaceutical products (Vasey and Feldman 1993:117).

Finally, to reduce the demand for breast augmentation and reconstruction, the "feminine beauty norms" (Davis 1991) that cause women to feel inadequate if they have small breasts or if they have undergone mastectomies needs to be deconstructed. In her research on breast cancer and reconstruction, Anne Kasper reports that

> . . . women themselves are admired, valued, viewed as objects of beauty, or not, in large measure because they have breasts. That the social status of women is linked to their breasts and that they derive a positive, negative, or ambiguous sense of their worthiness based on a body part is but one indicator of how little society has changed over centuries of treating women as objects or

property and of the continuing disdain with which women are viewed. (1995: 198)

As Kasper suggests, women are receiving powerful messages about their breasts. It should not be surprising then, that, for many women their self-esteem and self-worth are largely determined by their breast size and shape. How do we begin to address this problem that is so ingrained in our patriarchal society?

To begin, women's social status needs to be separated from the cultural valuation and objectification of their bodies. Specifically, media representations of women and women's bodies should be changed so that these images reflect the great diversity of body shapes and sizes that exist, including images of women who have had mastectomies. Moreover, media representations that seek to only sexually objectify women and women's bodies should be countered. In the short term, these solutions would make women far less vulnerable to social control by the medical establishment. These steps also, however, represent the beginnings of a longer process to substantially decrease the incentive for cosmetic surgery. To reach this goal, gender inequality needs to be eliminated in order to create a society where women are valued as individuals, as people who have important contributions to make to society, and not just as bodies with breasts.

NOTES

AUTHOR'S NOTE: I would like to acknowledge the work done by Alice Gates in helping me research and draft an earlier version of this chapter. I also want to thank Anne Kasper and Carla Talarico for their editing comments on later drafts.

1. See, for example, Diana Dull and Candace West, "Accounting for Cosmetic Surgery: The Accomplishment of Gender," *Social Problems* 38 (1991):54-70; and Anne S. Kasper (1995).
2. Panarites (1993:170) notes that this long latency period between exposure to silicone and the development of severe symptoms is especially problematic for women involved in litigating for financial compensation for health problems. The statute of limitations on many legal cases may expire before

the severity of potential health problems develop and before women get a chance to seek legal recourse.

3. The figure of $800 million dollars is calculated by taking the 132,378 breast augmentation surgeries performed in 1998 and multiplying that number by the estimated total cost of surgery at $6,000 each.

4. In 1992, Dow Corning withdrew from the silicone implant market but continued to supply silicone gel to one implant manufacturer. In 1994, Dow Corning was one of several companies that manufactured breast implants who were sued in a class action suit and agreed to pay into a $4.25 billion settlement fund for plaintiffs. Subsequently, that settlement fell apart and in 1995, Dow Corning filed for Chapter 11 bankruptcy (FDA 1999; Sharp 1999:1506).

REFERENCES

ABC. 9/1/99. "Breast Implant Commercial." Aired at 12:30 P.M. during a daytime soap opera.

American Society of Plastic and Reconstructive Surgeons (ASPRS). 1999. "ASPRS National Clearinghouse of Plastic Surgery Statistics." At http://www.plasticsurgery.org/mediactr/99stats.htm.

Angell, Marcia. 1994. "Do Breast Implants Cause Systemic Disease? Science in the Courtroom." *New England Journal of Medicine* 330:1748-49.

———. 1996. *Science on Trial.* New York: W. W. Norton.

"Beauty and the Breast." 1996. *Ms.* 5:45.

Berlin, Chester M. 1994. "Silicone Breast Implants and Breast-Feeding." *Pediatrics* 94:547-49.

"Body Work" 1994. *U.S. News and World Report* 117:15.

"Bosom Foe" 1954. *Time* 64:52.

Bridges, Alan J. 1994. "Silicone Implant Controversy Continues." *Lancet* 344:1451-52.

Bridges, Alan J. and Frank B. Vasey. 1993. "Silicone Breast Implants: History, Safety, and Potential Complications." *Archives of Internal Medicine* 153:2638-44.

Brink, Susan. 1995. "Pills, Balloons, and Now Tapeworms." *U.S. News and World Report* 119:48.

Bruning, Nancy. [1993] 1995. *Breast Implants: Everything You Need to Know.* New York: Hunter House.

"Building Up Bosoms." 1957. *Time* 70:59.

Burkholz, Herbert. 1994. *The FDA Follies.* New York: Basic Books.

Byrne, John A. 1996. "How Silicone Ended Up in Women's Breasts." *Ms.* 6:46-50.

Coco, Linda. [1993] 1994. "Silicone Breast Implants in America: A Choice of the 'Official Breast'." Pp. 103-32 in *Essays on Controlling Processes,* ed. Laura Nader. Berkeley: Kroeber Anthropological Society.

Conrad, Peter. [1992] 1996. "Medicalization and Social Control." Pp. 137-162 in *Perspectives in Medical Sociology,* 2nd ed., ed. Phil Brown. Prospect Heights, Ill: Waveland Press.

Conrad, Peter and Joseph W. Schneider. [1980] 1985. *Deviance and Medicalization: From Badness to Sickness.* Philadelphia: Temple University Press.

Council on Scientific Affairs, American Medical Association. 1993. "Silicone Gel Breast Implants." *Journal of the American Medical Association* 270:2602-06.

Davis, Kathy. 1991. "Remaking the She-Devil: A Critical Look at Feminist Approaches to Beauty." *Hypatia* 6:21-43.

DLR Research Note. 1994. "Health Insurance Practices Regarding Breast Implants." Annapolis, Maryland: Department of Legislative Reference.

Ehrenreich, Barbara. 1992. "Stamping Out A Dread Scourge." *Time* 139:88.

"Escalation." 1965. *Newsweek* 66:110.

Flick, Jonathan. 1994. "Silicone Implants and Esophogeal Motility: Are Breast-Fed Infants at Risk?" *Journal of the American Medical Association* 271:240-41.

FDA (U.S. Food and Drug Administration). 1994. *Breast Implants: An Information Update*. Rockville, Md: US FDA.

——. 1999. "Breast Implant Information on FDA's Website." At http://www.fda.gov/oca/breastimplants.

Frontline. 1996. "Breast Implants on Trial." PBS Video.

Gabriel, Sherine E., W. Michael O'Fallon, Leonard T. Kurland, C. Mary Bear, John E. Woods, and L. Joseph Melton. 1994 "Risk of Connective-Tissue Diseases and Other Disorders After Breast Implantation." *New England Journal of Medicine* 330:1697-1702.

Glatt, Brian S., Ghada Afifi, and R. Barrett Noone. 1999. "Long-term Follow-Up of a Sponge Breast Implant and Review of the Literature." *Annals of Plastic Surgery* 42:196-201.

Goldrich, Sybil Niden. 1988. "Restoration Drama: A Cautionary Tale by a Woman Who Had Breast Implants after Mastectomy." *Ms.* 16 (June):21-22.

Guthrie, Randolph H. with Doug Podolsky. 1994. *The Truth About Breast Implants.* New York: John Wiley.

Haiken, Elizabeth. 1997. *Venus Envy: A History of Cosmetic Surgery.* Baltimore: Johns Hopkins University Press.

Hatcher, Chris, Loren Brooks, and Candace Love. 1993. "Breast Cancer and Silicone Implants: Psychological Consequences for Women." *Journal of the National Cancer Institute* 85:1361-65.

"Hope for the Flat-chested." 1967. *Science Digest* 62:69.

Johnson, Judith A. 1992. *Breast Implants: Safety and FDA Regulation.* Washington, D.C.: Congressional Research Service, Library of Congress.

Kasper, Anne S. 1995. "The Social Construction of Breast Loss and Reconstruction." *Women's Health: Research on Gender, Behavior, and Policy* 1:197-219.

Levine, Jeremiah J. and Norman T. Ilowite. 1994. "Sclerodermalike Esophageal Disease in Children Breast-Fed by Mothers with Silicone Breast Implants." *Journal of the American Medical Association* 271:213-16.

Liau, M., S. Ito, and G. Koren. 1994. "Sclerodermalike Esophageal Disease in Children of Mothers with Silicone Breast Implants." *Journal of the American Medical Association* 272:769-70.

"Light on Breast Surgery." 1947. *Newsweek* 29:60.

Lorde, Audre [1980] 1987. *The Cancer Journals.* San Francisco: Spinsters/Aunt Lute.

Marcusson, Jan A., and Bolli Bjarnason. 1999. "Unusual Skin Reaction to Silicone Content in Breast Implants." *Acta Dermato-Venereologica* 79:136-38.

Mellican, Eugene R. 1995. "Breast Implants, The Cult of Beauty, and a Culturally Constructed 'Disease'." *Journal of Popular Culture* 28:7-17.

Miller, Susan Katz. 1993. "The Trouble with Implants." *New Scientist* 138:20-24.

Morgan, Kathryn Pauly. 1991 "Women and the Knife: Cosmetic Surgery and the Colonization of Women's Bodies." *Hypatia* 6:25-53.

Panarites, Zoë. 1993. "Breast Implants: Choices Women Thought They Made." *New York Law School Journal on Human Rights* 11:163-204.

Parker, Lisa S. 1995. "Beauty and Breast Implantation: How Candidate Selection Affects Autonomy and Informed Consent." *Hypatia* 10:183-201.

Regush, Nicholas. 1992. "Toxic Breasts." *Mother Jones* 17:24-31.

Riessman, Catherine Kohler. [1983] 1992. "Women and Medicalization: A New Perspective." Pp. 190-220 in *Perspectives in Medical Sociology*, 1st ed., ed. Phil Brown. Prospect Heights, Ill: Waveland Press.

Rohrich, Rod J., William P. Adams, Jr., Samuel J. Beran, Ranganathan Rathakrishnan, John Griffin, Jack B. Robinson, Jr., and Jeffrey M. Kenkel. 1998. "An Analysis of Silicone-gel-filled Breast Implants: Diagnosis and Failure Rates." *Plastic and Reconstructive Surgery* 102:2304-09.

Scully, Diana. [1980] 1994. *Men Who Control Women's Health: The Miseducation of Obstetrician-Gynecologists.* New York: Teacher's College Press.

Segal, Marian. 1992. "Silicone Breast Implants Available Under Tight Controls." *FDA Consumer* 26:6-9.

Shanklin, Douglas R., and David L. Smalley. 1998. "Additional Surgery After Breast Device Implantation." *Journal of Rheumatology* 25:2474.

Shapiro, Laura, Karen Springsteen, and Jeanne Gordon. 1992. "What Is It with Women and Breasts?" *Newsweek* (January 20) 57.

Shapiro, Michael M. 1999. "Assessing the Harm of Silicone-gel-filled Breast Implants." *Nurse Practitioner* 24:140-41.

Sharp, David. 1999. "'Bias' Challenge Fails in Breast Implant Cases." *Lancet* 353:1506.

Spiegler, Marc. 1996. "Breast Implants: Once is Not Enough." *American Demographics* 18:13.

Swartz, Mimi. 1995. "Silicone City." *Texas Monthly* 23:64-92.

Tavris, Carol. 1992. *The Mismeasure of Woman.* New York: Simon & Schuster.

Troutwine, Gayle L. 1993. "Breast Implants: A Beauty Fraud." *Trial* 29:48-51.

Vasey, Frank B., and Josh Feldstein. 1993. *The Silicone Breast Implant Controversy: What Women Need to Know.* Freedom, Calif: The Crossing Press.

Warren, Peter M. 1999. "Breast Implants at Top of Gift List for Some Teen Girls." *Des Moines Register,* May 23, A2.

Wartik, Nanci. 1993. "Removing Breast Implants." *American Health.* 12:28-30.

Washburn, Jennifer. 1996. "Reality Check: Can 40,000 Women Be Wrong?" *Ms.* 5:51-57.

Watson, Traci. 1995. "The New Skinny on Fat." *U.S. News and World Report* 119:45-48.

Wolf, Naomi. 1991. *The Beauty Myth: How Images of Beauty Are Used Against Women.* New York: William Morrow.

Wolfe, Sidney M. 1991. "Silicone Gel Breast Implants." In *Women's Health Alert,* ed. Sidney M. Wolfe with Rhoda Donkin Jones. Reading, Mass: Addison-Wesley.

Zimmerman, Susan M. 1998. *Silicone Survivors: Women's Experiences with Breast Implants.* Philadelphia: Temple University Press.

Zola, Irving Kenneth. [1971] 1994. "Medicine as an Institution of Social Control." Pp. 392-402 in *The Sociology of Health and Illness: Critical Perspectives,* ed. Peter Conrad and Rochelle Kern. New York: St. Martin's Press.

Zones, Jane Sprague. 1992. "The Political and Social Context of Silicone Breast Implant Use in the United States." *Journal of Long-Term Effects of Medical Implants* 1:225-41.

PART TWO

BREAST CANCER AS A SOCIAL PROBLEM

The Economics of Breast Cancer

Women, Their Bodies, and the Illness Experience

The Politics of Breast Cancer

Breast Cancer and the Evolving Health Care System: Why Health Care Reform Is a Breast Cancer Issue

Ellen R. Shaffer, M.P.H.

A former vice president of Genentech, described her first treatment for breast cancer:

> *I had world class health insurance. I was referred to an excellent general surgeon, who did not specialize in breast cancer. He recommended surgical biopsy and mastectomy, as soon as possible. He gave me no information about the illness or other options for treatment. I was terrified. I found my way to a breast cancer clinic in San Francisco, and paid out-of-pocket for a second opinion. This time the surgeon talked to me for over an hour. We discussed my particular condition, the pros and cons of various treatments, and the options for reconstructive surgery. She told me to take my time and make a decision I'd be happy with in ten years. (She also explained a new*

procedure that minimized the disabling side effects of diagnosing metastasis to the lymph nodes, a procedure the first surgeon didn't know about.) I quit Genentech and took a pay cut to get a job at the clinic, helping others get the kind of care I got. (Allen, 1998)

Breast cancer is a complex and deadly disease. Chillingly, although we know a great deal about who gets the illness and who dies from it, we do not know the causes of breast cancer, and we cannot prevent it.

Treating breast cancer is another matter. A great deal is known about high-quality medical care, and new research findings emerge continually. However, even wealth, insurance, and education do not guarantee acceptable odds of receiving treatment that is based on medical evidence and responsive to the patient's particular symptoms and personal preferences. Rarely is care coordinated among the multiplicity of providers inevitably involved in treating breast cancer, or across the continuum of services that include accurate and timely diagnosis, laboratory tests properly evaluated and communicated, medications appropriately scheduled and delivered, and a meaningful degree of psychosocial support.

For women with breast cancer, the fragmented organization and profit-driven financing of the U.S. health care system obstruct access to high-quality care. While many programs have succeeded in increasing screening for breast cancer, only a few policymakers and women's health advocates have turned their estimable efforts toward achieving a high-quality, accountable, and affordable health care delivery system.

A few model health care providers are demonstrating that deliberately organizing and providing patient-responsive, coordinated care, guided by the latest evidence, is also cost efficient. Unfortunately, their efforts have yet to become the standard.

Since 1994, there has been a dramatic shift to reliance on competitive market forces to control costs and organize health services. For women with breast cancer, the rise of corporate medicine has further undermined quality and access, and compounded inequalities based on gender, social class, race, and insurance status. Amid the longest economic boom in U.S. history, the proportion of people without health insurance continues to rise.

Women with breast cancer need good clinical care, and they need a health care system that is financed, organized, and accountable to provide it. Until we move decisively toward that goal, reform of the health care system will remain a breast cancer issue.

UPHEAVAL IN THE HEALTH CARE SYSTEM

With the defeat of national health care reform legislation in 1994, American businesses acted decisively to rein in spiraling costs by putting purchasers—those who buy health insurance plans or contract for health services directly—in control. Market restructuring of health care has entailed the emergence and consolidation of provider systems, such as hospital and physician networks, the growth of for-profit providers and managed care organizations (MCOs), and the restructuring and deskilling of the health care workforce. Cuts in health insurance benefits, such as dependent coverage, have shifted the financial burden of paying for health care away from groups of employers or health plans and onto individuals. The result has been less power for patients and clinicians, and growing disruption and inequality.

The most visible feature of market restructuring is managed care, which now covers 85 percent of people with employer-sponsored insurance. From their roots in the prepaid health plans of the 1930s and through a period of modest growth in the 1970s and 1980s, managed care organizations, at one time, seemed to offer solutions to many of the problems women with breast cancer face in the health care system regarding quality, coordination, and even affordability. Nevertheless, that promise has been undermined by the market-driven environment.

After 1994, a wave of mergers and acquisitions swept the health care industry, involving insurers, pharmaceutical companies, hospitals, and medical groups. All were seeking to compete more effectively for market share, usually by competing for contracts from MCOs. This trend has concentrated market power, leaving a handful of companies in control of the system. In 1996, the five largest health plans covered 88.3 percent of insured Californians, compared with 69 percent in 1990 (Managed Health Care Improvement Task Force 1997). Aetna Inc. became the nation's largest health insurer with 21 million enrollees in 1999, giving new meaning to the term single payer (Diamond 1999).

Many companies converted to for-profit status, most notably a majority of the Blue Cross and Blue Shield insurance plans, as well as a rash of investor-owned hospitals. For-profits divert funds from patient care, spending 20 to 30 percent of income on marketing and advertising, paying millions to corporate executives, and investing in other industries. Typical of other firms, in 1997, the CEO of United HealthCare Corporation earned $8.6 million in salary plus $61 million in stock options (Pollack and Slass 1998). That same year, compensation for the five top officers equaled half the deficit for the company.

The case of Columbia/HCA Healthcare is a glaring illustration of the harm that can result from putting shareholders' interests first. Columbia/HCA Healthcare grew in two years from a small regional chain into the owner of 311 hospitals—half of all the for-profit hospital capacity in the country (Sherrill 1995). Their mandate to turn a 20 percent profit led the CEO of one of the Columbia-owned hospitals to report the company to the federal government for fraudulent Medicare billing practices. Going after Columbia/HCA for Medicare fraud was reminiscent of putting Al Capone in prison for tax evasion. It was a real and costly problem, but Columbia/HCA's aggressively competitive tactics had more serious consequences, such as damaging access to care in many communities by systematically driving out community-based health care facilities that could present them with competition, turning away resource-needy patients, denying necessary care, and collaborating with health caregivers to elevate the interests of profit over medicine. The federal case against Columbia has chilled the pace of for-profit conversions by other hospitals. Nevertheless, 75 percent of all health plans were for-profit as of 1997, as were 13 percent of hospitals in 1996 (Levitt, Lundy, and Srinivasan 1999:46).

Analysts legitimately debate whether the new for-profits perform any worse than nonprofit providers that operated under the earlier perverse financial incentives of fee-for-service. Under the fee-for-service system that prevailed until recently, providers were paid a fee for every separate service delivered. Thus, doctors and hospitals had a financial incentive to provide expensive care, at least to those with good insurance, and there was little advantage to providing less costly and less aggressive treatments. The United States has the highest ratio of specialists compared to primary care doctors of any industrialized nation, further skewing resources toward the most interventionist care. There are many unjustified hospitalizations and surgical procedures, which not only are costly but also expose patients unnecessarily to the risks of morbidity and mortality that are associated with any surgery.

However, recent studies show that regions dominated by for-profit hospitals cost Medicare significantly more than nonprofit dominated areas (Silverman, Skinner, and Fisher 1999), and that for-profit health plans perform worse than nonprofits in providing preventive services (Himmelstein et al. 1999). David Himmelstein and his colleagues conclude that if all American women were enrolled in for-profit health maintenance organizations (HMOs) instead of nonprofits, 5,925 more would die annually from breast cancer due to lower rates of mammography (1999).

The upheavals in the health care industry are far from over, as the days of dramatic cost savings draw to a close. In 1998, physicians reported increasing failure to pay or delays in payment by health plans in financial crisis. Oxford Health Plan, one of the largest and most flexible preferred provider plans in New York State, declared bankruptcy. Over half of all HMOs lost money in both 1997 and 1998, and 100 failed to maintain recommended levels of monetary reserves (California Healthline 1999). Although many studies show that payments to MCOs have, in fact, been excessive, hundreds of MCOs pulled out of the federal Medicare program that covers the elderly and disabled, alleging inadequate reimbursements. The U.S. Department of Health and Human Services (HHS) predicts that health care inflation is set to resume in the coming decade (Smith, Heffler, and Freeland 1999). Medical and health market news outlets observe that plans are concentrating more directly on profits by cutting services and raising premiums, and they question whether managed care in its current form can long survive (Rauber 1998).

Market-based health care is producing more uninsured people daily. Many more are underinsured, facing high copayments or limited benefits. In 1998, 43 million Americans were uninsured at any time, about 16 percent of the population (U.S. Bureau of the Census 1998). Since people may gain and then lose insurance during the same year, the number of people without insurance over the course of a year is much higher. Rates of uninsured vary among states from about 8 percent in Wisconsin and Hawaii to approximately 24 percent in Texas, New Mexico, and California. Of the 34 million people living in poverty in 1998, about one-third had no health insurance (Campbell 1999). Since the 1980s, the percent of employed people and their families without insurance has been rising. Ironically, the uninsured includes many people in poor health (Vistnes and Zuvekas 1999).

Managed care has become an object of public backlash. Unable to find good care for her asthmatic son on a waitress's salary and health plan, Helen Hunt's character in the 1997 movie and Oscar-winner *As Good As It Gets* struck a responsive chord with cheering audiences when she muttered, "Managed care bastards." Paul Ellwood, an early proponent of managed care, contends that it has been a revolution driven by employers, resulting in "giant plans with overlapping networks that are largely in the hands of financial people" (Tokarski 1998:10). "Managed care has served as a different way to pay for medical care, not a better way to provide it," according to another observer (Kilborn 1998).

While the system fiddles with financial incentives, women with breast cancer are still looking for a better way to get care.

QUALITY, COORDINATION, AND CONTINUITY

QUALITY OF CARE

According to the Institute of Medicine's recent report on cancer care, good quality care should include appropriate services provided in a technically competent manner, with shared decision making and cultural sensitivity. Poor quality can mean the overuse, underuse, or misuse of services. However, the report notes a wide gulf between the ideal and the reality for many Americans with cancer (Hewitt and Simone 1999).

For example, a scant decade ago, feminist activists put to rest the practice of biopsy under anesthetic "followed by whatever the surgeon deemed appropriate" for diagnosing and treating breast cancer (Doyal 1995:217). For too long, surgeons had resisted the evidence that radical mastectomy—removing the entire breast and surrounding muscles—was no more likely to improve survival than more limited procedures that had the added advantage of leaving women with greater mobility and less disfigurement and disability. Scientists, policymakers, and activists prevailed, and today the practice is rare.

But inappropriate treatment still persists, illustrating underlying faults in the health care system. For example, breast conserving surgery (BCS) may still be performed too infrequently. BCS—lumpectomy followed by radiation—is less invasive, disabling, and disfiguring, and it exposes women to fewer complications compared to modified or simple mastectomy. A landmark study in 1985 demonstrated that survival rate is the same whether women undergo BCS or mastectomy (Fisher et al. 1985). According to clinical criteria, about 70 percent of women with breast cancer are candidates for BCS, and only 30 percent need a mastectomy. However, in the mid-1990s the actual proportions in the United States were reversed: 70 percent received mastectomies (Love 1997).

Geographic variations in the rate of BCS suggest that, in many cases, doctors rely on customary practices among other doctors they know, rather than on scientific evidence, to determine whether women receive BCS. In 1995, lumpectomies were performed for 41 percent of breast surgeries in the Northeast, compared with 20 percent in the South, 24 percent in the Midwest, and 23 percent in the West (Sugerman 1997). A 1990 study of Medicare patients with localized or regional breast cancer found that BCS was used for only 15 percent of cases, and the only geographic area that had an increase in BCS since 1986 was New England (Nattinger et al. 1996).

Older women and those covered by Medicaid, the state and federal program for low-income patients, are at greater risk for inappropriate care. Women over age 65 with nonmetastatic disease are more likely to receive BCS than younger women, but they are less likely to receive follow-up with radiation as recommended (Ballard-Barbash et al. 1996) or to receive chemotherapy (Hillner et al. 1996).

Some women may choose mastectomy over BCS, such as women in rural areas who may not have ready access to follow-up radiation treatments. In addition, some women have tumors that are not amenable to treatment with a lumpectomy. Some older women may prefer less aggressive therapy. There are several appropriate choices of treatment for breast cancer. However, inappropriate rates of treatment of this magnitude may reveal serious flaws in the health system.

Quality patient care requires accountable organizational systems and complementary financial incentives. In countries where the government finances most health care, government institutions can significantly influence the organization of services. However, the predominance of multiple individual health insurers in the United States has meant that no single entity has the clout to hold providers, or the system as a whole, accountable. The high rate of uninsured patients in the United States destabilizes financing and institutionalizes discrimination. Patients have had to fight for a role in making decisions ranging from the distribution of health care resources to whether to have breast conserving surgery. They have little information about which practitioners are conforming to recommended standards of care, and they have increasingly limited ability to select them.

While the fee-for-service system gave doctors and hospitals an incentive to overuse the most aggressive and invasive care, recent evidence suggests that the financial incentives of managed care may be no better at guiding treatment decisions. Patients in HMOs may be less likely to receive BCS because the cost of follow-up radiation may be more costly than a mastectomy (Hadley and Mitchell 1997/1998).

The core features of managed care, at one time, promised financial incentives to keep patients healthy and reduce unnecessary hospital stays, and organizational structures to reinforce those incentives. HMOs cover comprehensive care for a capitated fee—one fee paid in advance for each enrollee (per capita), whether or not the HMO and its clinicians provide a service. These plans are known as closed panel plans, where a full range of primary care doctors as well as specialists work exclusively for the HMO and the enrollee's choice is limited to these providers. With most clinicians under one roof, it is at least theoretically possible to create guidelines encouraging BCS when appropriate, to monitor and influence the quality of care provided, and to coordinate care. Early HMOs pioneered full payment for preventive services, such as mammograms. Some made important contributions to the development of systematic, population-based methods of follow-up, or borrowed methods from public health that vastly improved the rates of screening. Most were nonprofits.

Despite these considerable accomplishments, most HMOs never quite reached their optimal potential. In fact, in the market era, many of their actual and potential advantages have been subverted. Corporate managed care organizations (MCOs) compete for patients and profits. They are driven to attract health plan purchasers, who choose plans primarily based on price rather than quality. The majority of MCOs are network plans, unlike closed panel plans, such as preferred provider organizations (PPOs). These plans offer enrollees a choice of many physicians, and the doctors, in turn, contract with multiple MCOs, each ratcheting down payments, but none taking responsibility for quality or coordination of care.

Managed care organizations could encourage conformity to practice guidelines while reducing the cost of care (Winn 1995). Practice guidelines suggest standards for care and, often, decision-making pathways for clinicians, based on evidence supported by research. However, some MCOs use their clout in the market to impose rigid guidelines for clinical treatment that can become a mask for reducing benefits rather than a tool for quality improvement (Myerson 1995). Standards are often promulgated by accounting consultants, who rely on doctors' recommendations for one definition of illness and one ideal type of patient: young, healthy, and with strong support at home (Goodwin 1997). Some observers charge that for-profit managed care is transforming medical visits into commodities on a production line (Eisenberg 1996).

This practice can compromise care for an illness as complex and variable as breast cancer. In *One in Three: Woman With Cancer Confront an Epidemic* (Brady 1991), Simi Litvak reports finding little literature to help her decide whether to get chemotherapy after a mastectomy, and she was unsure about her HMO doctor's generic advice. With help from the Women's Cancer Resource Center (WCRC), a nonprofit organization in Berkeley, California, she decided to seek a second opinion from outside the HMO, although the HMO would not pay for it. The outside pathologist concluded she had a different type of cancer from that diagnosed by the HMO, leading to a new recommendation for treatment.

Thus, as evidenced by inappropriate rates of treatment and nonadherence to recommended standards for breast cancer care, the profit-driven nature of the U.S. health care system often translates into serious compromises in the quality, coordination, and continuity of care for women with breast cancer.

COORDINATED CARE CREATES BETTER OUTCOMES

According to Patricia Drury, Director of Research for the Buyers' Health Care Action Group in Minneapolis, "What makes the difference [in health care] is how the whole system works" (Sainbury et al. 1995). High-volume, multidisciplinary providers are able to bring together the necessary clinical disciplines and expertise across the full therapeutic range, and they are more likely to ensure that all relevant treatment methods are properly considered and deployed. Research shows that high-volume providers in multispecialty settings are most likely to give the best care and have the best outcomes for conditions such as breast cancer ("Women with Breast Cancer Fare Better at Multi-Disciplinary Clinics" 1997). For example, hospital volume— how frequently a hospital treats breast cancer patients—may influence appropriate use of breast conserving surgery. In 1990, 10 percent of hospitals performed 55 percent of conservative operations, and large urban hospitals or those with a cancer center were more likely to perform BCS (Nattinger et al. 1996). In addition, they can provide responsive, effective breast cancer care by coordinating a range of treatments and providers who can include oncologists, radiologists, and surgeons, as well as nurses, social workers, genetics counselors, and research coordinators (Costanza and Edmiston 1997). These sites provide faster diagnosis and treatment, and patients are more satisfied with care compared to women who must schedule separate appointments with numerous caregivers (Sainbury et al. 1995).

High volume also is associated with better quality for other aspects of breast cancer care. Doctors who treat a high volume of women with breast cancer are most likely to be able to evaluate a range of factors that affect which treatment, if any, should be considered. One study found that survival at five years was better for patients whose doctors treat more than 30 new cases of cancer a year (Sainbury et al. 1995).

The effect of volume on the outcome of breast cancer is a function of clinical organization as well as the skill of the doctor and surgical team. Research centers specializing in breast cancer can separate women into groups based on their type of breast cancer and follow them over a long period of time to differentiate between the courses of their illness and the distinctive treatments required. Here, complex treatment and outcome standards, based on the latest clinical evidence, can serve as a basis for reducing idiosyncratic variations in care.

In sum, research has shown that high-volume, multispecialty providers can effectively ensure the continuity of quality, coordinated care for women with breast cancer. However, market-driven managed care has focused on financial incentives rather than coordination, and market changes threaten continuity of care for women with breast cancer.

IT ISN'T MANAGED AND THEY DON'T CARE

Traditional HMOs had the advantage of relatively stable populations of providers and patients, offering a context to address systematic barriers to good care. The newest and most popular MCOs are network health plans with rotating rosters of clinicians. Employee enrollment in network plans, referred to as preferred provider organizations (PPOs) or point of service (POS) plans, grew 43 percent from 1993 to 1998, while enrollment in closed panel HMOs grew by just 13 percent (Levitt, Lundy, and Srinivasan 1999:18). Doctors are regularly recruited and dropped by these health plans. Health plans, themselves, are merging and reconfiguring, and medical groups and hospital networks have been realigning on an unprecedented scale. As health plans go out of business, enrollees may be left without a plan or a provider and, often, with a string of unpaid bills.

Continuity of care can disintegrate when there are changes in the choice of health plans and therefore the panel of available providers. In the current managed care environment, many employers bid for and change employee health care systems annually (Flocke, Stange, and Zyzanski 1997), with the result that a woman's regular provider may not be included in her health plan. MCOs restrict choice of primary care providers and access to specialists, a particular problem for a woman with breast cancer who needs to find not only one provider with whom she can communicate but a team of specialists whose care she often must coordinate herself. One in three enrollees in employer-sponsored plans changed plans between 1990 and 1993. Increasingly, privately insured managed care enrollees are offered only one health plan, further limiting options (Davis and Schoen 1997). Almost two-thirds of new Medicaid recipients lose coverage within 12 months; only 38 percent of new enrollees are still covered after a year (Carrasquillo, Himmelstein, and Woolhandler 1998).

Patients forced to change physicians due to changes in their health insurance have reported significantly lower quality of primary care than those who were not forced to change, particularly in the areas of interpersonal communication, doctors' personal knowledge, and coordination. Patients with PPO health insurance were four times as likely as patients with fee-for-service insurance to report a forced change in their primary care physician (Flocke, Stange, and Zyzanski 1997).

Services also can become fragmented due to contracting arrangements that call for laboratory work, radiology, and medical care from different providers. Dispersing sites of care means not only that seriously ill women have to travel over geographic distances to receive needed services, but also that caregivers are less likely to coordinate with each other. In a comparison of physician communication in managed care and nonmanaged care settings, primary care doctors reported they more often referred their patients to an unknown specialist in managed care, spoke personally with specialists less often, and sent a written summary to specialists less often (Roulidis and Schulman 1994). Thus, in a market environment, changes in health plans and providers as well as fragmented contracting for services, frequently lead to disintegration in the continuity and coordination of medical care for women with breast cancer.

DENIALS AND DELAYS OF CARE

The dynamics of capitation mean that managed care providers make more money by doing less. Under gatekeeper systems, primary care doctors have the responsibility—and may also face a financial loss—for referring patients to specialists. The President's Cancer Panel, convened by the National Cancer Institute (NCI), reported in 1996 that some primary care gatekeepers never referred cancer patients to an oncologist, inappropriately attempting to manage care themselves, including administering chemotherapy (President's Cancer Panel 1996). There are limited appeal rights when plans deny coverage for care that patients believe they need. Absent safeguards on accountability, and in the for-profit environment, capitation can be an inducement to underserve. Bureaucratic obstacles, such as unanswered, understaffed phone lines for making appointments, can also cause distressing delays in access to care. Congress, state legislatures, and the courts have responded to protests by taking steps to expand consumers' rights. In 1999, the U.S. House of Representatives passed the Norwood-Dingell bill that would allow patients to sue health plans. However, these measures have not been sufficient to alter the financial incentives of capitation.

Complex preauthorization processes can lead to inappropriate denials or delays in care, as the President's Cancer Panel further noted. Academic medical chairs, already overloaded with patient care and administration of their departments, have reported diverting 30 percent of their time to treatment approval and reimbursement issues. Particularly at issue has been access to experimental or investigational drugs and procedures, sometimes the only option for women in advanced stages of illness. By the time approval is secured, patients may be too ill to participate or to benefit.

Even routine treatments may be delayed, however. One report cited a managed care plan that "balked at paying for more than three of 33 radiation therapy treatments because the physician had failed to obtain additional authorization beyond initial approval" (Haas 1997:169). Diane Estrin, Executive Director of Berkeley's Women's Cancer Resource Center (WCRC), notes, "If women have their lymph nodes removed, it's common to get a swelling disease known as lymphedema. Women need to wear a special glove to keep down the swelling, just so they can function. But HMOs may provide only one per year, or even one per lifetime. It's ridiculous" (Estrin 1998).

Clinical trials involving cancer patients are the only way researchers can discover whether new, experimental treatments will be effective. MCOs generally have not covered these expenses, putting a damper on research and the hopes of patients with no other options. Legislation introduced in 1999 would require MCOs to cover the medical expenses associated with clinical trials, such as hospital stays and blood tests (Erikson 1999).

Plans may try to limit their costs by failing to include a sufficient number and range of specialists on a provider panel. If specialists are included but in short supply, long waits for care result.

Drug formularies, which restrict the choice of medications covered by a plan, can help solve a real problem: overuse of artificially expensive medications. However, inflexible plans that do not allow doctors to compensate for bad reactions to generic drugs, for example, have been linked to the use of more resources—

drugs and visits to the office, emergency room, and hospital—than where doctors had a wider choice of agents. Inflexible MCOs may also prevent patients from receiving needed drugs, such as anti-nausea drugs for women receiving chemotherapy (Kasper 1999).

Diane Estrin of WCRC says the cutbacks are noticeable. "Less services are covered. There is less in-home care, less emergency care, fewer social services like help with groceries. There's no coverage for the debilitating effects of most treatments when women may need nightly care, not just a few hours of help a week" (Estrin 1998). These restrictions on care by managed care plans undoubtedly have effects on women with breast cancer, ranging from the somewhat trivial to life threatening.

MANAGED CARE OUTCOMES: VARIATION CONTINUES

Coverage for disease prevention in general and for early detection in the case of breast cancer are among the features most often celebrated by MCOs (HMO Group 1998), and they have been the benefits noted most clearly by researchers (Wyn and Brown 1996). MCOs have removed most of the cost-related barriers to preventive care by charging only a small copayment or nothing at all for mammography screenings. Some have improved physician and patient reminder systems to increase adherence to yearly screen-ings. As a result, studies show that women in established HMOs are more likely to receive mammograms than those in fee-for-service plans, including women at higher risk of presenting with more advanced stages of cancer due to education, age, income, and race (Bernstein 1996; Kang and Bloom 1993).

In spite of this accomplishment, the high turnover among providers and patients in newer network arrangements, such as preferred provider organizations (PPOs), combined with shorter doctors' visits may present obstacles to successful early detection programs that rely on ongoing contact with enrollees. These include doctors' encouragement of breast self-exam (BSE), still the most efficacious method of detection to date for women under age 40 (Senie et al. 1982).

Numerous studies have explored whether, overall, quality outcomes are better under managed care or fee-for-service plans, and some of them have addressed breast cancer cases. Most have studied traditional HMOs, which are now the minority of managed care plans. Many have found lower satisfaction with the quality of care in managed care plans compared with fee-for-service enrollees, although higher satisfaction with costs of care (Miller and Luft 1994).

Most critically, the emerging answer seems to be that, whatever the method of financial incentive, there is still a high degree of random variation in all aspects of clinical care. Differences in treatment between MCOs as a group and fee-for-service plans as a group are not consistent. For example, a study by Riley et al. (1998) compares how Medicare patients with early stage breast cancer were treated between 1988 and 1993. In Seattle, San Francisco, and Oakland, HMO enrollees were more likely to receive BCS than were those in fee-for-service. The opposite was the case in Los Angeles. Nationally, they report, "Analyses at the individual plan level revealed that rates of BCS were significantly higher in some HMOs than in the local fee-for-service setting while in other plans, rates of BCS were significantly lower." This finding is consistent with other studies that have found mixed results in terms of mammography rates, survival, and rate of BCS (Hadley and Mitchell 1997/1998; Lee-Feldstein, Anton-Culver, and Feldstein 1994; Potosky et al. 1997).

Currently, there is simply too much variation among health plans, even those labeled MCOs, and the pace of change is too rapid, for carefully controlled studies to determine whether managed care is better or worse with regard to health outcomes. It is also possible that too many factors affect differences in provider practices to isolate the effects of managed care. For example, size, complexity, and fragmentation have been noted as barriers to high-quality care by large managed care organizations and hospitals, while some studies show better results in large hospitals (Barr 1995; Lee-Feldstein, Anton-Culver, and Feldstein 1994).

Regardless, it is clear that the market does not reward competition based on quality. Plans that advertise great care for breast cancer would suffer the financial consequences of adverse selection, attracting a disproportionate share of sick patients who need expensive care. It is more cost effective for providers, and the price-conscious purchasers they seek as customers, to attract healthy enrollees than to enhance systems of care for those who are ill (Angell and Kassirer 1996). Since purchasers generally do not factor quality into their choice of plans, providers who decide to invest in quality improvement are not likely to be able to charge more as a result (Segal 1996).

HOSPITAL CARE:
FEWER DAYS, FEWER STAFF, LOWER QUALITY

Since 1992, industrial reorganization of the hospital workforce has resulted in a sharp increase in administrative staff and cyclical declines in nursing staff (Woolhandler and Himmelstein 1998). Restructuring has involved efforts to replace skilled workers with those less skilled. There is growing evidence of the impact of short staffing on hospital deaths and adverse events, such as complications of early discharge and infections in the hospital (Kovner and Gergen 1998). Breast cancer activists and other consumers must, unfortunately, consider how to add this new burden to their long list of concerns.

For example, short hospital stays for mastectomy have been on the rise, and many states have enacted laws requiring adequate stays. Outpatient mastectomies or one-day stays may work well for some women. However, in the many cases when it does not, complications can be severe, including significant blood loss, infection, psychological trauma, or death. Elderly people who are dependent on wheelchairs and living alone require greater monitoring and more care, and HMO protocols may not cover a home health visit. Some injectable narcotic painkillers are too dangerous to administer at home, and safe oral medications may not be sufficient to control postoperative pain. Patients or their families may have to regularly clean surgical drains placed in wounds and measure body fluids. After a mastectomy, it can take weeks for a woman to look at the scar where the breast once was, let alone expertly change dressings the day after surgery (Goodwin 1997b). Finally, one-day stays practically eliminate the opportunity for visits from volunteer breast cancer outreach programs that combine patient education and psychosocial support, important aspects of care.

Hospital workforce shortages and restructuring have also had deleterious effects in the realm of cancer treatment, where attention to detail is crucial and where oncology has pushed the limits of drug therapy. With many anticancer drugs, a hair's breadth lies between a healing and a deadly dose. Research by Lucian Leape at the Harvard School of Public Health found that 28 percent of complications from drugs given in hospitals could have been prevented (Bates, Leape, and Petrycki 1995; Leape et al. 1995:35). Leape did not separate out cancer ward mistakes but saw from the data that mistakes in those wards caused more harm because the drugs are so toxic (Brink 1995). Betsy Lehman's shocking death at the elite Dana Farber specialty hospital in Boston resulted from doses of chemotherapy that were mistakenly quadrupled. A well-known science reporter, Lehman's death led to an investigation that uncovered other similar incidents. Dana Farber closed its inpatient services, keeping its clinics open. A state investigation concluded only that the structure in place for checking and double-checking was either ignored or inadequately followed (Brink 1995). A nurse at Dana Farber has said that there was, in fact, no system for checking pharmacists' work before delivering drugs to patients.

INEQUALITIES IN POWER
UNDERMINE DIAGNOSIS AND TREATMENT

Social inequality undermines access to quality health care. Being female, a racial or ethnic minority, of lower social class, of young or advanced age may all presage poorer care and poorer outcomes (Gordon et al. 1992; Hubbell et al. 1996; Lannin et al. 1998; Simon and Severson 1997). In a market-driven health care system, these factors are likely to predict a lack of health insurance or being underinsured, which are some of the most oppressive features of a pay-as-you-go health care economy.

Women also still have not achieved equality in the examining room. Approximately 50 to 80 percent of breast tumors are first detected by patients (Senie et al. 1982). However, the first and second largest number of malpractice liability suits are related to failure to diagnose breast cancer (especially in women under 50 years old) and to a lack of follow-up care, respectively. The most common explanation for failure to diagnose was that a patient's physical findings did not impress the doctor that cancer should be considered a risk (McCormick 1995). Asian Americans and Latinas have reported that doctors have discounted their symptoms, possibly misinterpreting the statistics to believe that women from these racial ethnic groups could not be at risk for breast cancer (Zaldivar 1998).

A diagnosis of breast cancer is frightening and devastating. Women vary in the amount of information they want and the degree of involvement in choosing treatments. However, those seeking the most active role are likely to be frustrated, according to several studies (Degner et al. 1997). Many also object to the rush to treatment. Most decisions about adjuvant therapy (treatments following surgery) were made by 82 percent of patients within the first clinic visit, which many considered too fast.

UNINSURED AND UNDERSERVED

In cases where health care could make a difference for women with breast cancer, the uninsured and those on Medicaid fare worse. Among women age 35 to 64 years old diagnosed with breast cancer from 1985 to 1987 in New Jersey, both uninsured women and those covered by Medicaid were diagnosed with more advanced disease than were those with private insurance (Ayanian et al. 1993). For those with localized or regional disease, the uninsured had a 49 percent higher risk of death within five to eight years of diagnosis, and Medicaid patients had a 40 percent higher risk than women who were privately insured. Medically indigent patients were diagnosed with higher stage disease and did not benefit from the general trend toward earlier stage at diagnosis, which occurred between 1983 and 1990.

The 1996 report by the President's Cancer Panel, fighting the War on Cancer in an Evolving Health Care System, notes the loss in funding for cancer care of the indigent, due to short-term and short-sighted cost containment. "The cost cutting achieved through strict utilization control and bare-bones provider contracting has all but eliminated the patient care surpluses that were the mainstay for indigent care in many institutions. No single organization, at any level, is financially poised to step into this breach" (President's Cancer Panel 1996:V). The public health system is challenged as never before, leaving little in the way of safety-net providers.

WOMEN OF COLOR:
LATER DIAGNOSIS, HIGHER MORTALITY

The incidence of breast cancer is higher among white women, but African American women are more likely to die from the disease (Collins et al. 1994). Poorer survival among African Americans is mostly explained by a later stage of disease at detection and diagnosis, when treatment is less effective, although this trend may be changing (Chevarley and White 1997). However, some studies have found poorer survival among women of color even with the same stage of the disease as whites (Hsu, Glaser, and West 1997; Simon and Severson 1997). There have been insufficient studies to determine whether worse survival rates reflect differences in medical care, environmental exposures, genetics, or other characteristics (Randolph 1995), but at least one study noted clinical differences in African American women, such as a higher rate of estrogen receptor negative tumors, that could contribute to their poorer prognosis (Simon and Severson 1996).

Women of color are less likely to have health insurance (Campbell 1999). In addition, they may be discouraged from seeking care even when they have insurance. In one study, nearly 99 percent of white women diagnosed with a breast abnormality visited a doctor for follow-up treatment; among African Americans, Asians, and Latinas, only 75 percent sought follow-up care (Stolberg 1998). A study of 246 women with advanced stages of disease at three closed panel HMOs found that African Americans were overrepresented among patients who missed appointments, which was, in turn, a key determinant of shorter survival (Howard, Penchansky, and Brown 1998).

These disparities are due, in part, to the attitudes, cultural beliefs, and practices of both providers and patients, which may vary among regions. A recent study of 34 African American women in rural North Carolina with late stage breast cancer found that some of their own beliefs (e.g., that cancer was caused by imbalances in the blood) contradicted conventional medical information. The women's attempts to reconcile their views with the diagnosis of cancer by telling stories were resented or dismissed by their doctors, who regarded the stories as irrational at best and as adversarial at worst. Some of the women felt rushed to discuss prognosis and treatment, as opposed to getting basic information, and six "walked out of the clinic and never returned" after they were diagnosed (Matthews, Lannin, and Mitchell 1994:796).

There are other structural barriers to care related to social class and race. For example, health care providers are less commonly located in minority communities. Minority health professionals, who often practice in solo offices as opposed to organized medical groups, have frequently claimed that managed care companies discriminate in contracting with them. Since the minority populations they treat are sicker and may, therefore, require more expensive treatments, providers also claim they may be dropped by health plans, even if they secure an initial contract (Dingle 1995).

MAKING IT WORK:
MODELS FOR DIAGNOSIS AND TREATMENT

Arguably, the triumph of purchasers and managed care plans imparts a responsibility to improve systems of care as much as possible. That is, providers and purchasers with relatively stable and sizable populations of patients *can* institute mechanisms proven to integrate and improve care and to attend to women's preferences. Purchasers can make exemplary plans and providers more available and affordable. Some employers, such as General Motors, are moving patients out of plans that perform poorly by freezing new enrollment and lowering cost sharing in high-scoring plans (Larkin 1997).

There is movement at the national level as well. The influential Institute of Medicine, part of the National Academy of Sciences, recently issued a blue-ribbon report calling for improvements in the quality of cancer care in the United States (Hewitt and Simone 1999). Congress is considering extending coverage for treatment to low-income women who have been able to get mammography screening through a federal program but then had nowhere to go for needed treatment. A federal agency, recently renamed the Agency for Healthcare Research and Quality, is continuing to fund both clinical and organizational health services research.

At the delivery system level—doctors and hospitals—some providers have identified meaningful standards of performance that go beyond mammography rates and have organized services to meet their standards. They have defined high-quality health care as responsive to patients (including a defined and active role for patients and advocates who want it), having flexible guidelines for clinical care that incorporate the most recent medical evidence, and providing care that is coordinated among continuous providers and psychosocial support. They also are demonstrating cost efficiency.

Some relieve the anxiety of long waits by streamlining care. For example, Henry Ford Breast Care Clinic, a multidisciplinary site, has documented that they provided definitive treatment within 29.6 days, compared to women seeing a specialist in traditional sequential fashion who began treatment after 42.2 days ("Improved Cancer Care Offered for Cancer Patients" 1997). The Breast Cancer Management System at Humana Health Care Plans in Chicago has reduced the turnaround time between screening and surgical treatment by 36 days, by spending only $50,000 for computer software and staff at each of three centers (Bloom et al. 1998).

At several sites, nurses coordinate care among physicians, social workers, and other professionals, track patients through their appointments, and provide education and counseling to patients and their families. Kaiser Permanente in Fontana, California, has sponsored a Breast Buddy Breast Care Program. Volunteer mentors offer support and information. Nurse coordinators connect patients with services available both within the medical center and in the community. There is a lending library. The program reports enhanced patient participation in treatment decisions, increased teamwork among clinicians, and better integrated and defined pathways of care for breast cancer patients (Bloom et al. 1998).

Furthermore, a program at the Johns Hopkins University Breast Center helps to make shorter hospital stays manageable for patients and their families (Goodwin 1997a). The team helps alleviate pain and nausea after same-day mastectomy by using a local anesthetic that lasts 12 hours and soft surgical drains to minimize discomfort. They teach patients how to avoid lymphedema, reducing their rate from the national average of six percent to three percent. A stress survey identifies families who are coping poorly, and counselors visit the same day; HMOs reimburse for the service.

Unfortunately, these providers are models in a system that has no routes for replicating them effectively or assuring that the women who need them can find and afford them. Ironically, Mt. Zion Medical Center in San Francisco was designated a specialty site for clinical cancer research by the National Cancer Institute the same week the financially troubled hospital's board announced its possible closure. Subsequently it did close only its in-patient services. What will it take to make model care available to everyone?

CONCLUSION:
HEALTH CARE REFORM IS A BREAST CANCER ISSUE

It is becoming increasingly clear that the United States cannot rely on private, for-profit insurance companies to underwrite and administer the health care system and expect serious progress on quality, accountability, affordability, and equity. The market is not an adequate system for achieving systemwide reorganization in the interest of coordinated services. It will not bring about universal financial coverage, and it will not even make health care more affordable for those who have coverage. This is hard news for the health-related corporations that siphon off 30 percent on every health care dollar for administration and profit (Himmelstein et al. 1999). It is important news, in a different way, for women with breast cancer.

Policymakers, advocates, providers, and purchasers must provide the impetus to reorganize health services on behalf of women with breast cancer. This means finding ways to advocate effectively for patients' health care concerns in the broadest sense, as well as focusing on specific issues related to breast cancer. Many of the barriers to optimal care faced by women with breast cancer are endemic to the social, political, and economic organization of health and medical care, and these areas are ripe for attention.

Most members of disease-based organizations, whether they have breast cancer, AIDS, or diabetes, want, above all, to feel better and to be healthier. Unfortunately, they are foot soldiers in the daily battles against hospital understaffing, denials of necessary treatment, and discrimination based on insurance status, age, social class, and race. For women with breast cancer, the environmental and social causes of disease and the efficacy of individual interventions are life and death issues. So is the way that health care in the United States is financed and delivered. An essential step is to recapture the focus on achieving access to high-quality health care that is accountable, affordable, and universally accessible for all.

NOTES

AUTHOR'S NOTE: Gratitude to Terri Owens for extensive editorial comments and guidance, to Karen Pollitz and Bernard Lo for reviews of earlier drafts, and to Bryan Lucena and Shalini Eddens for research assistance.

REFERENCES

Allen, Judi. 1998. Personal communication.

Angell, Marcia, and Jerome P. Kassirer. 1996. "Quality and the Medical Marketplace—Following Elephants." *New England Journal of Medicine* 335:883-85.

Ayanian, John Z., Betsy A. Kohler, Toshi Abe, Arnold M. Epstein. 1993. "The Relation Between Health Insurance Coverage and Clinical Outcomes Among Women with Breast Cancer." *New England Journal of Medicine* 329:326-31.

Ballard-Barbash, Rachel, Arnold L. Potosky, Linda C. Harlan, Susan G. Nayfield, and Larry G. Kessler. 1996. "Factors Associated with Surgical and Radiation Therapy for Early Stage Breast Cancer in Older Women." *Journal of the National Cancer Institute* 88:716-27.

Barr, Donald A. 1995. "The Effects of Organizational Structure on Primary Care Outcomes Under Managed Care." *Annals of Internal Medicine* 122:353-59.

Bates, David W., Lucian L. Leape, and S. Petrycki. 1995. "Incidence of Adverse Drug Events and Potential Drug Events: Implications for Prevention." *Journal of the American Medical Association* 274:29-34.

Bernstein, Amy B. 1996. "Women's Health in HMOs: What We Know and What We Need to Find Out." *Women's Health Issues* 6:51-59.

Bloom, Felicia B., Sharon J. Rolnick, Kristine K. J. Fortman, and Barbara D. Lardy. 1998. "Advancing Women's Health: Health Plans' Innovative Programs in Breast Cancer. Survey Results and Case Studies." *American Association of Health Plans,* New York, September.

Brady, Judy (ed.). 1991. *One in Three: Women with Cancer Confront an Epidemic.* Pittsburgh: Cleis Press.

Brink, Susan. 1995. "Tragedy at Dana-Farber: Betsy Lehman's Shocking Death is Still Roiling the Medical Community." *U. S. News and World Report* (July 24) 119:53.

California Healthline. 1999. "HMO Finances: Most Floundered in Red Last Year." *National Journal Group,* Washington, D.C., August 10.

Campbell, Jennifer A. 1999. "Health Insurance Coverage, Consumer Income, 1998." *Current Population Reports.* Rockville, Md: U.S. Census Bureau.

Carrasquillo, Olveen, David Himmelstein, and Steffie Woolhandler, 1998. "Can Medicaid Managed Care Provide Continuity of Care to New Medicaid Enrollees? An Analysis of Tenure on Medicaid." *American Journal of Public Health* 88:464-66.

Chevarley, Frances, and Emily White. 1997. "Recent Trends in Breast Cancer Mortality Among White and Black U.S. Women." *American Journal of Public Health* 87:775-81.

Collins, Karen Scott, Diane Rowland, Alina Salganicoff, and Elizabeth Chait. 1994. "Assessing and Improving Women's Health." Pp. 109-53 in *The American Woman 1994-9: Where We Stand,* ed. C. Costello and A. J. Stone. New York: W. W. Norton.

Costanza, Mary E., and K. L. Edmiston. 1997. "Breast Cancer Screening: Early Recognition." *Comprehensive Therapy* 23:7-12.

Davis, Karen, Karen Scott Collins, Cathy Schoen, and Cynthia Morris. 1997. "Choice Matters: Enrollees' Views of Their Health Plans." *Health Affairs* vol. 14, no. 2, 99-112.

Degner, Lesley F., Linda J. Kristjanson, David Bowman, Jeffrey A. Sloan, K. C. Carriere, John O'Neil, Barbara Bilodeau, Peter Watson, and Bryan Mueller. 1997. "Information Needs and Decisional Preferences in Women with Breast Cancer." *Journal of the American Medical Association* 277:1485.

Diamond, Randy. 1999. "Aetna Acquires Pru's HMO." *The Record Online,* August 7. At www.bergen.com/biz/aaetnaard199908071.htm.

Dingle, Lenox. 1995. "Testimony to Maryland State Legislature, House Economic Matters Committee, Regarding House Bill 1210, Health Care Provider Panels." *Criteria and Procedures,* February 28.

Doyal, Lesley. 1995. *What Makes Women Sick: Gender and the Political Economy of Health.* New Brunswick: Rutgers University Press and London: Macmillan.

Eisenberg, Leon. 1996. "The Social Construction of the Human Brain." *American Journal of Psychiatry* 153:1373-74.

Erikson, Jan. 1999. "HMO Directors Willing to Pay for Cancer Trials." *Arizona Daily Star,* August 16. At http://www.azstarnet.com/publicnews/127-6270.htm.

Estrin, Diane. 1998. Personal communication.

Fisher, Bernard, Madeline Bauer, Richard Margolese, Roger Poisson, Yosef Pilch, Carol Redmond, Edwin Fisher, Norman Wolmark, Melvin Deutsch, Eleanor Montague, Elizabeth Saffer, Lawrence Wickerhasm, Harvey Lerner, Andrew Glass, Henry Shibata, Peter Deckers, Alfred Ketcham, Robert Oishi, and Ian Russell. 1985. "Five-Year Results of a Randomized Clinical Trial Comparing Total Mastectomy and Segmental Mastectomy

With or Without Radiation in the Treatment of Breast Cancer." *New England Journal of Medicine* 312:665-73.

Flocke, Susan A., Kurt C. Stange, and Stephen J. Zyzanski. 1997. "The Impact of Insurance Type and Forced Discontinuity on the Delivery of Primary Care." *Journal of Family Practice* 45:129-35.

Goodwin, Jan. 1997a. "A Program that Takes the Stress and Pain Out of Same-Day Surgery." *Good Housekeeping* (July) 225:80-85.

———. 1997b. "Surgery to Go." *Good Housekeeping* (July) 225:80-85.

Gordon, Nahida H., Joseph P. Crowe, D. Jane Brumberg, and Nathan A. Berger. 1992. "Socioeconomic Factors and Race in Breast Cancer Recurrence and Survival." *American Journal of Epidemiology* 135:609-18.

Haas, Barbara K. 1997. "The Effect of Managed Care on Breast Cancer Detection, Treatment, and Research." *Nursing Outlook* 45:167-72.

Hadley, Jack, and Jean M. Mitchell. 1997/1998. "Breast Cancer Treatment Choice and Mastectomy Length of Stay: A Comparison of HMO and Other Privately Insured Women." *Inquiry* 34:288-301.

Hewitt, Maria and Joseph Simone, eds. 1999. *Ensuring Quality Cancer Care.* National Cancer Policy Board, Institute of Medicine and Commission on Life Sciences, National Research Council. Washington, D.C.: National Academy Press.

Hillner, Bruce E., Lynne Penberthy, Christopher E. Desch, M. Kathleen McDonald, Thomas J. Smith, and Sheldon M. Retchin. 1996. "Variation in Staging and Treatment of Local and Regional Breast Cancer in the Elderly." *Breast Cancer Research and Treatment* 40:75-86.

Himmelstein, David, Steffie Woolhandler, Ida Hellander, and Sidney M. Wolfe. 1999. "Quality of Care in Investor-Owned vs. Not-for-Profit HMOs." *Journal of the American Medical Association* 282:159-63.

HMO Group. 1998. "News Release: The HMO Group Plans Rank Among Best HMOs for Women, According to New Survey Data," January 21, New Brunswick, N.J.

Howard, Daniel L., Roy Penchansky, and Morton B. Brown. 1998. "Disaggregating the Effects of Race on Breast Cancer Survival." *Family Medicine* 30:228-35.

Hsu, Joe L., Sally L. Glaser, and Dee W. West. 1997. "Brief Communication: Racial/ Ethnic Differences in Breast Cancer Survival Among San Francisco Bay Area Women." *Journal of the National Cancer Institute* 89:1311-12.

Hubbell, F. Allen, Leo R. Chavez, Shiraz I. Mishra, and R. Burciaga Valdez. 1996. "Differing Beliefs About Breast Cancer Among Latinas and Anglo Women." *Western Journal of Medicine* 164:405-09.

"Improved Cancer Care Offered for Cancer Patients." 1997. *Cancer Weekly Plus* (June 30) 7.

Kang, Soo Hyang, and Joan R. Bloom. 1993. "Social Support and Cancer Screening Among Older Black Americans." *Journal of the National Cancer Institute* 85:737-42.

Kasper, Anne S. 1999. Personal communication.

Kilborn, Peter T. 1998. "Reality of the HMO System Doesn't Live Up to the Dream." *New York Times* (October 5) 1.

Kovner, Christine and Peter Gergen. 1998. "The Relationship Between Nurse Staffing Level and Adverse Events Following Surgery." *Image: Journal of Nursing Scholarship* 30:315-21.

Lannin, Donald R., Holly F. Mathews, Jim Mitchell, Melvin S. Swanson, Frances H. Swanson, and Maxine S. Edwards. 1998. "Influence of Socioeconomic and

Cultural Factors on Racial Differences in Late-Stage Presentation of Breast Cancer." *Journal of the American Medical Association* 279:1801-07.

Larkin, Howard. 1997. "Not All Health Plans Live Up to Potential." *American Medical News* (October 27) 40:1.

Leape, Lucian L., David W. Bates, David J. Cullen, Jeffrey Cooper, Harold J. Demonaco, Theresa Gallivan, Robert Hallisey, Jeanette Ivies, Na Laird, Glenn Label, Robert Numeral, Laura A. Petersen, Kathy Porter, Deborah Serve, Brian F. She, Stephen D. Small, Bobbie J. Switzer, B. Taylor Thompson, and Martha Vender Let. 1995. "Systems Analysis of Adverse Drug Events." *Journal of the American Medical Association* 274:35-43.

Lee-Feldstein, Anna, Hoda Anton-Culver, and Paul J. Feldstein. 1994. "Treatment Differences and Other Prognostic Factors Related to Breast Cancer Survival: Delivery Systems and Medical Outcomes." *Journal of the American Medical Association* 271:1163-68.

Levitt, Larry, Janet Lundy, and Srija Srinivasan. 1999. "Trends and Indicators in the Changing Health Care Marketplace: Chartbook." The Kaiser Changing Health Care Marketplace Project, Kaiser Family Foundation, Palo Alto, Calif.

Love, Susan. 1997. "A Surgeon's Challenge: We Need to do Better than the 'Slash, Burn and Poison' Approach to Breast Cancer." *Newsweek* (Feb. 24) 60.

Managed Health Care Improvement Task Force. 1997. Health Industry Profile, Background Paper, based on Interstudy Competitive Edge Survey, Sacramento, Calif.

Matthews, Holly F., Donald R. Lannin, and James P. Mitchell. 1994. "Coming to Terms with Advanced Breast Cancer: Black Women's Narratives from Eastern North Carolina." *Social Science and Medicine* 38:789-800.

McCormick, Brian. 1995. "Breast Cancer Still Top Liability Risk; Cost of Claims Rising." *American Medical News* (June 19) 38:23.

Miller, Robert H., and Harold S. Luft. 1994. "Managed Care Performance Since 1980." *Journal of the American Medical Association* 271:1512-19.

Myerson, Allen R. 1995. "Helping Health Insurers Say No." *New York Times* (March 20) D1.

Nattinger, Anne Butler, M. S. Gottlieb , Raymond G. Hoffman, A. P. Walker, and James S. Goodwin. 1996. "Minimal Increase in Use of Breast-Conserving Surgery from 1986 to 1990." *Medical Care* 34:479-89.

Pollack, Ronald, and Lorie Slass. 1998. *Premium Pay II: Corporate Compensation in American's HMOs.* Washington, D.C.: Families USA Foundation.

Potosky, Arnold L., Ray M. Merrill, Gerald F. Riley, Stephen H. Taplin, William Barlow, Bruce H. Fireman, and Rachel Ballard-Barbash. 1997. "Breast Cancer Survival and Treatment in Health Maintenance Organization and Fee-for-Service Settings." *Journal of the National Cancer Institute* 22:1683-91.

President's Cancer Panel, National Cancer Program. 1996. "Fighting the War on Cancer in an Evolving Health Care System, 1996 Annual Report." Advisory Boards and Groups, National Cancer Institute, Rockville, Md.

Randolph, Laura B. 1995. "Why Breast Cancer Kills More Black Women." *Ebony* (March) 50:122.

Rauber, Chris. 1998. "Evolution or Extinction? Experts Say HMOs Must Reinvent Themselves if They Are to Survive." *Modern Healthcare* (Oct. 19) 36.

Riley, Gerald F., Arnold L. Potosky, Carrie N. Klabunde, Joan L. Warren, and Rachel Ballard-Barbash. 1998. "State at Diagnosis and Treatment Patterns Among Older Women with Breast Cancer." *Journal of the American Medical Association* 281:720-26.

Roulidis, Zeses C., and Kevin A. Schulman. 1994. "Physician Communication in Managed Care Organizations: Opinions of Primary Care Physicians." *Journal of Family Practice* 39:446-51.

Sainbury, Richard, Bob Howard, Lesley Rider, Colin Johnston, and Caroline Round. 1995. "Influence of Clinician Workload and Patterns of Treatment on Survival from Breast Cancer." *Lancet* 345:1265-70.

Segal, David. 1996. "HMOs: How Much, Not How Well." *Washington Post* (January 19) F1, F3.

Senie, Ruby T., Paul Peter Rosen, Martin L. Lesser, and David W. Kinne. 1982. "Breast Self-Examination and Medical Examination Related to Breast Cancer Stage." *American Journal of Public Health* 71:583-90.

Sherrill, Robert. 1995. "Medicine and the Madness of the Market." *Nation* (January 9/16) 44-72.

Silverman, Elaine M., Jonathan S. Skinner, and Elliott S. Fisher. 1999. "The Association Between For-Profit Hospital Ownership and Increased Medicare Spending." *New England Journal of Medicine* 341:420-26.

Simon, Michael S., and Richard K. Severson. 1996. "Racial Differences in Survival of Female Breast Cancer in the Detroit Metropolitan Area." *Cancer* 72:308-14.

———. 1997. "Racial Differences in Breast Cancer Survival: The Interaction of Socioeconomic Status and Tumor Biology." *American Journal of Obstetrics & Gynecology* 176:S233-39.

Smith, Sheila, Stephen Heffler, Mark Freeland, and The National Health Expenditures Project Team. 1999. "The Next Decade of Health Spending." *Health Affairs* (July/August) 18:86-94.

Stolberg, Sheryl G. 1998. "Cultural Issues Pose Obstacles in Cancer Fight." *New York Times* (March 14) 1.

Sugerman, D. 1997. "New Treatments Offer Hope." *MPLS-St. Paul Magazine* (May) 25:108.

Tokarski, Cathy. 1998. "In the Hot Seat." *American Medical News* (March 23) 41:9-11.

U.S. Bureau of the Census. 1998. *Current Population Reports.* Washington, D.C.

Vistnes, Jessica P., and Samuel H. Zuvekas. 1999. "Health Insurance Status of the Civilian Noninstitutionalized Population: 1997. MEPS Research Findings No. 8; AHCPR Pub. No. 99-0030." Rockville, Md: Agency for Health Care Policy and Research.

Winn, Robert J. 1995. "The Role of Oncology Clinical Practice Guidelines in the Managed Care Era." *Oncology* 9(11 Suppl.):177-83.

"Women with Breast Cancer Fare Better at Multi-Disciplinary Clinics." 1997. *Cancer Weekly Plus* (June 9) 6-7.

Woolhandler, Steffie, and David U. Himmelstein. 1998. *For Our Patients, Not for Profits: A Call to Action. Chartbook and Slideshow, 1998 Edition.* The Center for Health Program Studies, Cambridge, Mass.

Wyn, Roberta, and E. Richard Brown. 1996. "Women's Health: Key Issues in Access to Insurance Coverage and to Services Among Non-Elderly Women," in *Changing the U. S. Health Care System,* ed. R. M. Andersen, Thomas H. Rice, and Gerald F. Kominski. San Francisco: Jossey Bass.

Zaldivar, R. A. 1998. "American Lifestyle Tied to Immigrant Health Woes." *HHS-HEO News,* #10, Part II.

Profits from Pain:
The Political Economy of Breast Cancer

Jane S. Zones, Ph.D.

AdWeek describes breast cancer as a "dream cause . . . it's the feminist issue without politics . . . without controversy" (Goldman 1997:70). Politicians may have adopted breast cancer issues to straddle the gender divide, but, in reality, breast cancer is an illness that is steeped in controversy. Breast cancer's visibility, accompanied by a bonanza of economic and political possibilities, has made the illness the province of entrepreneurs. Breast cancer has become a source of economic gain.

Breast cancer advocacy groups have successfully drawn attention to the disease in the past decade, lobbying to increase federal research spending, promoting screening programs to improve detection, and encouraging rapid approval of new treatments. Increased incidence and a relatively constant mortality rate have heightened fear of the disease. Other factors, too, have facilitated advocacy. Breast cancer represents a relatively comprehensible set of issues, unlike the more unwieldy problems posed by the chaos of the U.S. health care system that, in 1999, had 44.3 million uninsured individuals (Goldstein 1999:A1). The illness cuts across population subgroups and political constituencies, creating broad-based interest groups. Significantly, breast cancer is prevalent enough to have indirectly touched a majority of adult citizens through relatives, friends, and acquaintances.

Breast cancer, its origins, detection, treatment, and effects presents us with many scientific and clinical unknowns. Over the past decade, large sums of money have been invested in resolving some of the unanswered questions, with both beneficial and controversial outcomes. Government funding of breast cancer–related research by the National Institutes of Health (NIH) and by the Department of Defense (DOD) has increased dramatically, nearly six-fold since 1991, from $90 million to an estimated $600 million in 1999 (Breast Cancer Coalition 1999a; 1999b). While breast cancer advocates can be pleased by this marshaling of resources, investment on a large scale attracts opportunists as well as those committed to the eradication of this illness.

This chapter examines some of the ways that people and corporations, through the U.S. market economy, have benefited from the prominence of breast cancer as a means to create wealth. Profitability is a fundamental requirement of a capitalist economy, and cancer has many profit centers—detection, treatment, prevention, and even advocacy. Commercial ventures seek to increase their share of available dollars in a number of ways, including the introduction of new products or services to the marketplace, making claims for products that exaggerate their benefit or minimize their risk, expanding the market by creating demand, and cornering the market by reducing competition. Examples from a variety of enterprises related to breast cancer illustrate how these economic strategies shape what we know about the disease, who gets treated, and how.

INTRODUCTION OF NEW COMMODITIES OR PROCEDURES

The time-honored means to making money in a capitalist economy, of course, is to introduce a new commodity or way of doing things.

Americans have exalted inventors and new technologies throughout our history, and the arena of breast cancer is no exception. In recent years, we have witnessed the introduction of new treatments for advanced malignancies, innovative detection methods, less invasive biopsy techniques, and the use of a pharmaceutical treatment, tamoxifen, to reduce the risk of developing breast cancer in healthy women. Despite the profusion of innovative products and procedures, there has been only modest impact upon the death rate from breast cancer (Montague 1997).

CHEMOTHERAPY DRUGS USED IN BREAST CANCER

Chemotherapeutic drugs have generated the greatest profits and are the major arena for cancer research and investment. A recent magazine ad states "CANCER," in red letters that span the page's width against a black background, "It's a WAR. That's why we're developing 316 new weapons" ("Cancer. It's a War." 1999:61). Sponsored by "America's Pharmaceutical Companies," the advertisement highlights the astonishing array of cancer drugs that are in development, adding to an impressive number already on the market. Many of these so-called new drugs are minor reconfigurations of currently available medications (Marsa 1997).

Pharmaceutical manufacturing is clearly the nation's most profitable industry. With double-digit profit rates, in 1997, its top ten companies brought in more than $138 billion in revenue (Roush 1997:1039). Drug company CEOs earn an average of $12.7 million in annual compensation (Kealey 1999:5). In the United States individuals pay substantially more for their medications than people in European countries that have national health insurance. In this country, individuals pay an average of $15,000 to $40,000 for standard chemotherapy for advanced breast cancer (Napoli 1996:4).

Taxol, the largest selling cancer drug worldwide with estimated sales of $1.2 billion in 1998, has been used for years as a treatment for metastatic breast cancer. More recently, it has been shown to be beneficial for women with localized breast cancer that has spread to their lymph nodes (John 1999). Although taxol was discovered and developed by the federal government at taxpayers' expense, it is now produced and sold by Bristol-Myers Squibb (BMS), a major pharmaceutical manufacturer of chemotherapy and other drugs (Fellers 1998). BMS charges a wholesale price of nearly five dollars per milligram, although it costs less than 40 cents per milligram to manufacture, making the drug out of reach for many patients who may require several hundred milligrams per month over many months (John 1999:10).

HIGH-DOSE CHEMOTHERAPY (HDC)

Innovative procedures that use already available products are another means of generating new profits with anticipated improvement in breast cancer outcomes. For example, high-dose chemotherapy (about six to ten or more times the toxicity of standard chemotherapy) is a controversial procedure for treating breast cancer patients. High-dose chemotherapy (HDC) destroys bone marrow, which produces essential blood cells and platelets for the body's immune system. Consequently, to support the administration of HDC, doctors remove bone marrow (autologous bone marrow transplant) or blood stem cells (stem cell transplant) prior to treatment. Following the administration of the chemotherapy over several weeks, the bone marrow or stem cells are returned to the body to produce new cells. (For brevity, I will refer to the combined procedures as HDC.)

By the late 1990s, more than 6,000 women annually underwent this process, with a total expenditure estimated to be greater than half a billion dollars. HDC can cost up to $250,000, and, in the mid-1990s, had a survival rate of four percent at ten years (Napoli 1996:4). When first used to treat breast cancer in the mid-1980s, virtually all patients receiving HDC had metastatic (advanced) disease. It has been increasingly employed to fight less advanced breast cancers (Kelly and Koenig 1998:136-137). By 1999, over half of the women who received HDC had primary breast cancer with significant positive lymph nodes but without metastases in other parts of the body (National Institutes of Health 1999).

In the late 1980s, the NIH began sponsoring research to assess the long-term effectiveness of HDC. Physicians and their patients, eager for promising treatments, had high expectations for its benefits. However, physicians were reluctant to encourage their breast cancer patients to enter these NIH research trials (in which subjects are randomly assigned to either the experimental treatment or to a conventional treatment), because participants had a 50 percent chance of being randomly assigned to conventional chemotherapy rather than the experimental HDC. In addition, entrepreneurs, such as Tennessee's Response Oncology, opened up centers around the country to support the administration of HDC, further decreasing the likelihood of referral to major medical centers where women could enter research trials. Fewer than 10 percent of the women who were treated with HDC did so as part of a randomized clinical trial (Smigel 1995:954).

In April 1999 the NIH released preliminary findings from two of the HDC trials (corroborating findings from randomized studies from Sweden and France), indicating that the procedure is no more effective than conventional therapy in preventing relapse or prolonging survival (National Institutes of Health 1999). The NIH studies corroborated findings of an earlier multistudy analysis (ECRI 1996). Although two smaller studies from South Africa showed significant benefit for HDC, they were shown to be fraudulent in early 2000, and advocacy for HDC has diminished (Weiss et al. 2000).

GENETIC TESTING FOR BREAST CANCER

Genetic testing exemplifies another type of new technology that is being marketed to women concerned about breast cancer. In 1994, scientists identified the BRCA1 breast and ovarian cancer gene that is associated with increased breast cancer risk. A year and a half later, a second gene sequence implicated in increased risk of breast cancer, BRCA2, was described. Since that time, a multimillion-dollar enterprise has been built up around testing women with family histories of breast and ovarian cancer. Although an estimated 600,000 U.S. women carry a mutated form of the BRCA1 gene (Angier 1994:C12), heredity accounts for the development of only about five percent of all breast cancers. Genetic mutations can be inherited or acquired as a result of radiation, diet, environmental toxins, or other unknown assaults on the body (National Cancer Institute 1998).

BRCA1 was discovered by Mark Skolnick and his research colleagues at the University of Utah three years after he cofounded Myriad Genetics to generate funding for discoveries of genetic links to major diseases. Myriad filed for and won patents that allowed them virtual monopoly rights to genetic tests and therapeutic uses of BRCA1. Myriad's patent application created controversy. As one scientist put it, "the human genome project should be a cooperative search for new knowledge rather than a self-interested search for profits" (Butler and Gershon 1994:272). It appeared that profits from BRCA1 would go to a private company although the discovery had been heavily subsidized by taxpayers. The NIH, which contributed one-third of the funding for BRCA1's discovery, challenged the patent, which did not credit NIH's funding or contributing discoveries by its government scientists (Garaghan 1994). The dispute was settled when Myriad and the University of Utah agreed to include the names of the NIH scientists and to allocate a quarter of future royalties to the federal government (Marshall 1995).

In 1996, when Myriad announced the availability of its $2,400 BRCA1 screening test, scientists expressed concern that, because genetic studies had been carried out on families with high rates of breast cancer, risk estimates were inflated. Epidemiologist John Hopper, who helped develop criteria for BRCA screening in Australia, worried that commercial testing would "make money out of raising anxiety and exploiting women. We should all take a deep breath and wait until there are decent data on the general population" (Kahn 1996:496).

Genetic testing can offer women only probabilities of developing the disease; it cannot provide certainty that breast cancer will develop, or how dangerous it would be if it does occur (Hubbard 1995). Risks of unregulated genetic testing include the possible failure of physicians to provide correct information, inaccurate DNA analysis, generation of apprehension leading to overutilization of screening tests and surgery, and discrimination in employment and insurance (Cunningham 1997). Despite these facts, groups of women are being encouraged to undergo testing. One gene test provider, a surgeon marketing to Ashkenazi Jewish women (who have a higher risk of having the BRCA1 mutation), placed an advertisement in the *Hartford Jewish Ledger* that stated, "if you carry damaged breast cancer genes and you live long enough, you are almost guaranteed to develop breast cancer" ("The Future Is Now" 1997:9). This type of hyperbole provokes fear that can distort an individual's ability to think clearly about alternatives.

Those women who are found to have genetic risk are offered the option of aggressive screening to catch potential cancers at an early stage, tamoxifen to lower risk, or prophylactic mastectomy—amputating healthy breasts to reduce the risk of developing breast cancer. Along with mastectomy, surgeons generally suggest reconstruction of the breasts, usually with saline- or silicone-filled implants. For many women, genetic testing can open the door to additional procedures, pills, and products that, in turn, come with their own controversial risks.

EXAGGERATING CLAIMS OF BENEFIT

While new technologies, such as high-dose chemotherapy and genetic testing, are generating large profits for their manufacturers, companies also aim to increase sales by putting the best light on their products. Advertising and other marketing tools are very effective at increasing demand for commodities and procedures that industries want to sell; however, exaggerating benefit is not limited to industry. In the cancer field, it is often the scientists who are doing the selling. Every decade or so, the cancer establishment is asked to assess the progress in the War on Cancer, which President Richard Nixon declared in 1971. To show that the huge investment is worthwhile, cancer agencies tout their work as effective, despite continued high mortality from the disease. In 1985, the National Cancer Institute (NCI), the largest source of federal funding for cancer research, declared that the United States was about to attain a five-year survival rate of 50 percent for all cancers. However, to obtain this statistic required excluding the nonwhite population (Bailar and Smith 1986). Recent celebration of the decline in breast cancer mortality since 1990 has made little mention of the increasing death rate for African American women during this period (Brenner 1997).

MAMMOGRAPHY

For years, mammography campaigns have actively recruited women by claiming that early detection of breast cancer greatly increases chances of survival. This argument has been questioned for premenopausal women (Ernster 1997). A national advertising campaign featuring Whoopi Goldberg claimed, "Nine in ten will survive [breast cancer] if they follow a program of detection by having a mammogram" (Napoli 1994:3). In 1994, the Center for Medical Consumers successfully challenged the veracity of this claim, and its sponsors voluntarily removed all statistics rather than report the actual low success rate of mammography in younger women.

DIET

Another example of exaggerated claims is found in a popular book entitled *The Breast Cancer Prevention Diet—The Powerful Foods,*

Supplements and Drugs That Combat Breast Cancer (Arnot 1998). This book urges women to adopt a diet rich in soy, flaxseed, and fish oils to prevent breast cancer. Research on diet and breast cancer indicates that societies that consume a low-fat diet (such as Japan) have lower rates of breast cancer. However, the complexity of the many other factors that differentiate societies makes the relationship inconclusive. For Arnot to attribute lifestyle factors, such as a specific diet, to eradicating breast cancer is presumptuous. Capitalizing on women's fears, Arnot's unfounded claims that "[n]utrition is emerging as the most important way to prevent breast cancer" (1998: 4) wrought such an onslaught of criticism that he has since agreed that risk reduction would be a more appropriate term than prevention to characterize his perspective (Brown 1999:85).

TAMOXIFEN

Similar exaggerated claims surrounded the world's leading breast cancer drug, tamoxifen (Paulsen 1994). AstraZeneca, the manufacturers of tamoxifen, urged the Food and Drug Administration's (FDA) Oncologic Drugs Advisory Committee in September 1998, to approve tamoxifen for breast cancer "prevention" in healthy women at high risk. The Breast Cancer Prevention Trial, funded with $60 million from the NCI, announced its results five months earlier at a press conference, showing a nearly 50 percent reduction in the incidence of invasive breast cancer (cancer that infiltrates surrounding tissue) among women in the study who took tamoxifen (Cimons 1998). The trial was ended prematurely because of the positive results, so that women in the control arm of the study, who were receiving a placebo, could avail themselves of tamoxifen.

Publicizing results of the study at that stage was controversial for several reasons. First, curtailing the study precluded the opportunity to determine whether tamoxifen has time-limited effectiveness, as it does in the treatment of breast cancer (five years). Second, usually the results of a large federally funded clinical trial are published in a scientific journal prior to soliciting media attention. Third, the press conference that preceded the announcement of the success of a new rival drug, raloxifene, by several weeks gave the appearance of a preemptive strike to focus attention on tamoxifen. Further, the serious side effects of tamoxifen were downplayed.

The FDA advisory committee recommended approving the use of tamoxifen to "lower [the] risk" of developing breast cancer in healthy women at high risk. However, because the drug may simply delay the development of the disease, the FDA did not allow AstraZeneca's proposed change in the labeling to portray tamoxifen as "preventing" breast cancer (Okie 1998:A3). Nevertheless, a report of the FDA meeting in the *Journal of the National Cancer Institute* opened with the sentence: "Tamoxifen moved another step closer to approval for breast cancer *prevention* [emphasis added] when the [FDA advisors] recommended approval of its use to reduce the risk of breast cancer in women at high risk for the disease" (Reynolds 1998:1428). Clearly, AstraZeneca is winning the commodity war, even if it is losing the FDA battle.

STATISTICS

Statistics also are used to exaggerate benefits. Rates of prophylactic mastectomy are surging because of the widespread and successful marketing of BRCA genetic susceptibility testing. The drastic option of amputating healthy breasts has been held out as an option for women at high risk of developing breast cancer. In 1999, a follow-up study reported that prophylactic mastectomy effectively reduces the risk of developing cancer by 90 percent (Hartmann et al. 1999:81). This statistic made headlines in virtually every daily newspaper in the United States. Buried in the story was a more telling fact—that for every woman who was "saved" from a breast cancer death (an estimated 18 of 639), 35 who suffered the trauma of mastectomy would have survived even if they had kept their breasts and developed breast cancer (Eisen and Weber 1999:138).

Maryann Napoli (1999:2) points out that "whether it's chemotherapy or radiotherapy, overtreatment of the majority to save a small minority has been the story of breast cancer treatment for decades."

RESEARCH AND TREATMENT BIASES

Breast cancer research has been characterized by biases that enhance outcomes, making treatments appear to be more effective than they actually are. For example, lengthening survival times of women with breast cancer have been attributed to early detection and successful treatments, but these statistics are compromised by lead time bias, that is, detection of tumors earlier in their development. Women survive approximately the same length of time they would have had their cancers been diagnosed at a later date, but with longer awareness that they have the disease and longer length of treatment (Bailar 1976). Since women with breast cancer are arbitrarily considered "cured" if they are alive (even if dying) five years after diagnosis, lead time bias has lent an aura of progress.

Similarly, length bias refers to the effect of slowly progressing disease. Slow-growing tumors have the best prognosis (Plotkin 1996). They also remain in a detectable but nonthreatening state much longer than rapidly growing cancers, and therefore are more likely to be identified by mammography. "The very neoplasms [tumors] with the most favorable disease progression rates are the ones most likely to be found while in the asymptomatic phase" (Bailar 1976:77). Consequently, screening mammography appears to be more effective than it actually is.

Selection bias refers to self-referral or preferential choice of subjects in a study. Women who comply with mammography screening requests, for example, have higher incomes, which is generally associated with better health status and health care utilization (Stein, Fox, and Murata 1991). These qualities mean women are more likely to survive breast cancer regardless of screening benefits. Moreover, research on high-dose chemotherapy

(HDC) has been more likely to include women who are considered strong enough to withstand the extremely toxic treatment, responsive enough to chemotherapy to benefit from the high dosage, and insured or financially capable of paying for this expensive procedure. When compared to women in conventional treatment who are not selected with the same standard, this comparison biases the study outcomes in favor of HDC. Moreover, much of the literature does not describe patient characteristics, making accurate comparisons between therapies difficult. (Selection bias is not a factor when women are randomized in experimental trials.)

The elimination of participants after they have already been enrolled in a research study constitutes another form of selection bias. For instance, some studies of HDC exclude women from the outcome statistics if they die during the chemotherapy administration phase. Although deaths attributed to immediate treatment have been declining in recent years, as many as 5 to 17 percent of patients had been estimated to die during HDC treatment (ECRI 1996; Jaggar 1996). Removing from the analysis those who died of the treatment has the effect of making treatment outcomes appear to be more positive.

CHEMOTHERAPY

The advantages of standard chemotherapy have been exaggerated as well. While it is clear that chemotherapy helps some women, clinicians and researchers are still unable to determine who those women are. Of the approximately 70,000 U.S. women who are diagnosed each year with breast cancer without lymph node involvement, an estimated 5,000 will be free of the disease for a longer time period with chemotherapy. However, it is not yet clear whether this treatment improves their chances of survival. About 65,000 of these women do not benefit from the treatment, but many of them suffer the consequences of side effects such as chemotherapy-related illness and discomfort, time lost from work, and a collective expense that amounts to nearly a half-billion dollars a year (Moss 1995:91).

MINIMIZING RISK

The counterpart to exaggerating the benefit of a product or service is to dismiss or minimize its costs or hazards. Examples of this practice can be seen with chemotherapy, tamoxifen, and screening mammography. The usual side effects of chemotherapy are well known—nausea, vomiting, hair loss, and mouth sores. (Side effects, of course, generate their own armory of symptom-alleviating drugs.) The intensity of the effects of chemotherapy can be inferred from this warning to oncological nurses, who are merely preparing the drugs: "cytotoxic [chemotherapy] agents pose a 'significant risk' of damage to the skin, reproductive abnormalities, hematologic problems, and of liver and chromosomal lesions" (Moss 1995:67). Even so, many oncologists downplay the difficulties that are a part of chemotherapy. In one report of an experimental high-dose regimen for metastatic breast cancer, ICE (ifosfamide + cyclophos-phamide + etoposide, a combination chemotherapy), patients experienced enteritis (inflammation of the intestine), central nervous system and lung complications, liver toxicity, ear damage, kidney toxicity, and damage to the heart. One patient went into a coma and eight percent of the group died from the effects of the drugs. Nevertheless, the article that reported on this regimen concludes, "In summary, ICE is well tolerated, with acceptable hematopoietic [affecting the formation of blood cells] side effects and predictable organ toxicity" (Moss 1995:69).

Former National Cancer Institute clinical director Dr. Vincent DeVita stated, "[C]ancer patients today are *hugely* better off—not modestly better off, *hugely* better off . . . Our ability to control nausea, vomiting, and pain has gone from virtually no ability to a remarkable degree of control" (Skolnick 1995:526). However, Rose Kushner, one of the first breast cancer advocates, noted early on

that many physicians are removed from the side effects of chemotherapy. "Most of the time, oncologists do not even see their patients
during regular, routine appointments. In the United States, bald-
ness, nausea, vomiting, diarrhea, clogged veins, financial problems,
broken marriages, disturbed children, loss of libido, loss of self-
esteem, and body image are nurses' turf" (Kushner 1984:345).

The immediate side effects of high-dose chemotherapy are
similar to conventional chemotherapy but much more extreme
(Groopman 1998). Patients receiving HDC are typically confined
to a hospital isolation room for several weeks in order to reduce the
risk of infection. Contacts with friends and family are limited. Up
to 10 percent of the transplantations fail, making it impossible for
the body to generate new blood cells. Those who survive beyond
the first month after transplantation are at greater risk for developing secondary leukemias (ECRI 1996:42-43). HDC patients have
eight times the risk of cognitive impairment (affecting memory,
concentration, language, and thought) than do women with breast
cancer who are not treated with chemotherapy at all (van Dam et
al. 1998:216).

TAMOXIFEN

Tamoxifen, a hormonal breast cancer treatment whose side effects
are much less severe than most chemotherapies, can be used for up
to five years to reduce the risk of recurrence. However, in an early
NCI-sponsored study of approximately 4,000 women being treated
for breast cancer, 23 of the women given tamoxifen contracted
uterine cancer, and four of them died of it. Despite this fact, healthy
women volunteering in the Breast Cancer Prevention Trial were
told initially in informed consent statements that "no deaths from
uterine cancer were reported" (Paulsen 1994:41). Consent statement forms were subsequently altered to reflect more accurate
information after pressure on the NCI from the National Women's
Health Network. Other side effects of tamoxifen include liver

disease, blood clotting disorders, eye damage, and menopausal symptoms (Fugh-Berman and Epstein 1992). Although tamoxifen is being widely advertised in magazines and on television to healthy women to lower their chances of developing breast cancer, the drug's risks continue to be minimized.

SCREENING MAMMOGRAPHY

Even widely heralded measures for healthy women carry unacknowledged problems. During the debates over screening mammography for premenopausal women, it became clear that there are serious risks related to this type of x-ray screening that are not generally communicated to women. These include radiation exposure, inaccurate assessments leading to large numbers of negative biopsies, unnecessary mastectomies, and an increasing number of *in situ* diagnoses that have complex repercussions for women and the health care system.

Radiation, including x-rays, is known to be associated with risk of early onset breast cancer. This risk has been shown in studies done on women who experienced different levels of radiation exposure as child survivors of the atomic bomb explosions (Land et al. 1993), women treated for pulmonary tuberculosis (MacKenzie 1965), and women given radiation for benign breast disease (Fackelmann 1993). In 1976, in the wake of the establishment of the National Cancer Institute (NCI)/American Cancer Society (ACS) breast screening program, a landmark article by the editor of the *Journal of the National Cancer Institute* questioned the lack of research scrutiny of radiation effects from mammography. He argued that promotion of mammography as a general public health measure was premature, and "regretfully" concluded that there was a possibility that "screening asymptomatic women may eventually take almost as many lives as it saves" (Bailar 1976:82).

In 1977, three NCI advisory committees on screening mammography concluded that "routine x-ray mammography for breast cancer is apparently of little value and is quite possibly dangerous" (Greenberg 1977:1015). The former president of the American Cancer Society (ACS), in an article in *Reader's Digest,* sought to allay fears by predicting that "science will have learned to control the disease" by the time radiation-induced cancers developed in the distant future (Greenberg 1977:1016).

The amount of radiation exposure resulting from mammography has declined dramatically over the past 40 years, and most health providers discount hazards of radiation from the procedure. In 1972, the United Nations Scientific Committee on the Effects of Atomic Radiation (UNSCEAR) reported that 10 to 35 rads was the mammographic dose in the 1960s. In 1977, UNSCEAR claimed that it was technically possible to obtain clear images with 0.2 rads or less (Gofman 1995). By the 1990s, the lowest effective dose for mammography was considered to be about 0.04 rads, and the maximum recommended dose was 0.4 (Kuester and Wolfe 1991:19).

Variation between machines has been extreme, with some machines using over 100 times the radiation of others for the same task (Kuester and Wolfe 1991). The Mammography Quality Standards Act (MQSA), passed by Congress in 1992, required the FDA to set comprehensive standards for the nation's mammographic facilities, certify facilities, conduct an annual inspection, and limit the average dose to 0.3 rads for a single exposure mammography (Skolnick 1994:735). By the time the law was implemented, the number of facilities had declined to approximately 10,000 from an estimated 14,000. Because of an oversupply of mammography facilities, access to services was not affected. Most of those that were closed were located near other, certified facilities (Pasquier and Ku 1997:12).

Other mammography risks include errors in assessment. Finding abnormality when the breast is cancer free (a false-positive result) requires follow-up procedures. This is particularly problematic for premenopausal women, whose breasts have denser tissue and whose mammographic images are more difficult to read than those of older women (Kerlikowske et al. 1996). Over half of premenopausal women will receive a false positive reading after a decade of annual screening mammography and nearly 20 percent will undergo biopsy—which can create scarring and further obscure results of future mammograms (Elmore et al. 1998). Younger women have approximately two-and-one-half times as many biopsies for every diagnosed cancer compared to women over 50 years old (Kerlikowske et al. 1993:2449).

Approximately 15 percent of cancerous tumors of the breast are not identified by mammograms that preceded a breast cancer diagnosis (false-negative results) (Leopold 1998). There is a wide range in the accuracy of radiologists' interpretation of mammograms, with differences increasing in the assessment of breasts with dense tissue (Kerlikowske et al. 1998). In one study, 10 community radiologists examined 150 mammograms; all of the doctors came to the same conclusion in only 10 of the cases (Elmore et al. 1994:1495). Failure to discern a tumor at the time of screening mammography is a major cause of liability claims for malpractice. A 1990 study by the Physician Insurers Association of America (PIAA), a trade group whose member organizations cover about half of all physicians in the United States, showed that two-thirds of malpractice claims involved delays in breast cancer diagnosis for premenopausal women. A disproportionate share of the total (40 percent) were the youngest group, under 40 years old. Five years later, breast cancer remained the most common condition for which women filed malpractice claims. By 1995, 80 percent of those with delayed diagnosis claims were premenopausal women with false negative or equivocal mammograms. PIAA attributed this to the increase in screening of asymptomatic younger women (Leopold 1998).

In addition, there have been cases of cancer-free women who were mistakenly given mastectomies. In the late 1970s, an investigation into outcomes of the NCI/ACS-sponsored mammography screening program found that 48 women who underwent screening in the early 1970s had "had their breasts removed needlessly or hastily because of misdiagnosis" ("Most Women Who Had Breasts Removed Had Cancer" 1977:7). The NCI decided not to inform these women directly of any mistaken results, but told their physicians and asked them to give the news to their patients. No follow-up was done, and it is not known whether these women were ever told that they did not have cancer. Withholding this information has repercussions not only for them, but for their families' peace of mind ("Women Misdiagnosed with Breast Cancer" 1983:5).

As mammography becomes more sensitive, it is picking up smaller and smaller lesions. Ductal carcinoma *in situ* (DCIS) is a lesion, considered precancerous, that often forms soft thickenings or shows up as clusters of small calcifications discernable in a mammogram. Although relatively little is known about how DCIS progresses if it is left untreated, it is clear that women with DCIS are at higher risk of developing invasive breast cancer. It is also known that a large proportion of women who have DCIS would not be affected by it if it remained undetected. Small studies indicate that about 20 to 25 percent of women with untreated DCIS go on to develop invasive cancer (in which the malignant cells break through the walls of the milk ducts) within 10 years (Love and Lindsey 1995:227). On the other hand, DCIS is commonly found during autopsy in women who died of other causes, never knowing that they had the condition (Ernster et al. 1996).

From 1973, just as screening mammography was becoming institutionalized by the ACS and the NCI, to 1992, the rate of reported cases of DCIS grew over sixfold, from 2.4 to 15.8 per 100,000 women. Most of this increase came during the 1980s and is heavily associated with screening mammography of healthy women. Virtually all cases were treated by surgery. In 1992, 54 percent of women with DCIS had a lumpectomy, and about half of these women had radiation treatment as well. Fewer were treated with mastectomy (44 percent), a procedure considered to be over-treatment. Follow-up of women diagnosed with DCIS between 1983 and 1991, treated or not, showed that as a group they had the same life expectancy as women in the general population (Ernster et al. 1996:915, 917).

Since DCIS is not defined as cancer, but as an indicator of increased risk, Virginia Ernster and her colleagues categorize detection of DCIS in premenopausal women as "a definite potential risk of screening," possibly including decades of needless anxiety, unnecessary surgery, or other cancer treatments with their own attendant risks (1996:918). A clear picture of DCIS remains to be elucidated.

EXPANDING EXISTING MARKETS

Once a product or service has made its way into the marketplace, sales may be increased by appealing to new consumers. The incidence of breast cancer has been slowly rising for many years (Landis et al. 1999), but it is the much larger market of women *without* breast cancer, particularly the baby-boom population, now age 35 to 55 years old, who are the major target for breast cancer industries looking to enlarge the demand for what they have to sell.

It is no accident that the visibility of breast cancer as a disease feared among healthy women has grown dramatically, and that women overestimate their risk of getting breast cancer (Kelly 1996). In 1928, President Calvin Coolidge's personal physician, James Coupal, stated that "[c]ancer will never be cured unless the medical profession starts a *cancer panic*" (Payer 1992:203). The American Cancer Society (ACS) has been generating fear for decades and, simultaneously, reassuring the public with news of progress, in order to increase contributions and their significance as a charitable organization (DiLorenzo and Bennett 1994). For example, breast cancer incidence is tragically high, but the ACS disseminates the one-in-eight risk figure with its ring of doom, not noting that this is a risk spread out over a lifetime of 80 years. Fear, in turn, increases demand for services.

Screening mammography for premenopausal women is the most successful example of expanding markets to increase profits. In 1972, the ACS funded 12 mammography centers in an effort to reach 60,000 women. The NCI then financed an expansion of the ACS program, and by 1975 there were 29 centers that had enrolled more than 280,000 women aged 35 to 74 years old (Gofman 1995). This program, in addition to the widely publicized 1974 diagnoses of breast cancer in such high-profile women as Betty Ford and Happy Rockefeller, institutionalized screening mammography as an important component of breast cancer containment. With mass education campaigns hailing victory, the number of U.S. women who had mammograms rose 30 percent between 1989 and 1995 ("Joy at Increase in Mammograms" 1997).

Although fewer than 20 percent of all breast cancers occur in premenopausal women, this is the group that has been most heavily targeted for routine screening. Early detection of breast cancer through screening mammography has been shown to reduce mortality in postmenopausal women (Welch and Fisher 1998:1391), but its utility for premenopausal women has been questioned for many years. "Screening is a lottery. Any winnings are shared by the minority of women—about one in 60 or 70—who are diagnosed with breast cancer in their forties. The overwhelming majority of women experience no benefit" (Berry 1998:1437). Some women die even if their breast cancer is very tiny when first detected by mammography. In a multistudy analysis of eight randomized trials, Donald Berry found that after about 15 years, there were 29 breast cancer deaths for each 10,000 women assigned to receive mammography screening, and 36 per 10,000 for controls who did not receive mammography screening (1998: 1437).

In 1997, a NIH Consensus Conference on mammography screening for premenopausal women weighed the evidence and concluded that the benefit of screening this group was so small that the decision to have mammograms should be left to women in consultation with their doctors. A large and vocal lobby, convinced of the value of mammography for younger women, rallied Congress and the president and prevailed upon the NIH hierarchy to disregard the panel's conclusions and to recommend guidelines urging women in their forties to be screened every year or two.

At the same time, the ACS, which already had such guidelines in place, altered them to recommend *annual* screening for this cohort. Proponents of screening, including spokespersons for the American College of Radiology, contend that annual mammography would be more likely to catch fast-growing tumors (Feig 1996). However, evidence from controlled trials does not support this contention, and annual screening would double the already prevalent risks (Berry 1998).

Why was scientific evidence largely disregarded in this significant and expensive policy decision? Many premenopausal women who are diagnosed with cancer following mammography are told that their survival is due to early detection of the cancer. Evidence suggests, however, that a large number of these women would have survived even if their tumors had been diagnosed at a later stage (Love and Lindsey 1995; Plotkin 1996) because of great variation in types of tumor and the rates at which tumors grow. At the Consensus Conference, many younger women testified in moving speeches about their belief that mammography saved their lives. There were no comparable statements, of course, from women whose breast cancer, though detected early, had not been contained by treatment, or from women whose surgical biopsies followed false positive mammograms. Reports from researchers citing data from large samples do not carry the forcefulness of personal testimonials and are less compelling.

In addition, many of the proponents of more frequent screening at younger ages have a vested interest in expanding the market for mammography services. Although advocates of early and frequent mammography blame managed care's cost containment ethic as the motivation to limit screening of premenopausal women (Sickles and Kopans 1993), there is little evidence to support that claim. Most private insurance, Medicare, and Medicaid programs cover guideline-based mammograms (Gordon, Rundall, and Parker 1998). Screening mammography for women in their forties is zealously endorsed by several powerful groups, including radiologists, manufacturers of mammography film and machines, and institutional providers.

Radiologists have also been leaders in swaying public policy decisions in this area. "The experts who believe screening should be officially recommended to women in their forties are mainly radiologists . . . Those who are skeptical . . . are mainly epidemiologists and public health physicians versed in the science of evidence-based medicine" (Taubes 1997:1056). If premenopausal women were to comply with ACS guidelines that recommend annual screening for this group, at $100 per mammogram, annual revenues would be close to two billion dollars. This estimate does not include the cost of follow-up tests for the 7 to 10 percent of women with abnormal findings, few of whom have breast cancer (Ernster 1997).

Another group that has a vested interest in broadening the market for mammography services is the major manufacturers of mammography equipment: General Electric (GE) and DuPont. GE has sales of over $100 million a year in mammography machines, and DuPont produces the film used to make mammographic images of the breast. An NCI report concludes that the approximately 14,000 mammography machines installed in the United States in 1990 represented two to three times the needed number (Brown, Kessler, and Rueter 1990), the consequence of an "aggressive industry vigorously promoting and willing to sell the equipment to anyone regardless of qualifications" (McLelland 1990:491). Purchasing machines necessitates a need for users, and GE, DuPont, and health care providers who purchase their products direct their advertising appeals to younger women. Writer Monte Paulsen cites a DuPont television ad that lauds its new mammography film as making it "safer to start mammography early" (1994:41).

Institutional providers have a stake in policy decisions as well. At the 1997 NIH Consensus Conference, the director of X-Ray Associates of New Mexico, a radiologist, was quoted as saying "I fear this document [the panel's draft that left the decision whether or not to undergo mammography screening to premenopausal women in consultation with their physician] *is tantamount to a death sentence* [emphasis added] for thousands of women. I grieve for them" (Marwick 1997:520).

DEFENDING CORPORATE STATUS

Information is the foundation of the modern Women's Health Movement, and access to knowledge has allowed women to make sound decisions about their own health care. Many arenas of the health care world have become sources of breast cancer information, products, and services. In each of these domains, commercial interests may conflict with the best interests of women in relationship to breast cancer. Nowhere is this more clear than in the arena of breast cancer prevention.

Many agree that preventing breast cancer should be our highest priority. The trend in breast cancer research is toward increasingly expensive and technical solutions. However, a public health perspective calls for prioritizing research and programs that would eliminate the causes of this disease before it develops. Despite the investment of billions of dollars into research since President Richard Nixon declared the War on Cancer in 1971, little progress has been made in lowering mortality in the more common forms of the disease (Sporn 1996). Treatments have alleviated painful symptoms and extended years of life for some, but they have not brought us even close to the NCI's 1985 goal of halving age-adjusted mortality from cancer by the year 2000. Given this situation, many leaders in the field have recommended shifting the current emphasis on treatment to prevention in order to realize substantial progress against cancer (Bailar and Smith 1986; Cairns 1997; Sporn 1996; Weiss 1995).

In the twentieth century, public health preventive measures, including environmental, social, behavioral, and nutritional improvements, have had a far greater impact on survival than medical technologies, including penicillin and vaccination. In this age of amazing medical innovation and expenditure, it is difficult to comprehend that less than five percent of the total decline in mortality since 1900 is a result of disease-specific medical measures. Mortality rates from influenza, pneumonia, diphtheria, whooping cough, and even polio achieved their steepest declines in the decades prior to innovative medical measures that were hailed as their conquerors (McKinlay and McKinlay 1997:20).

One preventive measure is focused on by John Gofman, a molecular biologist and physician, who discusses the role of ionizing radiation in the development of breast cancer in his book *Preventing Breast Cancer: The Story of a Major, Proven, Preventable Cause of this Disease* (1995). Gofman contends that this form of radiation causes about 75 percent of new cases of breast cancer in the United States. Since exposure to ionizing radiation comes primarily from medical sources, Gofman suggests that we can prevent a substantial number of future breast cancers by eliminating unnecessary x-rays and by monitoring and lowering dosages.

Moreover, in 1992, Greenpeace released a report that implicates environmental organochlorines with increasing incidence of breast cancer (Thornton 1992). Organochlorines are industrial chemicals, many of which are known carcinogens, including DDT, PCBs, and dioxin. Organochlorine compounds that have weak estrogen-like effects (xenoestrogens) are strongly associated with an increased risk of breast cancer. Three of four major studies of the effects of these compounds as potential carcinogens in breast cancer found a positive link (Høyer et al. 1998; Hunter et al. 1997; Krieger et al. 1994; Wolff et al. 1993). (For more discussion of environmental links to breast cancer, see chapter 9 of this volume.)

As long as corporate interests have a large monetary interest in breast cancer detection and treatment, they have little to gain by preventing breast cancer and much to lose from the regulation of toxic products, manufacturing by-products, and waste disposal. Efforts to encourage research and advocacy into possible environmental causes—including corporate pollution—have met with stiff resistance and meager funding, not to mention potential conflict of interest. Harvard University's Center for Cancer Prevention declared in a 1997 report that a mere two percent of cancers were attributable to environmental pollution. Companies that have provided funding for the Harvard School of Public Health, home of the Center, include the Chemical Manufacturers Association, Chevron, Dow Chemical, DuPont, Monsanto, Shell Oil, and Texaco, and a number of drug companies (Shapiro 1998:1).

In another case, the *New England Journal of Medicine* published a scathing review of Sandra Steingraber's *Living Downstream—An Ecologist Looks at Cancer and the Environment* (Steingraber 1997). The reviewer, whose affiliations were not identified by the journal, was an official of W. R. Grace, a major chemical company. W. R. Grace also was implicated in a popular book and movie, *A Civil Action*, for its role in toxic dumping and contamination of the water supply of Woburn, Mass., alleged to have caused a cluster of childhood cancers. The prestigious medical journal was forced to apologize for publishing a review with such clear conflict of interest and for not acknowledging the conflict upon publication.

In health care as elsewhere, public relations is a major vehicle for influencing public perception of corporate behavior. Corporations that produce environmentally damaging products, whose manufacturing processes have questionable environmental effects, or whose products are priced at a premium are acutely cognizant of the importance of a good image in creating good will and public acceptance in the marketplace. Moreover, major industries assist in shaping public image. In 1994, the top 15 public relations firms in the United States netted one billion dollars. The largest, Burson-

Marsteller, netted $192 million from 1,700 employees in 63 offices in 32 countries; their stated mission is to help "clients manage issues by influencing . . . public attitudes, public perceptions, public behavior, and public policy" (Stauber and Rampton 1995:208).

Each October brings the breast cancer public relations drive. During Breast Cancer Awareness Month (BCAM), the cancer establishment, hand in hand with the media, disseminate their breast cancer messages. The cancer establishment includes the interdependent political and economic entities of the major cancer research institutions, the pharmaceutical industry, government agencies, such as the NCI, and the cancer nonprofits, notably the ACS (Moss 1989). BCAM-distributed model proclamations are signed by government officials, announcing National Mammography Day. No mention is made of a possible connection between environmental toxins and breast cancer (Hightower 1997).

Breast Cancer Awareness Month was conceived and funded in 1985 by Imperial Chemical Industries (ICI), a British conglomerate that spawned Zeneca Pharmaceuticals in 1993. While its best-selling drug, tamoxifen, brings in approximately a half-billion dollars a year, Zeneca (which merged with Sweden-based Astra Pharmaceuticals to become AstraZeneca in 1999) also has sold pesticides and herbicides, some of which are thought to be carcinogens (Paulsen 1994). Now the principal corporate sponsor of BCAM, AstraZeneca retains authority to approve or disapprove all printed material used in BCAM (Paulsen 1993). The main message is "Early Detection is your best protection—get a mammogram now!" (Paulsen 1993:558; Proctor 1995:255). AstraZeneca also owns Salick Health Care, a managed care company that operates 11 cancer centers in the United States. Profits are made at each stage of the process: possible causes, therapies, and care providers. As ethicist Arthur Caplan has remarked, "Having your doctor, your clinic, your pharmacy, and your testing lab all owned by the same person is not the optimal structure for health care" ("Treatment Trouble: Zeneca Takes Over Salick Health Care" 1997:1).

WHAT IS TO BE DONE?

Corporate influence distorts our understanding of breast cancer, which can lead to decisions that are not in the best interests of women affected by the disease. The power of corporations continues to surge. The 1996 combined sales of the largest 200 U.S. corporations were greater than the combined gross national products of all except the largest nine nations of the world (Derber 1998). The growth of corporate profits is particularly great in the health sector. Between 1965 and 1990, "corporations found money in health services at a pace *almost 20 times greater* [emphasis added] than profits in general" (Andrews 1995:27). Wealth and political power are rapidly shifting from citizens to corporations that have limited accountability and massive global influence.

What are some solutions to this situation? Breast cancer advocacy groups have done well in raising women's awareness about treatment alternatives and requiring providers to alter some practices, such as unnecessary radical surgery. However, advocates must critically assess new breast cancer technologies and reassess the old, including who stands to gain or to lose from their adoption and widespread usage.

Individuals who seek to elicit responsible behavior from those who provide the technical expertise, products, and equipment used to detect and treat breast cancer have two main avenues of recourse within the current system: first, assuring the strength of regulatory agencies, particularly the FDA, that oversee the safety, efficacy, and quality of drugs, devices, products, and providers that women rely on to contain breast cancer; and second, maintaining the ability of the legal system to bring individuals and corporations to task when their improper behavior has resulted in unnecessary harm to those affected by breast cancer. Both of these avenues of recourse, regulation and litigation, have been under attack in the United States, most recently in the guise of FDA reform and tort reform (limiting product liability suits). Changes have been proposed and implemented that have strengthened the position of manufacturers and weakened consumer protection.

For truly effective change to take place, breast cancer must be viewed in a larger context. Reform and recompense is more easily realized than fundamental alteration of the distribution of wealth and power that will eventually be required to shape a health care system that works well for all citizens. (See chapters 3 and 6 of this volume.) Although meaningful change can be implemented at the personal and the institutional levels, the ways that the profit system dominates health care in the United States will require grander interventions for widespread benefit to the population. The health sector is generating phenomenal wealth for relatively few entrepreneurs at the expense of those who are patients in the health system and of many who provide direct services. As long as health care is fragmented by private health insurance, heavily bankrolled vested interests will continue to control the direction of research and the application of new knowledge.

The far-reaching agenda for breast cancer advocates is social change that will provide universal access to safe and effective health care and a system of governance that renews and protects the physical environment. Detection and treatment issues can be addressed more effectively in a health system that provides quality care, independent from market-driven greed. These are worthy goals for the breast cancer community.

NOTES

AUTHOR'S NOTE: Thanks go to Anne Kasper and Susan Ferguson, who assisted in the surgical strengthening of this chapter, and to Ellen Shaffer, who provided the introductory quote from *AdWeek*. Esther Rome, my friend and colleague and a cofounder of the Boston Women's Health Book Collective, would have loved to write this chapter with me. She died of breast cancer in June 1995.

REFERENCES

Andrews, Charles. 1995. *Profit Fever—The Drive to Corporatize Health Care and How to Stop It*. Monroe, Maine: Common Courage Press.

Angier, Natalie. 1994. "Vexing Pursuit of Breast Cancer Gene." *New York Times* (July 12) C1.

Arnot, Bob. 1998. *The Breast Cancer Prevention Diet—The Powerful Foods, Supplements and Drugs That Combat Breast Cancer.* Boston: Little, Brown.

Bailar, John C., III. 1976. "Mammography: A Contrary View." *Annals of Internal Medicine* 84:77-84.

Bailar, John C., III and Elaine M. Smith. 1986. "Progress Against Cancer?" *New England Journal of Medicine* 314:1226-32.

Berry, Donald A. 1998. "Benefits and Risks of Screening Mammography for Women in Their Forties: A Statistical Appraisal." *Journal of the National Cancer Institute* 90:1431-39.

Brenner, Barbara A. 1997. "The Government's Numbers Game." *Breast Cancer Action Newsletter* (December 1996/January 1997) 1.

———. 1997. "The Future Is Now." *Breast Cancer Action Newsletter* (Feb./March) 2, 9.

Brown, Jennifer. 1999. "Debunking Health Book Hype." *Self* (June) 84-85.

Brown, M. L., L. G. Kessler, and F. G. Rueter. 1990. "Is the Supply of Mammography Machines Outstripping Need and Demand?" *Annals of Internal Medicine* 113:547-52.

Butler, Declan, and Diane Gershon. 1994. "Breast Cancer Discovery Sparks New Debate on Patenting Human Genes." *Nature* 371:271-72.

"Cancer. It's a War." 1999. *New Yorker* (February 22 and March 1) 61.

Cairns, John. 1997. *Matters of Life and Death—Perspectives on Public Health, Molecular Biology, Cancer, and the Prospects for the Human Race.* Princeton: Princeton University Press.

Cimons, Marlene. 1998. "Breast Cancer Study Offers Hope but No Easy Answers." *Los Angeles Times* (April 7) A1.

Cunningham, George C. 1997. "A Public Health Perspective on the Control of Predictive Screening for Breast Cancer." *Health Matrix* 7:31-48.

Derber, Charles. 1998. *Corporate Nation.* New York: St. Martin's Press.

DiLorenzo, James T. and Thomas J. Bennett 1994. *Unhealthy Charities—Hazardous to Your Health and Wealth.* New York: Basic Books.

ECRI. 1996. "High-Dose Chemotherapy with Bone Marrow Transplant for Metastatic Breast Cancer—Patient Reference Guide." ECRI, Plymouth Meeting, Pa.

Eisen, Andrea, and Barbara L. Weber. 1999. "Prophylactic Mastectomy—The Price of Fear." *New England Journal of Medicine* 340:137-38.

Elmore, Joann G., Carolyn K. Wells, C. H. Lee, Deborah H. Howard, and Alvan R. Feinstein. 1994. "Variability in Radiologists' Interpretations of Mammograms." *New England Journal of Medicine* 331:1493-99.

Elmore, Joann G., Mary B. Barton, Victoria M. Moceri, Sarah Polk, Philip J. Arena, and Susan W. Fletcher. 1998. "Ten-Year Risk of False Positive Screening Mammograms and Clinical Breast Examinations." *New England Journal of Medicine* 338:1089-96.

Ernster, Virginia L. 1997. "Mammography Screening for Women Aged 40 through 49—A Guidelines Saga and a Clarion Call for Informed Decision Making." *American Journal of Public Health* 87:1103-5.

Ernster, Virginia L., John Barclay, Karla Kerlikowske, Deborah Grady, and I. Craig Henderson. 1996. "Incidence of and Treatment for Ductal Carcinoma In Situ of the Breast." *Journal of the American Medical Association* 275:913-18.

Fackelmann, K. A. 1993. "Weighing Risks, Benefits of Mammography." *Science News* (October 23) 262.

Feig, Stephen A. 1996. "Strategies for Improving Sensitivity of Screening Mammography for Women Aged 40 to 49 Years." *Journal of the American Medical Association* 276:73-74.

Fellers, Li. 1998. "Taxol Is One of the Best Cancer Drugs Ever Discovered by the Federal Government. Why Is It Beyond Some Patients' Reach?" *Washington Post* (March 31) W10.

Fugh-Berman, Adriane, and Samuel Epstein. 1992. "Tamoxifen: Disease Prevention or Disease Substitution?" *Lancet* 340:1143-45.

Garaghan, Helen. 1994. "NIH Files Counter-Patent in Breast Cancer Gene Dispute." *Nature* 372:118.

Gofman, John W. 1995. *Preventing Breast Cancer: The Story of a Major, Proven, Preventable Cause of this Disease.* San Francisco: Committee for Nuclear Responsibility.

Goldman, D. 1997. "Illness as Metaphor." *AdWeek* (November 3) 70.

Goldstein, Amy. 1999. "More Americans Lack Health Coverage." *San Francisco Chronicle* (October 4)A1.

Gordon, Nancy P., Thomas G. Rundall, and Laurence Parker. 1998. "Type of Health Care Coverage and the Likelihood of Being Screened for Cancer." *Medical Care* 36(5):636-45.

Greenberg, Daniel S. 1977. "X-Ray Mammography: Silent Treatment for a Troublesome Report." *New England Journal of Medicine* 296:1015-16.

Groopman, Jerome 1998. "A Healing Hell." *The New Yorker* (October 19) 34-39.

Hartmann, Lynn C., Daniel J. Schaid, John E. Woods, Thomas P. Crotty, Jeffrey L. Myers, P. G. Arnold, Paul M. Pety, Thomas A. Sellers, Joanne L. Johnson, Shannon K. McDonnell, Marlene H. Frost, and Robert B. Jenkins. 1999. "Efficacy of Bilateral Prophylactic Mastectomy in Women with a Family History of Breast Cancer." *New England Journal of Medicine* 340:77-84.

Hightower, Jim. 1997. *There's Nothing in the Middle of the Road but Yellow Stripes and Dead Armadillos.* New York: HarperCollins.

Høyer, Annette Pernille, Philippe Grandjean, Torben Jørgensen, John W. Brock, and Helle Bøggild Hartvig. 1998. "Organochlorine Exposure and Risk of Breast Cancer." *Lancet* 352:1816-20.

Hubbard, Ruth. 1995. *Profitable Promises.* Monroe, Maine: Common Courage Press.

Hunter, David J., Susan E. Hankinson, Francine Laden, Graham A. Colditz, JoAnn E. Manson, Walter C. Willett, Frank E. Speizer, and Mary S. Wolff. 1997. "Plasma Organochlorine Levels and Risk of Breast Cancer." *New England Journal of Medicine* 18:1253-58.

Jaggar, Sarah F. 1996. "Health Insurance: Coverage of Autologous Bone Marrow Transplant for Breast Cancer." General Accounting Office, Washington, D.C.

John, Lauren 1999. "High-priced Taxol Becoming First-line Breast Cancer Drug." *Breast Cancer Action Newsletter* (April/May) 1.

"Joy at Increase in Mammograms." 1997. *San Francisco Chronicle* (October 10) A4.

Kahn, Patricia. 1996. "Coming to Grips with Genes and Risk." *Science* 274:496-98.

Kealey, Maura. 1999. "Drug Industry Takes Aim at Medicare and Consumers." *Public Citizen News* (January/February) 5.

Kelly, Patricia T. 1996. "Cancer Risk Information Services: Promise and Pitfalls." *Breast Journal* 2:233-37.

Kelly, Susan E. and Barbara A. Koenig. 1998. "'Rescue' Technologies Following High-Dose Chemotherapy for Breast Cancer: How Social Context Shapes the Assessment of Innovative, Aggressive, and Lifesaving Medical Technologies." Pp. 126-51 in *Getting Doctors to Listen—Ethics and Outcomes Data in Context,* ed. P. J. Boyle. Washington, D.C.: Georgetown University Press.

Kerlikowske, Karla, Deborah Grady, John Barclay, Steven D. Frankel, Steven H. Ominsky, Edward A. Sickles, and Virginia Ernster. 1998. "Variability and Accuracy in Mammographic Interpretation Using the American College of Radiology Breast Imaging Reporting and Data System." *Journal of the National Cancer Institute* 90:1801-9.

Kerlikowske, Karla, Deborah Grady, J. Barclay, Edward A. Sickles, A. Eaton, and Virginia Ernster. 1993. "Positive Predictive Value of Screening Mammography by Age and Family History of Breast Cancer." *Journal of the American Medical Association* 270:2444-50.

Kerlikowske, Karla, Deborah Grady, John Barclay, Edward A. Sickles, and Virginia Ernster. 1996. "Effect of Age, Breast Density, and Family History on the Sensitivity of First Screening Mammography." *Journal of the American Medical Association* 276:33-38.

Krieger, Nancy, M. S. Wolff, R. A. Hiatt, M. Rivera, J. Vogelman, and N. Orentreich. 1994. "Breast Cancer and Serum Organochlorines: A Prospective Study Among White, Black, and Asian Women." *Journal of the National Cancer Institute* 86:589-99.

Kuester, Gerald F., and Sidney M. Wolfe. 1991. "Health Research Group Report on Screening Mammography." Public Citizen's Health Research Group, Washington, D.C.

Kushner, Rose. 1984. "Is Aggressive Adjuvant Chemotherapy the Halsted Radical of the '80s?" *CA—A Cancer Journal for Clinicians* 34:345-51.

Land, Charles, Masayoshi Tokunaga, Shoji Tokuoka, and Nori Nakamura. 1993. "Early-Onset Breast Cancer in A-Bomb Survivors." *Lancet* 342:237.

Landis, Sarah H., Taylor Murray, Sherry Bolden, and Phyllis A. Wingo. 1999. "Cancer Statistics, 1999." *CA—A Cancer Journal for Clinicians* 49:8-31.

Leopold, Ellen. 1998. "Not Every Picture Tells a Story." *Women's Community Cancer Project Newsletter* (Summer) 1-7.

Love, Susan M., and Karen Lindsey. 1995. *Dr. Susan Love's Breast Book.* New York: Addison-Wesley.

MacKenzie, Ian. 1965. "Breast Cancer Following Multiple Fluoroscopies." *British Journal of Cancer* 19:1-8.

Marsa, Linda. 1997. *Prescription for Profits.* New York: Charles Scribner.

Marshall, Eliot. 1995. "NIH Gets a Share of BRCA1 Patent." *Science* 267:1086.

Marwick, Charles. 1997. "NIH Consensus Panel Spurs Discontent." *Journal of the American Medical Association* 277:519-20.

McKinlay, John B. and Sonja M. McKinlay 1997. "Medical Measures and the Decline of Mortality." Pp. 10-23 in *The Sociology of Health and Illness—Critical Perspectives,* ed. P. Conrad. New York: St. Martin's Press.

McLelland, R. 1990. "Supply and Quality of Screening Mammography: A Radiologist's View." *Annals of Internal Medicine* 113:490-91.

Montague, Peter 1997. "Cancer Trends." *Rachel's Environment and Health Weekly* (July 12) 1-5.

Moss, Ralph W. 1989. *The Cancer Industry—Unraveling the Politics.* New York: Paragon House.

————. 1995. *Questioning Chemotherapy.* Brooklyn: Equinox Press.

"Most Women Who Had Breasts Removed Had Cancer, Study Says." 1977. *Los Angeles Times* (November 22) I:7.

Napoli, Maryann. 1994. "Misleading Ad Campaign by Mammography Clinics." *HealthFacts* (April) 3.

———. 1996. "Cancer Treatment: High Profits, Conflict of Interest, Little Efficacy." *HealthFacts* (April) 1,4-5.

———. 1999. "Breast Removal: The Latest in Cancer Prevention." *HealthFacts* (February) 1-2.

National Breast Cancer Coalition. 1999a. "15 Percent Increased Appropriations for Breast Cancer Research at the National Institutes of Health." Washington, D.C.

National Breast Cancer Coalition. 1999b. "$175 Million for the Department of Defense Peer-Reviewed Breast Cancer Research Program." In *Briefing Paper, Legislative Priority #1* Washington, D.C.

National Cancer Institute. 1998. "Genetic Testing for Breast Cancer Risk: It's Your Choice." Washington, D.C.

National Institutes of Health and American Society of Clinical Oncologists. 1999. "The Role of High-Dose Chemotherapy and Bone Marrow Transplant or Peripheral Stem-Cell Support in the Treatment of Breast Cancer." At www.asco.org.

Okie, Susan. 1998. "FDA Panel Endorses Breast Cancer Drugs." *Washington Post* (September 3) A3.

Pasquier, Frank and Sophia Ku. 1997. "Mammography Services—Impact of Federal Legislation on Quality, Access, and Health Outcomes." U.S. General Accounting Office, Washington, D.C.

Paulsen, Monte. 1993. *Nation* (November 15) 557-58.

———. 1994. "The Cancer Business." *Mother Jones* (May-June) 41.

Payer, Lynn. 1992. *Disease-Mongers—How Doctors, Drug Companies, and Insurers Are Making You Feel Sick.* New York: John Wiley.

Plotkin, David 1996. "Good News and Bad News About Breast Cancer." *Atlantic Monthly* (June) 53-82.

Proctor, Robert N. 1995. *Cancer Wars—How Politics Shape What We Know and Don't Know About Cancer.* New York: Basic Books.

Reynolds, Tom. 1998. "Tamoxifen Debate Hinges on Whose Risk is High Enough." *Journal of the National Cancer Institute* 90:1428-30.

Roush, Wade. 1997. "On the Biotech Pharm, A Race to Harvest New Cancer Cures." *Science* 278:1039-40.

Shapiro, Renee 1998. "The Link Between Organochlorines and Breast Cancer—A Response." *Women's Community Cancer Center Newsletter* (Winter) 1, 4-5.

Sickles, Edward A. and Daniel B. Kopans. 1993. "Deficiencies in the Analysis of Breast Cancer Screening Data." *Journal of the National Cancer Institute* 85:1621-24.

Skolnick, Andrew A. 1994. "Interim Federal Quality Standards for Nation's Mammography Facilities Acquire Force of Law." *Journal of the American Medical Association* 271:735-36.

———. 1995. "Leader in War on Cancer Looks Ahead." *Journal of the American Medical Association* 273:525-27.

Smigel, Kara. 1995. "Women Flock to ABMT for Breast Cancer Without Final Proof." *Journal of the National Cancer Institute* 87:952-55.

Sporn, Michael B. 1996. "The War on Cancer." *Lancet* 347:1377-81.

Stauber, John and Sheldon Rampton. 1995. *Toxic Sludge is Good for You!—Lies, Damn Lies and the Public Relations Industry.* Monroe, Maine: Common Courage Press.

Stein, Judith A., Sarah A. Fox, and Paul J. Murata. 1991. "The Influence of Ethnicity, Socioeconomic Status, and Psychological Barriers on Use of Mammography." *Journal of Health and Social Behavior* 32:101-13.

Steingraber, Sandra. 1997. *Living Downstream—An Ecologist Looks at Cancer and the Environment.* New York: Addison-Wesley.

Taubes, Gary. 1997. "The Breast-Screening Brawl." *Science* 275:1056-59.

"Treatment Trouble: Zeneca Takes Over Salick Health Care." 1997. *Breast Cancer Action News* (June/July) 1.

Thornton, Joe. 1992. "Breast Cancer and the Environment: The Chlorine Connection." Washington, D.C.: Greenpeace.

van Dam, Frits S. A. M., Sanne B. Schagen, Martin J. Muller, Willem Boogerd, Elsken v. d. Wall, Maria E. Droogleever Fortuyn, and Sjoerd Rodenhuis. 1998. "Impairment of Cognitive Function in Women Receiving Adjuvant Treatment for High-Risk Breast Cancer: High-Dose versus Standard-Dose Chemotherapy." *Journal of the National Cancer Institute* 90:210-18.

Weiss, Raymond B., Robert M. Rifkin, F. Marc Stewart, Richard L. Theriault, Lori A. Williams, Allen A. Herman, and Roy A. Beveridge. "High-Dose Chemotherapy for High-Risk Primary Breast Cancer: An On-Site Review of the Bezwoda Study." *Lancet* 355:999-1003.

Weiss, Rick. 1995. "How Goes the War on Cancer? Are Cases Going Up? Are Death Rates Going Down?" *Washington Post* (January 28) Z12.

Welch, H. Gilbert and Elliott S. Fisher. 1998. "Diagnostic Testing Following Screening Mammography in the Elderly." *Journal of the National Cancer Institute* 90:1389-92.

Wolff, M. S., P. G. Toniolo, E. W. Lee, L. M. Rivera, and N. Dubin. 1993. "Blood Levels of Organochlorine Residues and Risk of Breast Cancer." *Journal of the National Cancer Institute* 85:648-52.

"Women Misdiagnosed with Breast Cancer." 1983. *National Women's Health Network News* (January/February) 5.

Women's Experiences of Breast Cancer

Marcy E. Rosenbaum, Ph.D., and Gun M. Roos, Ph.D.

Women's experiences of breast cancer go beyond managing the physical issues of disease progression, treatment, and recovery. These experiences are inextricably woven with their social worlds. In confronting breast cancer, women must grapple with pervasive cultural meanings that surround this illness. For most women, there are a limited number of meanings from which to choose when trying to make sense of their encounters with breast cancer. The available models come to women through the media, social interactions, implicit cultural values, and individual experiences. Three areas of meaning consistently stand out in women's stories about breast cancer. These include perceptions of (1) breast cancer as equated with death or, alternatively, as manageable and survivable; (2) treatment for breast cancer as compromising to a woman's identity, femininity, and self-worth; and (3) breast cancer as an experience that should not be openly discussed. Most of these perception models bring with them implications that can compromise women's ability to maintain feelings of hope, self-worth, and the power to share their experiences in the context of breast cancer. While some women readily embrace these available models, many struggle with the incongruence between their personal experiences and societal expectations. In order to convey what it is like to be a woman with breast cancer, this chapter focuses on women's experiences of breast cancer and the influences that dominant cultural models have on that experience.

The first model relates to the meaning of cancer for a woman's life. In this realm, rather than one culturally prevailing model of meaning, women are confronted with two competing models of cancer. One model equates breast cancer with suffering and death. While treatments may temporarily alleviate or remove cancer from the body, having breast cancer means facing inevitable death (Balshem 1991; Matthews, Lannin, and Mitchell 1994). In contrast, the other major model focuses on breast cancer as treatable, manageable, and even curable. This model, often found in media accounts and biomedical approaches to breast cancer, emphasizes that one can overcome and survive breast cancer (Saillant 1990). Each model reflects the reality of breast cancer, in part. Many women survive breast cancer and even perceive it as just a temporary medical crisis. However, many women also die from breast cancer. Thus, part of the lived experience of breast cancer entails trying to reconcile these competing meanings. How women relate to breast cancer is not only influenced by perceptions of the disease process, but also strongly influenced by the implications of the current standards of treatment.

A second model of meaning suggests that one of the major aspects of the breast cancer crisis for women is treatment that involves surgical alteration or removal of the breast or breasts. In this context, women must grapple with the meaning of their breasts as defined through their experiences and society. For most women, the messages they have received throughout their lives are that women are defined by, and primarily valued for, their appearance, and that a woman's appearance is largely defined by her breasts. As Iris Young notes, "In the total scheme of objectification of women, breasts are the primary things." (1990:190). The values placed on breasts and their assumed link to femininity, sexuality, identity, and self-worth are consistently presented to women through the media, through social interactions, and through their experiences in the medical realm. Consequently, the surgical alteration or removal of the breast as part of treatment for breast cancer is viewed as significantly decreasing a woman's femininity, sexuality, and over-all self-esteem. Women facing treatment for breast cancer are forced to deal with these pervasive ideas regarding women and their bodies. Moreover, women often must face these concerns alone because societal values limit open expression of these issues.

A third perception model relates to the way, historically, the experience of breast cancer has been shrouded in silence and viewed as an intensely private matter. Discussing breast cancer outside of the medical realm has been considered taboo; women have been encouraged to hide their conditions with prostheses and recon-struction and to move on with their lives. This emphasis on silence reflects both the stigma of having a potentially fatal disease and of having an illness whose treatment involves the alteration of such a value-laden body part. Hence, women with breast cancer are confronted with the implicit societal rules that they should control where, how, and to whom they speak about their illness. Through the writings, speeches, and actions of breast cancer survivors and health care personnel in the past two decades attempts have been made to empower women to discuss their experiences more openly. Women facing breast cancer must negotiate between these compet-ing standards of appropriate communication.

BREAST CANCER IN THE LITERATURE

Up until the early 1970s, women wanting to know about breast cancer had little available information beyond what could be learned from health care practitioners and resource literature that focused primarily on the technical aspects of breast cancer.[1] Since 1970, there has been a burgeoning of research focusing on psycho-social aspects of the breast cancer experience. These works, primarily by psychologists and health care practitioners, focus on the emotional and attitudinal reactions of women to breast cancer and breast cancer treatment.[2]

These academic works have done much to further our understanding of some of the parameters of women's experiences of breast cancer. However, most of these studies have used quantitative measures of women's moods, attitudes, and coping behaviors and are thus limited in their ability to capture the depth and complexity of women's perceptions and experiences.[3] In general, by relying on numerical ratings, this type of research presents women with an already defined framework of meaning and measures how women fit within this framework. The concepts and categories that are considered salient by the researcher, rather than those of women with breast cancer, are measured. Hence, this research method often precludes the gathering of the patient's perspectives on the issues being examined.

In addition, this type of investigation fails to include women's voices in illuminating the breast cancer context. For women and others seeking to understand the experience, this quantitatively based literature is often unable to portray the personal context of living with breast cancer. Thus, in the early 1970s, what was missing from the available literature were accounts of women describing, in their own words, the lived experience of breast cancer.

PERSONAL NARRATIVES

In the mid 1970s, a few women set out to address the gaps in the literature regarding breast cancer. The desire to humanize and personalize the experience and explore the myriad of feelings that accompany breast cancer served as a catalyst for these women to write about their own encounters with breast cancer. They also sought to expose and often criticize the dominant cultural meanings surrounding breast cancer. In the first published personal narrative on breast cancer, *Breast Cancer: A Personal History and an Investigative Report*

(1975),[4] Rose Kushner, a journalist, candidly takes the reader through her experience from diagnosis to recovery and also provides information about breast cancer and treatment in nontechnical terms. Kushner recognizes that the experience of breast cancer is deeply embedded in social meaning. She is especially critical of the importance placed on breasts in the context of breast cancer and in the culture in general, and she is also critical of the male dominance of biomedicine and the silence that surrounds the illness.

Another pioneer, Audre Lorde, an African American lesbian poet, provides a much more radical criticism of the silence that surrounds breast cancer in *The Cancer Journals* (1980). In sharing her experiences with diagnosis and recovery, Lorde argues that the wearing of prostheses or having breast reconstruction disempowers women by hiding "survivors" of the breast cancer "war" from each other and from themselves (pp. 52-53). Lorde provides one of the most powerful indictments to date of the oppressive nature of societal views surrounding breast cancer. Her book is also one of the few published breast cancer biographies in the voice of a nonwhite, nonheterosexual woman.[5]

Following these pioneering works,[6] a number of women have told their own stories of breast cancer in published biographies. These stories, produced mainly by white middle-class writers, push beyond the earlier histories by examining more deeply both the internal processing of breast cancer in their lives and the social and political implications of breast cancer incidence and treatment.[7] While the early writings were produced by women with early stage cancer, many of the later biographies explore the range of experiences with advanced and metastatic breast cancer and with dying. Included in these works are the perspectives of partners, friends, and family members. These later writings, rather than overemphasizing courage and triumph over illness, delve deeply into the challenges women face in coping with breast cancer. Although they vary in perspective, all of these works echo one another in identifying salient issues that women struggle with in the face of breast cancer diagnosis and treatment. All either implicitly or explicitly address the dominant cultural constructions surrounding breast cancer.

OTHER VOICES

The narrative works on breast cancer cited thus far were produced primarily by women who were professional writers. However, the majority of women with breast cancer are not writers. This chapter introduces three women who have been diagnosed and treated for breast cancer. Their previously untold stories both echo and expand upon the groundwork laid by those women who published their own stories.

The three women's stories presented in this chapter were chosen out of the stories of 40 women who participated in a longitudinal research study examining women's adjustment to breast cancer (Rosenbaum 1994).[8] Women were recruited into the study through the department of surgery at a major southeastern university medical center. The women in the study ranged in age from 32 to 70 years old when they were first diagnosed with breast cancer.[9] Semistructured, open-ended interviews were conducted by the first author with each woman within a few weeks of diagnosis and then at approximately six weeks, three months, and six months following surgical treatment. Thirty of the women also participated in interviews four to five years after their initial diagnosis.

The following three stories reveal how women confront the meanings of breast cancer that exist in their social worlds. Most often, women must negotiate different meanings that arise in the context of cancer and weigh the cultural values and opinions expressed by others against their own experiences and perceptions. As the following stories demonstrate, women with breast cancer vary widely in the extent to which they accept or reject pervasive cultural models regarding cancer, breasts, and communication. The stories presented portray the range of responses to cultural meanings surrounding breast cancer that were expressed by the majority of participants in the study.

THE MEANING OF BREAST CANCER

Much of the literature on breast cancer acknowledges that cancer is equated with death in American culture. This notion, that death from cancer is inevitable, in part reflects the historical reality of breast cancer prior to development of better treatment approaches; it also reflects the ongoing reality that many women still die from breast cancer. However, this notion is pervasive even in the face of increasing numbers of breast cancer survivors. More recently, at least in biomedical and breast cancer support contexts, the discourse has shifted to emphasize that breast cancer is manageable and survivable. As Saillant (1990) points out, disseminating the notion that "we can beat cancer" has been an increasing focus of health care groups. Hence, women are faced with potentially contradictory cultural meanings of breast cancer: cancer as inevitably fatal versus cancer as controllable and curable. In the following excerpts we see how struggling with these competing meanings of cancer can be an ongoing part of living with breast cancer.

SARAH[10]

Sarah was 70 years old when she was diagnosed with breast cancer after finding a lump in her breast. She is African American and married; neither she nor her husband completed high school. At the time of her diagnosis, Sarah cleaned houses and also helped her husband clean hotels. They had no medical insurance other than Medicare. Sarah underwent a modified radical mastectomy and had chemotherapy. Sarah is a soft-spoken woman who believes in what she describes as Christian values and treating people with respect. She dresses in practical clothing and keeps a modest household with her husband and granddaughter. She watched her mother and one sister die from breast cancer. These deaths undoubtedly shaped the meaning of cancer for her.

In Sarah's case, she initially accepted the perception of a cancer diagnosis as being "handed a death sentence." Sarah recounts her feelings when she was told her diagnosis: "*. . . it just shocked me so. I mean all I could think of was dying. You know, 'I'm going to die. I've got cancer now.'*" Three months following her surgery, Sarah reflects on the impact breast cancer has had on her life: "*I can't exactly explain it except all my thinking is different . . . planning and the way I kept house, and the way I dressed. It's all different. I can't just get up and go on. It's like I'm waiting for this thing to come back.*" These feelings of despair and inertia stayed with Sarah for a long time through surgery, chemotherapy, and recovery. Six months after surgery, she tells of her struggles with the uncertainty of her future and fears of recurrence, especially in the context of being confronted with notions about cancer in the media and in her community. "*Worst of all is the waiting game . . . and thinking and wondering if it's gonna come back. And it seems like it's all you hear everywhere you go. You read about it, and you see it on TV. People say they think they are going to die with cancer. I don't know what kind of person you'd have to be, to be strong enough to say, 'Well, it won't happen to me.'*" She recounts a conversation with one family member that was often echoed in her social circles:

> [She] sat over there one day and said, "Nobody gets cured from no cancer. If you have cancer, you are gonna die anyway." She said, "It's gonna come back." And I said, "It may not." And she said, "Well, it always do. I don't know nobody get cured." And I said, "Well, there's a lot of people that has gone for years, and it didn't come back." I just said it that way and just went on. But I still thought about it.

Sarah finds it especially difficult to maintain hope around her family and friends who hold the model of cancer as incurable. Her comments demonstrate the extent to which Sarah is consistently confronted with the pervasive model equating cancer with death.

Sarah's narrative also reveals that the experience of breast cancer is not static but a process of gradually changing perspectives. In an interview four years after her diagnosis, Sarah reflects on this process.

> For a long time, I just kind of gave up and waited to die because I didn't know any better. I just worked and tried to forget it, and the doctor said that at chemotherapy they examined me and said "now as far as we know, you're free of cancer." I didn't believe it for a long time. I didn't get over it that quick, that easy. I just felt like it was the end of my life, and I could not pick it back up and get going. It took me two years and over to be sure that it was really gone. They [the doctors] convinced me that it really was gone.

Although Sarah came to embrace the model of cancer promoted by the medical community and believes that the cancer itself is gone, four years after diagnosis she notes that cancer is still a part of her mental life. "It's just there, and I can't get it out of my brain, and it's just something that I've just learned to live with. It's just like sometime you wished you could just put your brain under a faucet and just wash the kinks out because it's just sticking there."

Like Sarah, most participants in the study and most breast cancer biographers had initial reactions to a breast cancer diagnosis that focused on death. However, the persistence of this notion for Sarah is connected with the primary messages she receives in the world around her. Even though, increasingly, biomedical and activist information focuses on breast cancer management and becoming a survivor, for many women these messages are not pervasive. Sarah notes that in her immediate social world, and even in the media, she is consistently confronted with the concept that one does not survive breast cancer, that it always comes back. It appears that the stories of women dying from breast cancer are much more available in Sarah's world than stories of people surviving the disease. Believing in her survival thus requires explicit resistance to the messages Sarah receives from her surroundings. Other women in the study vary in the extent to which contemplating death is viewed as a major part of having breast cancer.

GLORIA

Gloria was 52 years old when she was diagnosed with breast cancer that was found through a routine mammogram. She is well educated, works in human services, and is politically active. She is European American, lower-middle class, widowed, and has two adolescent children. She had private health insurance through her work. Gloria had a modified radical mastectomy and underwent chemotherapy. She is an intense and dynamic woman of small stature who reflects deeply and critically on her life experiences. She is passionate about her human service and political work, which is personally fulfilling but has consistently made her struggle financially.

Like Sarah, Gloria reflects on being faced with the meaning of cancer when she received her initial diagnosis.

> There were two weeks in the beginning of all this I really felt like I was an ill person. I just was overwhelmed by the word "cancer." Cancer does mean "life threatening, death." And until the surgery is done . . . I think that fear of cancer also is kind of there. It's cancer, but I'm going to take this a step at a time. So I'm remembering and looking for all the stories about the women who had their surgery 25 years ago and ten years ago. And those are the stories I want to focus on. Of course, I've had fears of dying. But I'm not going to deal with it that way. I keep talking about getting well. But all around me I hear, once you have cancer you are never the same.

Similar to Sarah, Gloria is confronted with conflicting messages regarding the impact of cancer on her life. Gloria explicitly chooses to seek out women's experiences that do not fit with the cultural notion that equates breast cancer with death.

In comparison with Sarah, Gloria much more confidently sees the treatment for breast cancer as immediately and effectively controlling the cancer. Three months after surgery she says: *"I talk about, 'I had breast cancer,' because somehow in the surgery, the removal of the breast represents the taking of my cancer."* At six months after surgery, Gloria relates that the meaning of cancer changed significantly upon being diagnosed and treated for it: *"Cancer was a much more frightening term until it was said to me about me. It changes when you have it, the fear of this dreadful cancer. Or the feeling I would have had, 'What will happen if I have cancer?,' has really changed. I just adjusted those feelings to say, 'I've had cancer, but I'm still here, and it's okay.'"*

Gloria's perspective contrasts with the persistent fear Sarah reports having experienced. Gloria directly acknowledges the pervasive idea that cancer equals death and explicitly rejects it. Although this perspective is shared by many women in the study, most did not necessarily come to it as quickly as Gloria. Gloria's narrative, like Sarah's, raises the issue of the availability of different models of breast cancer. She is aware of these models in the lives of long-term survivors of breast cancer. As Gloria notes, she chooses to focus on these stories, however few, rather than those that reinforce the notion that cancer always leads to death. Thus, Gloria falls at the opposite end of the spectrum from Sarah, emphasizing survivorship and embracing the idea that one can live through cancer. However, as the next narrative demonstrates, not all women comfortably accept either of these models.

CLAIRE

Claire was 32 years old when first diagnosed with breast cancer. As a result of this first diagnosis, she had a lumpectomy and underwent chemotherapy. A year and a half later she was diagnosed with a recurrence. During both diagnoses, she was a graduate student at the local university, lived with roommates, and had a semisteady boyfriend. For treatment of her recurrence she underwent a modified radical mastectomy with immediate breast reconstruction. Claire is a tall slender European American woman with striking features, who accentuates her appearance with conscientious fashion choices. Claire has a sparkling sense of humor.

In an interview with Claire three months after her surgery for the recurrence, she talked about how the meaning of having breast cancer is different for her now than it was the first time she had breast cancer:

> The last time I almost didn't think that I had cancer. I had chemo for a year, but after it was over I didn't feel too different. It didn't really change me. It was just over. But this time, even though I am not having chemo, every day I look in the mirror and I can really tell the difference. When I thought I was finished with cancer and it came back, I had to deal with it right from square one . . . all over again.

Six months after surgery for the recurrence, Claire continues to compare her two experiences with breast cancer. She also reflects on how her emotions have changed since surgery. Her change in feelings is not just the result of the physical difference resulting from the more drastic surgery, but it also relates to the meaning of cancer in general.

> I have felt this bout of cancer much more deeply than I felt the other one. In a way, I think it has really changed me quite a bit. Before, it just washed right away. And this time there was the shock of having the cancer to deal with and then there was the shock of the changes in my body. I'm just very glad that the surgery worked. I'm beginning to feel like a whole person. I compare it to being raped, actually. You go through the process of trying to escape, trying to deny it. And then you say, "My God, I really have this. This is really happening to me."

And then there is a lot of depression. And you see a changed life. But being the optimist that I am, I think that it will continue to get better.

Claire expresses ambivalence about trying to believe that her cancer is gone and that it will not lead to death. This statement demonstrates that she is aware of both primary cultural models of breast cancer. However, for Claire, neither model sits comfortably, and her only way to reconcile them is to focus not on those external models but, rather, on her own experience. Thus, Claire is much more internally focused in making sense of breast cancer.

Each of these narratives demonstrates that women confront two models of cancer meaning in adjusting to diagnosis, treatment, and recovery, although the extent to which the women in the study embrace one model or the other appears to vary. In most instances, the equation of cancer with death is most salient at initial diagnosis and then over time is replaced, at least to a certain extent, with the model emphasizing the manageability of the illness. However, like Sarah, most women in the study and in breast cancer biographies note that awareness of the potential for recurrence never completely disappears from women's consciousness.

The three narratives also clarify the extent to which different models of cancer meaning influence women as they develop their own personal understandings of breast cancer. While some, like Gloria, were able to find examples of breast cancer survivors, for Sarah and several other women in the study, stories of women dying from breast cancer were the ones that dominated their social worlds. Available models for relating to breast cancer involve not only the meaning of the illness, but also the impact of treatment on women's lives.

THE MEANING OF BREASTS

Because the treatment for breast cancer involves surgical removal or alteration of breasts, women diagnosed with breast cancer often face the question, "what meaning do breasts have?" Prevailing cultural attitudes about breasts specifically, and women's bodies and feminine identity in general, provide the filter through which women relate to the impact of breast loss on their lives and feelings about themselves. As Susan Bordo (1993) notes, American culture emphasizes women's bodily appearance over other qualities as determinants of social acceptability and self-worth. As a consequence, women undergoing mastectomy are faced with socially pervasive ideas that they will be "less a woman," less feminine, not a "whole person," and somehow "damaged goods" as a result of breast cancer treatment.[11] The following narratives demonstrate the ways that women grapple with the cultural meanings surrounding breasts in the context of breast cancer.

SARAH, 70, AFRICAN AMERICAN

Prior to surgery, Sarah talks about the impact she thinks mastectomy will have on her life.

> *I am desperately afraid. And wondering how am I going to stand at the mirror and see myself in that shape. It really takes a lot from me. I'm just kind of a type that likes everything perfect, so it's going to make a big difference. I don't feel very feminine anyway. And I always thought my breasts were the only part about me that really looked [feminine] anyway at all. I probably would feel not feminine at all without them. It'll affect me, my femininity. I feel like it's been damaged.*

These statements reflect Sarah's concerns about having a body part removed and the resulting disfigurement. And, beyond this general conception, her concerns reflect her adopting the predominant model that links breasts with femininity.

Following surgery, Sarah talks about the impact of the surgery on her feelings about herself and how she is confronted with the meanings of breasts in her everyday life.

I didn't think for a 70-year-old woman I looked so bad and I just think
with your breast gone, you can't help feeling bad about it. I see people
on TV dancing and all that stuff and bosoms. I notice them all the
time now. Now that mine's gone, I don't feel like a "whole person."
And I feel like I'm always gonna be not exactly whole anymore.

Sarah expresses strong sentiments about the impact of mastectomy on her feelings about herself. These feelings are echoed by many women in the study. Because Sarah essentially embraces the dominant model, what results are feelings of less self-worth, loss of womanhood, and damage to her sense of herself as a whole person.

Sarah initially expressed interest in having immediate reconstruction but was discouraged from pursuing it by some breast cancer survivors with whom she talked. The message she received was that older women should not care about beauty and breasts.[12] As her narrative demonstrates, regardless of her age, these issues are important to her and missing a breast has had an impact on her.[13] Sarah's narrative demonstrates how pervasive ideas about feminine appearance can influence the way women relate to breast cancer surgery; the next narrative shows that not all women give priority to these concerns.

GLORIA, 52, EUROPEAN AMERICAN

Beyond the initial diagnosis, women diagnosed with breast cancer are usually confronted with the need to make treatment choices, particularly regarding the type of surgery they will undergo—lumpectomy, mastectomy, or mastectomy with immediate reconstruction.[14] In the context of trying to make these choices, Gloria reflects deeply on the meaning of breasts.

I think that I assumed that should I ever have a diagnosis of breast
cancer that I would just say "off with the breast, take it away." But
obviously it wasn't this clear because I had trouble making my

*decision about the form of treatment I would choose. I find that I'm
thinking more about the significance of breasts. They're part of my
body, and they've been with me for a pretty long time. I nursed both
of my children and was very comfortable with it. When involved in
a physical relationship, [they were] a source of arousal or satisfaction. And yet, I really feel I am interested in doing what I can to save
my life, to prolong my life, but within reason. I think mastectomy is
a reasonable choice. I don't feel I'll be any less a mother or any less
a woman.*

Gloria acknowledges pervasive messages that imply that her
womanhood will be tainted by mastectomy. Her last statement
indicates a direct and conscious rejection of these notions. It also
points to the challenge of balancing concern over appearance
with one's overall health. Anne Kasper (1995) has written
eloquently about the struggle women with breast cancer face
between preservation of physical appearance and preservation of
one's health and life. She argues that in the medical realm there
is often more emphasis given to fixing a woman's appearance
through reconstruction in spite of women's more pressing concerns related to ridding themselves of the cancer.

Gloria reiterates these sentiments during interviews following
her surgery and explicitly responds to popular notions that mastectomy compromises one's femininity:

*It's just my femininity, my womanhood, and my sense of self are not
embodied in my breasts. My femininity is my caring, my nurturing,
my warmth . . . It's an emotional kind of thing. I mean somebody with
small breasts, or very flat chested, is not less feminine because of that.
And I have always felt strongly about that.*

Gloria puts forward an alternative model of femininity that
emphasizes her interactions with others and her overall perspec-

tive on the world rather than limiting the definition of femininity to aspects of appearance.

Gloria recounts how being confronted with treatment choices in the medical system brings out more explicit expressions of the cultural values placed on breasts.

> *I wonder about the doctors who offered me choices and seemed kind of irritated that I didn't immediately jump at lumpectomy or, in the case of the plastic surgeon, reconstruction. But in both cases they were men, and I think it's their perception of the female and the female body. What I'm trying to say is, the loss of the breast has a significance, yet I maintain that some of these doctors who are talking about reconstruction are doing it in terms of their maleness and their images about women and tits, as opposed to great concern for a woman's emotional state.*

Gloria's criticism echoes the viewpoints of writers, such as Anne Kasper (1995), Rose Kushner (1975), and Audre Lorde (1980), with regard to the impact of male perspectives and sex role stereotypes on the context of breast cancer treatment choices. Gloria's narrative indicates that the prevailing model of breast meaning does not capture her experience and concerns. Again, we see that Gloria falls at the opposite end of the spectrum from Sarah as to how she relates to primary ideas about breast meaning. In contrast to Sarah, Gloria completely rejects these dominant notions. As a result, mastectomy appears to have had much less impact on Gloria's perception of herself. Like Lorde, Gloria states that mastectomy somehow made her feel "more whole" because it reinforced that her identity was not contained in or determined by her body. About one-quarter of the women in the study join Gloria in strongly rejecting the equation of breasts with femininity and self-worth; however, many find that rejection of these notions is a difficult task. The next narrative demonstrates the challenge that resisting these ideas presents.

CLAIRE, 32, EUROPEAN AMERICAN

Claire chose to have immediate reconstruction of her breast. Her statements during an interview prior to her surgery indicate her struggle with concerns about her breasts and self-image: *"I feel a certain determination to try to be as unaffected by it as possible. I'm afraid I might not succeed at that . . . I'm afraid that my one breast might mean more to me than I think it should. I'm afraid I might feel sorry for myself for a long time."* In her use of the word "should," Claire suggests an awareness of alternative ideas that de-emphasize the importance of breasts and appearance. She points to how difficult truly embracing these alternative ideas can be, and in this sense, she struggles with attempting to isolate her feelings and expectations from the culture and its influences. This reflects what Carole Spitzack (1990) identifies as the double bind in which many women find themselves. At the same time that women receive messages that they are valued primarily for their appearance, they also receive messages that attention to appearance is frivolous and vain. Claire's statements reveal this bind, indicating an awareness that she is valued for her appearance and breasts, but also that she should not care about these issues and that breast cancer should have little impact on her.

Claire also discusses how having cancer and surgery have affected her feelings about intimacy, which she links specifically with her femininity. Three months after surgery she says:

> In clothes I feel very good. But as a naked person, I definitely feel different from an unaltered state, a presurgery state. Even though I tell myself I shouldn't. In casual relationships my feminine sense of myself really hasn't changed. But, in intimate relationships it has changed. I feel kind of fragile. I could be hurt easily. I just feel more inhibited.

Like Sarah, Claire accepts a model of femininity that is defined by a woman's appearance, but she also echoes Gloria by indicating that femininity is more than just appearance. Claire defines femininity as both an emotional sense of herself and as related to her appearance. She defines femininity in relation to her internal thoughts and feelings while Gloria defines her femininity in terms of her social relationships with others.

Claire expressed little regret in having the reconstruction as part of her surgery. When asked if she would have felt different without the reconstruction she says:

> *Oh, yes. I think I would feel very inhibited about how I looked in clothes, bathing suits, sports activities, in bed. Just in every way. I'm afraid it's true, but I think that I identify too much with my breasts. I think it's normal for this culture, but I think it's too much. The culture is wrong. It's like you are more than your breasts, or more than your nose, or your whatever.*

Thus, even though Claire is aware of the limitations and oppressiveness of the societal equation of breasts with identity and self-worth, she finds it difficult to fully reject these notions in her own breast cancer experience.

In each of these women's narratives, the women respond to the dominant cultural model, which emphasizes the importance of breasts in defining a woman's identity, femininity, and self-worth. They differ in the extent to which they either embrace or challenge these meanings: Sarah seems to accept this meaning most fully, Gloria adamantly rejects it, and Claire tries to balance between the dominant and other models. Sarah is primarily aware of the dominant model that emphasizes the importance of breasts and appearance to self-worth. Many women in the study who lost a breast experienced some of these feelings of lack of wholeness and decreased femininity. However, as Gloria demonstrates, this response is not universal. Drawing on her own experience, but also on other women-centered notions of women's bodies and women's worth, Gloria argues that women do not have to accept that they are somehow less valued as women because they have lost a breast, but she admits that rejecting these notions can be a consistent challenge. While different models of breast meaning may be available to women, Claire's narrative strongly points to limitations of the women-centered perspectives in capturing her experience. For Claire and other women, just knowing that there are different, potentially less-oppressive ways to relate to breast loss does not necessarily make it easier to reject pervasive social notions. Rather, Claire gives the sense that she feels pressure from both sides to conform to a particular model of breast meaning.

BREAST CANCER AND SILENCE

Historically, society has discouraged open discussion of the breast cancer experience. In spite of the efforts of many who work in the health care field, particularly women's health advocates and breast cancer survivors, to bring the subject into the open, many women still experience a sense that their discussion of breast cancer should be constrained. In general, limited discussion about breast cancer can be attributed to two major issues. The first is the pervasive notion that cancer should not be publicly discussed. Susan Sontag (1977) points to the powerful metaphor that somehow in talking about cancer it could be transmitted or caused to develop in other people.[15] Talk about cancer also has been controlled because cancer itself is perceived as uncontrollable (Balshem 1991). This belief ties into notions that cancer is inevitably equated with death. The other primary obstacle to open discussion of breast cancer reflects the way talk about breasts is constrained in general. This control is paradoxical. On one level, breasts are viewed as inappropriate for discussion because they are perceived as sexual organs. However, the only socially acceptable way to talk about breasts has been in talking about them as sexual objects ("tits" as noted by Gloria). Expression of other breast meanings outside of their function as sexual objects is systematically muted (Rosenbaum 1994; Young

1990). In the following narratives, the three women react to social standards they perceive with regard to talking about their breast cancer experiences. They also identify additional issues that reinforce the silence surrounding breast cancer.

SARAH, 70, AFRICAN AMERICAN

Sarah consistently reports feeling that she gets very little social support from her family and friends in adjusting to breast cancer. Regarding her husband, she comments that they have never talked about it and that he has "never said nothing." She notes feeling self-conscious and embarrassed around others because of her mastectomy. She also witnesses a certain taboo in talking about breast cancer with others. *"I was really panicked for awhile. It was awfully hard because I was mostly alone. Nobody wanted to talk about it. If I said something about it to my people, they would say, 'Oh, why do you want to talk about it? Why don't you just don't think about it.'"*

Sarah speaks fondly of the local breast cancer support group that provided her with a place to talk about her experiences and to be understood.

> *I think that's really when I started getting strong, when I started going there and realizing that I wasn't by myself. If the rest of them can live through it, I ought to be able to live through it. It taught me that . . . I wasn't the only one that had cancer. You feel comfortable around those people because they all know what I'm going through, and I know what they're going through, where outside people just don't know. They just have no idea and they don't want to talk about it.*

For Sarah, the support group not only provides an acceptable context for her to speak about her feelings but also, by hearing other survivors' stories, makes her aware of different ways to approach her own experience. Having access through support groups to different women's stories regarding the lived experience of breast cancer reveals the wide range of ways women can respond to this crisis. Outside the support group, as Sarah indicates, the main messages she receives are that talk about breast cancer is not acceptable. Many women in the study, especially those who did not have access to formal support groups, echo Sarah in noting that they had no one with whom to discuss their feelings and experiences.

GLORIA, 52, EUROPEAN AMERICAN

Through her actions, Gloria explicitly responds to and rejects notions that talking about breast cancer is taboo.

> I'm very open in talking about my experience. I'm not ashamed about it. I say, "I had breast cancer." Because I think that is really okay, to use the word breast, and to say breast cancer. I really feel, if I can talk about it openly, I can help somebody else should they ever face this in the future. And I've had several experiences now where because I've come out about my breast cancer, somebody else will acknowledge that they've had surgery but felt uncomfortable talking about it. I just think it's something we need to talk about.

Gloria also talked about the reactions of some individuals when she would discuss her feelings about the breast cancer. As an example, she recounts that a colleague at work criticized her for talking about her cancer too much and not "getting over it" quickly enough.

> I mean if I express my frustrations and I express my fears, does that mean then that you say to yourself, "Oh, God, this woman is out of control." It's not an indication to me [that I'm not coping], but I am fearful that it might be to someone else. I think the fact that I can express those concerns is an indication that I am coping, dealing.

In these statements, Gloria rejects two predominant beliefs that encourage women to stay quiet about breast cancer. She acknowledges that women receive the message that they should be ashamed of having breast cancer, both because of cancer, but even more because it involves breasts. In Gloria's view, talking about breast cancer provides the opportunity to help other women, and it also empowers other women to share their breast cancer stories. Hence, Gloria identifies open expression as an important part of making sense of the lived experience of breast cancer. This notion is Gloria's rejection of cultural standards of coping behavior that include not discussing the experience, and where women are perceived as failing to effectively manage their emotions if they talk about their breast cancer experiences.

CLAIRE, 32, EUROPEAN AMERICAN

Claire also reflects on the implications of the extent to which one talks about the breast cancer experience. *"I think that I am able to talk to some people. I get some relief from talking to people. It's about all I can talk about. Which is another sign to me that I am not coping too well."* Like Gloria, Claire is aware of the standard of coping that emphasizes not talking openly about the illness but, in contrast to Gloria, Claire more readily adopts this standard rather than rejecting it. Although she finds talking about breast cancer helpful, she is self-conscious about what this action indicates in terms of managing her feelings. Claire also talks about feeling constrained in other ways.

> *I'm not too able to talk to my family. They will ask me questions. My feeling is they want to hear the good side of the story. What do you call it? "The bright side." And I'm encouraged to keep my chin up. And one of my family members thinks or acts like the whole thing is not really serious. They don't want to feel [the things I'm feeling]. I*

think they are terrified of feeling it. And I'm wondering . . . what I
am going to do about that. If I'm going to feel compelled to support
them in their illusions, or if I'm going to feel like I want to talk to
them about it. I feel like I have to protect them. Or help them protect
themselves is really what it comes to.

Claire perceives that talk about breast cancer needs to be controlled in order to spare others the emotional distress of sharing the experience. Many women in the study express a desire to not burden their loved ones with their true feelings about how difficult it is to have breast cancer and to undergo treatment.[16]

The three women varied in the extent to which they refrained from talking about breast cancer because of expectations in their social worlds. For Sarah, the only acceptable place to discuss cancer was with other breast cancer survivors. Gloria believed that speaking openly about breast cancer benefited both herself and other women. She did this consciously and in direct opposition to social expectations to keep silent, in part because of her social and political consciousness. Claire's choice of when and when not to discuss breast cancer was much more personal than political. She considered her talk about breast cancer in the context of personal relationships and coping. In sum, all of these narratives reveal that the burden of having breast cancer can extend beyond issues of mortality and treatment to being challenged with pervasive social notions regarding when and how to talk about breast cancer.

CONCLUSION

The three women presented in this chapter all started their breast cancer journeys in different locations with regard to dominant models of breast cancer meaning. Sarah most clearly represents women who embrace the equation of cancer with death, breasts with femininity and self-worth, and breast cancer as a taboo topic. Her narrative demonstrates how these meanings and conceptions change over time, especially with support and influence from other breast cancer survivors. In contrast, Gloria began as consciously critical of prevailing cultural meanings and brought this criticism into play as she lived with breast cancer. Her conceptions and feelings about herself changed little through the experience of breast cancer—rather, she continued to apply her critical consciousness to the issues surrounding the experience. It thus provided a basis for her to question and speak out against social beliefs surrounding women's bodies and women's discourse both inside and outside the breast cancer context. Claire's narrative shows a woman struggling between embracing or rejecting dominant conceptions of cancer, breast meaning, and communication. While she is aware of more critical perspectives and pressures to reject preeminent models, she finds it difficult to completely disregard these societal values and meanings. Threaded through her narrative is the ambivalence she feels in facing these competing models.

These three women's stories raise two important issues. First and most important, regardless of individual experiences, part of the breast cancer experience entails facing persistent cultural meanings related to cancer, breasts, and appropriate communication. Breast cancer is not just a personal process but rather an experience filtered through the meanings constructed by the social context. For some, these meanings can limit the range of choices women feel they have in responding to and coping with breast cancer. For others, rejection of these meanings provides the basis for defining women-centered and less-oppressive ways of relating to the breast cancer crisis.

The second issue illuminated in the exploration of these women's stories is that each woman's experience of breast cancer can indeed be unique. Not all women experience breast cancer as ultimately fatal or as compromising to their identity and femininity. Conversely, neither do all women find themselves able to comfortably reject these prevalent notions by embracing other models of breast cancer meaning. Rather, each woman weighs these dominant meanings against her personal and social experiences of breast cancer. Many find that the available models do not adequately capture their own feelings and experiences. However, the pervasive nature of these social models serves to mute expression of the myriad ways women can and do respond to breast cancer.

The more we learn about women's personal experiences with breast cancer the clearer it becomes that we need models that reflect the diversity of women's experiences and address breast cancer from different ethnic, socioeconomic, cultural, and sexual orientations. We need models that value women for more than just their bodies. We need models that empower women to talk openly and critically about breast cancer and the meanings that surround the illness. Only when more individuals, including those from underrepresented groups,[17] begin to talk about and question the meanings of breast cancer, will the available models through which women make sense of their experiences be expanded.

EPILOGUE

During our last official interview, six months following her surgery, Claire talked with some ambivalence about the meaning of the breast cancer experience:

> How do I describe this experience? In some ways, like any tragedy . . . it's had some good points like bringing me closer to my dad. [However], the good that came wasn't worth the price. So, it has really been an awful thing in my life. I guess in my coping I try to see the good and the bad. But this has been really bad. I don't care that I learned that beauty isn't important. So I was shown that lesson. And it is true that beauty isn't important. But I would rather not have learned that lesson and not have my body mutilated, my health threatened. Some of the cares of the world have left me. I've lost some of the carefreeness of youth, I feel older. There's some regret. There's also a lot of peace. Bittersweet.

Claire lived for two years after this last interview. She got married and continued school for a while. She then had metastases to her bones and brain, went through radiation, chemotherapy, and a bone marrow transplant. She died quietly surrounded by her family and friends.

NOTES

AUTHORS' NOTE: We are grateful to "Claire," "Gloria," "Sarah," and the rest of the participants in the study for sharing their stories and lives with us. We also thank Dan Jaffee, Andrea Spagat, Jonathan Haas, John F. Wilson, Eileen Scherl, Louise Rosenbaum, and Irene Rosenbaum for their editorial support.

1. For exceptions see Fosket, Chapter 10, in this volume.
2. Examples of review articles of psychosocial literature include: Glanz and Lerman 1992; Meyerowitz 1980; and Wainstock 1991.
3. For examples of critiques of these type of methods see Kasper 1994; Waxler-Morrison, Doll, and Hislop 1995.
4. It is interesting to note that the book's publishers insisted that Kushner change the title of the book to *Why Me: What Every Woman Should Know About Breast Cancer to Save Her Life* for its second printing in 1977 so women would not be afraid or embarrassed to be seen reading it.
5. Works featuring perspectives of nonwhite or nonheterosexual women include Matthews, Lannin, and Mitchell 1994; and Butler and Rosenblum 1991.
6. These early works also include biographies by Rollin 1976 and Metzger 1983.
7. Examples of these later works include: Mayer 1993; Middlebrook 1996; Butler and Rosenblum 1991; Wadler 1992; and Wittman 1993.
8. This research was funded in part by the Elsa Pardee Foundation. Investigators included John F. Wilson, Eileen Scherl, and Marcy E. Rosenbaum.
9. Three of the women were African American, 36 were European American, and one was born in Asia but raised in the United States. Twenty-five percent of the women had Medicaid benefits and the remainder had private insurance or Medicare as their primary insurance. Sixty-five percent of the women were married. Twenty-five percent had not completed high school, 25 percent had completed high school, and the remaining had at least some college. All of the women in the study were diagnosed with an early form, Stage I, of breast cancer. Sixty-five percent of the women chose mastectomy with immediate reconstruction and 35 percent chose mastectomy alone. Twenty-five percent of the participants received postoperative chemotherapy.
10. The women's names used in this paper are pseudonyms. Narrative quotes have been lightly edited to remove grammatical lapses and extraneous content information; however, the direct meaning of each narrative has been preserved in the quotes presented. Parentheses indicate the context or

subject the woman is talking about when not made explicit within the sentence.

11. Many authors identify and are critical of these pervasive notions about the impact of mastectomy including: Kahane 1990; Kasper 1995; Kushner 1975; Lorde 1980; Meyerowitz 1980.

12. Sarah recounted a conversation she had with a woman from a local breast cancer support group about reconstruction, ". . . *another lady called me [and] said that if it was left to her she wouldn't have one. She said, "How old is your husband?" And I said, "Seventy-four." And she said, "Well, how old are you?" And I told her. And she said, "Well if I were you I wouldn't worry about it at that age." And I said, "Well, I just don't want to be lookin' at myself without one, it don't make no difference how old I am "*

13. Dr. Susan Love mentions being appalled at instances where surgeons tell elderly patients "you don't need your breasts anymore " (1990:243).

14. Not all women are offered this range of treatment choices. Whether choices are offered depends on both medical issues, e.g., stage and specific site of cancer, as well as on socioeconomic and geographic issues. In the current study, all participants were offered the choice of immediate reconstruction.

15. It is also worth noting that, historically, women have been discouraged from discussing cancer openly because they risked being discriminated against in employment situations.

16. Many women identified the research interview as an important opportunity to talk about things they could not share with loved ones for fear of causing them worry and distress.

17. "Underrepresented groups" in this context refers to, for example, women of color and poor women who have had little or no voice in the construction of dominant models of breast cancer experience.

REFERENCES

Balshem, Martha. 1991. "Cancer, Control and Causality: Talking About Cancer in a Working-Class Community." *American Ethnologist* 18:152-72.

Bordo, Susan. 1993. *Unbearable Weight: Feminism, Western Culture, and the Body.* Berkeley: University of California Press.

Butler, Sandra, and Barbara Rosenblum. 1991. *Cancer in Two Voices.* San Francisco: Spinsters.

Glanz, Karen, and Caryn Lerman. 1991. "Psychosocial Impact of Breast Cancer: A Critical Review." *Annals of Behavioral Medicine* 14:204-12.

Kahane, Deborah. 1990. *No Less A Woman: Ten Women Shatter the Myths about Breast Cancer.* New York: Prentice Hall.

Kasper, Anne S. 1994. "A Feminist, Qualitative Methodology: A Study of Women with Breast Cancer. *Qualitative Sociology* 17:263-81.

————. 1995. "The Social Construction of Breast Loss and Reconstruction." *Women's Health: Research on Gender, Behavior, and Policy* 1:197-219.

Kushner, Rose. 1975. *Breast Cancer: A Personal History and an Investigative Report.* New York: Harcourt Brace Jovanovich.

————. 1977. *Why Me? What Every Woman Should Know About Breast Cancer to Save Her Life.* New York: New American Library.

Lorde, Audre. 1980. *The Cancer Journals.* London: Sheba Feminist Publishers.

Love, Susan. 1990. *Dr. Susan Love's Breast Book.* Reading, Mass.: Addison-Wesley.

Matthews, Holly F., Donald R. Lannin, and James P. Mitchell. 1994. "Coming to Terms with Advanced Breast Cancer: Black Women's Narratives from Eastern North Carolina." *Social Science and Medicine* 38:789-800.

Mayer, Musa. 1993. *Examining Myself.* Boston: Faber & Faber.

Metzger, Deena. 1983. *Women Who Slept with Men to Take the War Out of Them and Tree.* Berkeley: Wingbow Press.

Meyerowitz, Beth E. 1980. "Psychosocial Correlates of Breast Cancer and Its Treatments." *Psychological Bulletin* 87:108-31.

———. 1981. "The Impact of Mastectomy on the Lives of Women." *Professional Psychology* 12:118-27.

Middlebrook, Christina. 1996. *Seeing the Crab: A Memoir of Dying.* New York: Basic Books.

Rollin, Betty. 1976. *First You Cry.* New York: J. B. Lippincott.

Rosenbaum, Marcy. 1994. "Cultural Analysis of Women, Breast Cancer Surgery and the Meaning of Breasts." Ph.D. dissertation, Department of Anthropology, University of Kentucky, Lexington.

Saillant, Francine. 1990. "Discourse, Knowledge and Experience of Cancer: A Life Story." *Culture, Medicine and Psychiatry* 14:81-104.

Sontag, Susan. 1977. *Illness as Metaphor.* New York: Farrar, Strauss and Giroux.

Spitzack, Carole. 1990. *Confessing Excess: Women and the Politics of Body Reduction.* Albany: State University of New York Press.

Wadler, Joyce. 1992. *My Breast: One Woman's Cancer Story.* Reading, Mass.: Addison-Wesley.

Wainstock, J. M. 1991. "Breast Cancer: Psychosocial Consequences for the Patient." *Seminars in Oncology Nursing* 7:207-15.

Waxler-Morrison, Nancy, Richard Doll, and T. Gregory Hislop. 1995. "The Use of Qualitative Methods to Strengthen Psychosocial Research on Cancer." *Journal of Psychosocial Oncology* 13:177-91.

Wittman, Juliet. 1993. *Breast Cancer Journal: A Century of Petals.* Golden, Colo.: Fulcrum.

Young, Iris M. 1990. *Throwing Like a Girl and Other Essays in Feminist Philosophy and Social Theory.* Bloomington: Indiana University Press.

Barriers and Burdens:
Poor Women Face Breast Cancer

Anne S. Kasper, Ph.D.

Little is known about breast cancer among economically disadvantaged women, except for two generally accepted facts: Low income women are more likely to be diagnosed with a later stage of the disease and to have higher mortality rates. In the United States, assumptions run high that the lack of health insurance among the poor may explain these two dismal facts. Being uninsured may preclude access to health services, thereby creating delays or even the absence of screening, diagnostic, and treatment services. This lack of access, in turn, may account for women diagnosed when the cancer is more advanced, reducing the women's chances of survival.

A study I conducted of urban poor women with breast cancer demonstrates that being uninsured is but one factor that explains more advanced disease and lowered survival. The multiple and persistent features of poverty that precede and follow the women's breast cancer diagnosis and treatment are of greater consequence than whether or not they are insured. Women who are poor and diagnosed with breast cancer face barriers and burdens not encountered by women who are not poor. Furthermore, these difficulties determine if and when the women are treated, whether or not they receive optimal or even appropriate treatment, the quality of the health services they receive, and how they manage their lives during the breast cancer crisis. In sum, the barriers and burdens of poverty shape these women's experiences of breast cancer.

This chapter explores what it means to be poor and have breast cancer from the vantage point of 24 women who spoke at length with me in narrative interviews. Excerpts of their own words, their breast cancer experiences, and descriptions of their life circumstances illustrate how poverty shapes both their lives and their breast cancer experiences.

THE SOCIAL CONTEXT

To better understand the larger social context in which the 24 study participants live, a few social factors relevant to their status as poor and underserved women are briefly reviewed. These features of society may affect us all to some degree, but they have far greater salience in the lives of economically disadvantaged women with breast cancer.

HEALTH INSURANCE

In 1998, 43 million Americans or more than 16 percent of the population had no health insurance—the highest proportion in a decade (U.S. Bureau of the Census 1998). The simple fact is that the majority of the uninsured lack coverage because it is too costly for them. More than half of uninsured adults delay getting care because of cost, and the fear of debt is why many report not getting the care they need (Henry J. Kaiser Family Foundation 1998). For the majority of those who are insured, health insurance is obtained through the workplace. However, most low-paying service sector and small business jobs, where women frequently work, do not offer health insurance to their employees. The growth of this sector of the economy in recent years explains, in part, the increase in the uninsured.

Women are more likely to have health care coverage than men, but they rely on public programs, such as Medicaid and Medicare, rather than on employment-provided coverage (Reisinger 1996). According to a national survey, more than 30 percent of Latinas, 22 percent of black women, and 13 percent of white women are not insured (Vistnes and Monheit 1998). Moreover, less than 40 percent of women with Medicaid or uninsured women reported having a mammogram in the past year as compared to 67 percent of women with workplace-provided insurance (Reisinger 1996).

A study of women with breast cancer and the link between their insurance status and health outcomes showed that uninsured women and those with Medicaid were diagnosed with more advanced disease than privately insured women. Survival rates were far worse for the uninsured women and those with Medicaid (Ayanian et al. 1993). Reviewing the study, Jean Hardisty and Ellen Leopold argue in *Cancer and Poverty: Double Jeopardy for Women* that women with Medicaid fared no better than their uninsured counterparts despite having medical coverage. Hardisty and Leopold state, "In other words, the provision of a safety net in the form of guaranteed payment could not, on its own, overcome the more pervasive and persistent consequences of economic disadvantage on the course of disease" (1996:220-21).

Lack of health insurance is but one of several reasons why economically disadvantaged individuals and their families do not receive needed health care services.

UNMET NEEDS AND UNCOMPENSATED CARE

In 1994-1995, one-third of poor people reported an unmet need for health care as compared with 7 percent of high income people. Poor women with health problems were almost three times as likely not to have seen a doctor as high income women (U.S. Department of

Health and Human Services [HHS] 1998). Increased competition and cost containment in the health care marketplace have eroded the ability of traditional safety-net providers to pay for the uncompensated health care of those without insurance who cannot pay out of their own pockets. An example of safety-net providers in many communities are clinics offering low-cost mammograms.

The number of individuals without a usual place to go for health care has increased in recent years, with ten million more in these circumstances in 1992 than in 1987. This is a far larger change than the increase in the uninsured during the same time period (Agency for Health Care Policy and Research 1998). Without a place to go when health care is needed, many individuals resort to emergency rooms, when they should be seen by a primary care provider whose role is to evaluate nonemergency health conditions. The use of expensive sources of care, such as emergency rooms, instead of lower-cost primary care providers leads to health care cost increases, further curtailing the ability of all of these institutions to provide uncompensated care.

In 1988, Ruth Zambrana wrote, "The major issue for poor and racial/ethnic populations, especially the women, is access and availability of services." She argued at that time that medical care cost containment, the loss of funding for public health facilities, and reduced services all affect the underserved and that "the preeminent need is to lower the barriers that continue to limit access of the poor and racial/ethnic populations to essential human services" (pp. 155-56). These circumstances are all the more true today.

POVERTY

Poverty and its effects on the lives of people is not much discussed in the United States, the richest and most powerful nation in the world. Yet poverty has enormous and varied negative consequences on health and well-being. Over a third of the U.S. population lives in or near poverty (HHS 1998). More than 30 percent of female-headed households live below the poverty line. Twenty-seven percent of white, 44 percent of African American, and more than 50 percent of Latina headed households live below the poverty line (Rawlings 1998). In recent years, poverty has increased for those who are already poor, despite strong national economic growth and low unemployment, in part because of the loss of public assistance programs such as Aid to Families with Dependent Children (AFDC). Additionally, remaining social programs are paying out less to individuals and families entitled to benefits today than in the past because of reduced social service budgets (Center on Budget and Policy Priorities 1998).

Hardisty and Leopold, in their work on women, cancer, and poverty, state that poverty and related factors, such as cultural barriers, limited education, as well as job and income insecurity, make poverty a "powerful predictor of late diagnosis, poor treatment, and high mortality" for breast cancer (1996:1). Economic discrimination coupled with racial and ethnic discrimination limit the financial and emotional resources that women diagnosed with breast cancer may call upon to be assured of diagnostic and treatment services when they need them.

INCOME INEQUALITY

Poverty has been exacerbated in recent years by the growth of national income inequality. Income inequality is the difference between those individuals who are economically privileged and those who are poor or with low incomes. Income inequality continues to increase in the United States and is currently at an all time high (Center on Budget and Policy Priorities 1998). Adults with low incomes are more likely to be sick than those with higher incomes. They also are less able to afford out-of-pocket health costs but more likely to incur these costs than high income people. Out-of-pocket costs are a known barrier to the use of timely and appropriate health services (HHS 1998).

Income inequality has a myriad of consequences. For example, income inequality is associated with low levels of social capital (mutual trust and cooperation in neighborhoods and communities), which in turn has been shown to increase mortality (Kawachi et al. 1997). There has been a general decline in civic trust in the last thirty years, leaving people to fend for themselves and, as a result, they report declines in personal health (Kawachi 1999). Moreover, income inequality and poverty intersect in ways that affect health. Individuals who are socially isolated and living alone have higher poverty rates today than in the past (Center on Budget and Policy Priorities 1998). They also are more likely to live in socially disrupted neighborhoods with inadequate housing and other lower standards of public health, increasing the likelihood of ill health and fewer resources to cope with it.

For example, a review of 42 studies on social class differences in cancer survival showed that patients in low social classes had poorer survival rates than those in high social classes. Breast cancer was one of the cancers in which the differential was greatest (Kogevinas and Porta 1997). Moreover, social class can exert an influence on survival regardless of access to health care, as reported in a Finnish study where women in the lowest social class had a risk of death from breast cancer that was 1.3 times greater than women in the highest social class. Since Finland has universal health care, access was not a factor (Karjalainen and Pukkala 1990). The Finnish study demonstrates that even when an entire population has equal access to health care services, lower social class still results in poorer health outcomes.

THE WOMEN

Twenty-four women with breast cancer were participants in a study funded by the U.S. Agency for Health Care Policy Research and conducted in two cities, Washington, D.C., and Chicago, Illinois.[1] All the women were poor or low income as defined by federal poverty thresholds (U.S. Bureau of the Census 1999). Eighteen of the women lived on annual incomes of their own of $8,000 or less. Participants included ten black women, eight Latinas, and six white women. Their ages ranged from 39 to 73 with the median age at 51 years. Although they were seriously economically disadvantaged, the majority were surprisingly well educated, demonstrating a wide gap between educational attainment and earning power. Fifteen women held a high school diploma or higher, including two women with master's degrees and three with bachelor's degrees.

Eleven of the 24 women were employed, while five were unemployed, five retired, and three were homemakers. In addition to working as homemakers, the women worked variously as waitresses, housekeepers, stock clerks, legal secretary, cook, nanny, professor, billing clerk, factory worker, educator, and receptionist. Despite their low incomes, only half of the women received some form of public assistance or social insurance, such as Medicaid, Medicare, medical assistance, state or local aid for hospitalization, welfare, food stamps, housing support, Social Security, Supplemental Security Income (SSI), public aid, and unemployment compensation. The recent dissolution of welfare does not explain the surprising lack of public assistance for many of these women as they were diagnosed with breast cancer and treated prior to welfare's cutbacks.

Perhaps even more startling, 11 of the 24 women had no health insurance of any kind, public or private. Only three of the 24 women had health insurance through their jobs. Four women were Medicaid eligible, four Medicare eligible, and one woman was eligible for both. Despite their low incomes, their relatively high levels of education, and full-time employment, the women were inadequately insured for primary and preventive health care, much less for costly cancer care. And, unlike middle- or upper-class women, they were frequently unable to fall back on their own incomes, if necessary, to pay for health services they needed. All the women, save one whose job-based insurance paid for all her care, were obliged to find alternate means or piece together ways to be treated and pay for breast cancer care. Strikingly, one woman was untreated, for reasons related to poverty, lack of access to care, and the failure of health and social service providers to attend to her circumstances. The next section will look at the difficulties this woman and many of the other women in the study faced as they attempted to find breast cancer services.

BARRIERS TO CARE

WHO PAYS?

Of the three women insured through their jobs, only one had breast cancer treatment paid for in full and without difficulty. A second woman, Jean,[2] a single mother of two dependent children, had health insurance that left her with $3,800 in medical bills to pay out of her annual income of $19,000. The third woman, Maria, was told by her insurer that she had a preexisting condition even though she had never been previously diagnosed with breast cancer nor had she ever made a claim on the policy. The insurance company sent her account to a collection agency, and she continues to get bills from them, which she tries to pay in small monthly installments.

Two women, Estela and Josefina, were insured through their husbands' work but their coverage lapsed when their husbands lost their jobs, interrupting continuing care and affecting their health outcomes. Several other women with private insurance had supplemental insurance policies on which they were unable to make any successful claims for their cancer treatments when their main insurance policies did not cover their costs. These women never received adequate explanations for these refusals. These accounts illustrate the tenuousness of insurance for those women who are insured.

For two uninsured women, state medical assistance paid for some of their care. One of the women, Gloria, was advised by a social worker to lie about her income in order to qualify and receive treatment. When she forgot to lie again when renewing the assistance, she was cut off and had to pay for continuing care out of her own pocket. Another woman, Lorraine, received temporary state hospitalization that paid her in-hospital costs but left her with $10,000 to $13,000 in bills to pay herself. She sold her life insurance policy and depleted her savings to pay immediate medical costs, including a $2,000 down payment before she was permitted to have surgery for the breast cancer. She also asked her physicians to accept payment plans, and several did so. She borrows from her mother to pay her doctors. For these two women, medical assistance programs were insufficient to compensate for their being uninsured and left them with medical costs neither woman had the resources to absorb.

Although the women in the study were strapped financially, ten women were obliged to pay some or all of their care out of their own pockets, ranging from several hundred to many thousands of dollars. Susana is attempting to pay all but $2,000 of her $34,000 in treatment costs on monthly installments of $475 out of the family income of $24,000. Although she teaches at the college level, she has no insurance and was at one time denied coverage because she is mildly overweight. During our interview she said, *"I think that as a human being you have the right for some basic needs if you work and you are honest. When I need help, it is denied.* After five months of going here and there saying *"'please listen, please can I speak with someone, please!,'"* the only help Susana was able to find was $2,000 from a cancer organization. Susana's plight, as well as Gloria's and Lorraine's, illustrate what we know about low-income individuals: They are less able to afford out-of-pocket health costs, but more likely to incur them than those with high incomes.

Similarly, Victorine was treated under Medicare, but Medicare refused to pay in full for her radiation treatments, leaving her with a $1,200 bill she could not afford to pay out of her lean retirement income. She said she was "tortured" for more than two years by collection agencies, Medicare, and the hospital calling her several times a week, both late at night and early in the morning. She recalled that they were rude and threatening: *"Every time you see it* [the letters in the mail]*, your heart just . . . sank."* Victorine lived in constant fear of these threats and said, *"It was torture and you are sick already."*

No insurance company, state or local aid plan, charity, hospital, program, or clinic had to pay for Donna's medical care. At the time of our interview, Donna was still untreated one year after being diagnosed with breast cancer. She had no health insurance, was ineligible for Medicaid or Medicare, and no one at the clinic where she was diagnosed told her how to apply for medical assistance or charity care. No social worker saw her and no one referred her to any voluntary cancer organizations or support groups. During our interview she said, *"Like I was in it all by myself. That's the way it sound to me. And that's the way it felt."* Donna's assessment of her circumstances reflects the difficulties the majority of the women encountered. While the other 23 women in the study generally fared better than Donna in finding needed services, her circumstances cast in sharp relief the obstacles encountered by these poor women with breast cancer. Donna's circumstances illustrate the data that poor individuals are more likely to have an unmet need for health care, and echo all too clearly Ruth Zambrana's call for access and availability of health services for the poor.

Fifteen of the 24 women depended on their treatments being arranged and paid for through national or local programs designed to help those who are economically at risk. These programs included Medicaid, Medicare, state and local breast cancer partnership programs for low-income women,[3] and public hospitals. For some of these women, their health care was paid for in full, was well coordinated, and appropriate. For instance, two women treated through the Medicaid program, Diana and Geraldine, were properly diagnosed, allowed second opinions, given choices among treatment options, had a team of physicians, received the full complement of treatments they chose, and were offered breast reconstruction and psychotherapy. They continue to receive follow-up care paid for by Medicaid. Both women had been patients at free clinics whose personnel acted as advocates for them once they were diagnosed. Neither woman felt that being low income made a difference in their care. Diana's and Geraldine's experiences were examples of how well a program designed to help the economically disadvantaged and medically underserved can work to provide breast cancer services.

Several women were treated through breast cancer partnership programs or at public hospitals where most of their care was paid for. One woman, Margaret, was treated in a partnership program and wanted breast reconstruction, especially since cancer was found in both breasts and she had to have a bilateral mastectomy. However, the program did not cover reconstruction and she mortgaged her home to pay for the reconstructive surgery. Jeannie, treated in the same program, was pleased with her care, and she was able to go to the hospital nearest her home and choose a surgeon she knew. She also is pleased that the program pays for her continuing use of the anticancer drug tamoxifen since, although she is now Medicare eligible, Medicare does not pay for prescription drugs.

Some of the women sought help at public hospitals. Public hospitals were a haven for several women who reported they did not know what they would have done or where they would have gone if the hospitals were not available to them. Carrie knowingly said, "Everyone that's there [in the public hospital] is there because they don't have any health insurance." Although several women received bills from the hospitals that they could not afford to pay, when they ignored them or called the hospitals, the bills were forgiven.

Charity was not a source the women found they could turn to. One exceptionally fortunate but uninsured woman had long been a patient at a free clinic and, when she was diagnosed with breast cancer, the director of the clinic arranged for a religious charity to pay for all her treatment costs. She was the only woman in the study to receive charity care.

DELAYS IN DIAGNOSIS AND TREATMENT

Delays prior to being diagnosed with breast cancer or receiving treatment were a perilous but all too common occurrence for these women. Half the women in the study faced considerable delays before being diagnosed or treated after they found a breast lump. These delays ranged from three months to eight years. Sarah was confronted with an eight-year delay both because her physician dismissed a growing breast mass and because, after paying for doctor visits, she had no money left for mammograms for several intervening years. She said, *"The expense of the mammogram kept me from going every year."* Another woman, Estela, went five years from the time a suspicious finding was seen on a mammogram to being treated. Her husband lost his job and the health insurance that covered her, so that she had no means of paying for follow-up care. When her breast enlarged, a friend told her of a low-cost community health center where she was seen. By then five years had elapsed since the initial breast mass was detected. Although both these women had received some health services, because they were uninsured and were unable to pay for costs out of their own pockets, their remaining unmet needs for health care resulted in serious delays, risking their health and lives. Their accounts demonstrate another well-known feature of those without health insurance: Uninsured individuals delay getting care because of cost.

Ellie was treated at a public hospital, but there was a seven-month delay between diagnosis and treatment because the hospital could not give her an earlier appointment. Fatalistic about the long delay, she said, *"They don't need me. I need them. So I have to be patient and wait my turn."* Others treated at public hospitals were not so sanguine. For instance, Carrie recalled that six months had elapsed before the results of a mammogram and biopsy were finally reported. She said, *"I mean if you're getting optimal care, all this could have been done in like three or four weeks. I believe a lot of people's health is compromised."* Although she was treated at the public hospital because she had no other choice, Carrie knew that she had received deficient cancer care. Ellie's and Carrie's delays illustrate the decline in the number of traditional safety-net providers giving timely medical care because changes in the health system have resulted in public hospitals receiving fewer dollars to meet the needs of the populations they try to serve.

Sue's treatment was delayed five months because she lost her job, had no health insurance and no money to pay for care, and was unable to find a location for low-cost or charity care. She finally found her way to a public hospital more than two hours from her home where she was seen at no cost. Asked what she would have done if she had not learned about the hospital or had not been admitted there, she replied, *"I suppose open up a phone book and start calling doctors— that idea really scared me."* The clinic in her home town where she had been diagnosed had no advice to offer her other than to try to find a doctor who would treat her on a payment plan. This solution was a highly improbable one given that she had no job and no income. Even if she did find both a willing doctor and a job, it is unclear how she would have paid the high costs of breast cancer treatment out of her usual annual salary of $8,000.

Gloria faced a three-year delay both because her doctor advised her not to worry about a lump she had found and because she had no health insurance. When she saw a doctor in her home country of El Salvador, he advised her to have a mammogram as soon as she returned to the United States. By that time, three years had elapsed and she was forced to pay out of pocket for a mammogram and biopsy, and she worried how she would pay for cancer treatment. Similarly, Jeannie encountered a delay because her supplemental health insurance would not pay for the treatment services she needed and she was advised to wait until she would become eligible for Medicare three months later. In the interim she learned about and entered a local breast cancer partnership program for low-income women, which paid for her treatment costs. Although Jeannie's circumstances may be seen by some as a gap in coverage, she was insured at the time of diagnosis but the insurer refused to pay for treatment. Gloria's and Sue's delays, however, were not only the result of being uninsured; they were women with breast cancer for whom there was no apparent access to the treatments they clearly needed. These three women's accounts illustrate the gaps in the health system through which poor women's lives can fall.

QUALITY OF CARE

In addition to the barriers of locating care and facing lengthy delays, the women in the study also confronted health care services of inferior quality. When asked about the quality of the care they received, the women generally replied in terms of how they assessed the health personnel who cared for them. More than half the women reported that they felt that their care was less than adequate and often inexcusably inferior. However, some women were quite pleased with the care they received. Margaret, treated in a partnership program for low-income women, stated, *"They were all beautiful people. I mean they would help you in any way, shape, or form. It didn't make any difference where you came from, they were there to take care of you."* June, whose medical care was paid for by a charity, said of the physicians and nurses who treated her in a private hospital, *"They treat you like royalty. Money or no money, they treat people very kind."*

Several women reported being very pleased with the care they received at a public hospital. Sarah stated emphatically, *"I do not believe that low income means that you have lesser qualified doctors. Nor are you treated any differently."* She said, *"I don't think anybody could do any better than Dr. M. She has never not had time for me. She has never not explained everything that was going to happen to me. I would put her against any doc in any other hospital."* Note, however, that Sarah was the woman whose long-time family physician ignored a growing mass in her breast for eight years. She believes that her health was seriously imperiled by his negligence.

Although they often encountered long delays getting appointments or waiting to be seen, some of the women still felt good about the quality of the care they received at public hospitals. For women like Ellie, a public hospital is far more than the stereotyped hospital-of-last-resort. Now in her seventies, she says, *"That is the only place I know and like. They have good doctors there. They got my record ever since I was a teenager."*

Carrie, on the other hand, was dismayed by the long waits to get an appointment, to be seen at the hospital, or to pick up the free prescriptions at the public hospital. She recounted waits of six to eight hours just to see a physician: *"You thought you worked a job when you leave there, you just that tired."* Similarly, Eleanor decided not to go back to the public hospital, where she was treated, to pick up the tamoxifen prescription she needs each month. Recalling the long hours standing in line to have a prescription filled, she said, *"It's like waiting for next spring."*

Other women in the study who believed they received less than adequate care included Susana, the woman who continues to pay the near total cost of her care out of her own pocket. She was obliged to shop around for lower-cost services, was unable to pay for a second opinion, and could not afford an overnight stay in the hospital following surgery. She was refused treatment at several hospitals because she was uninsured and like Lorraine she was forced to make a $2,000 down payment she could barely manage before the hospital would admit her for surgery. In the process of shopping around for the best prices for tests, surgery, and radiation, Susana became a patient at three different hospitals in two different metropolitan areas—hardly a prescription for well-coordinated care. Susana's perspective on her health and medical care were that both were seriously jeopardized by the complications of multiple financial woes. Her circumstances demonstrate not only the enormous financial burden to the poor of out-of-pocket costs but the ways in which such costs can jeopardize the quality of their medical care.

Compromised quality of care comes in many versions. For instance, Victorine, who was treated at a private hospital, was dismayed that hospital personnel made no provisions for her to return home safely and comfortably after surgery. After same-day, outpatient breast cancer surgery, she was sent home without painkillers or transportation. Age 69 and in serious postoperative pain, Victorine was obliged to take two buses and travel for over an hour to reach her home. At one point she was forced to stop at a pharmacy on the way to fill a prescription and take a painkiller in order to make it home. She later recounted an episode of waiting at a public hospital from 8 A.M. to 10 P.M. to see a physician for pain in her arm; told it was her nerves, she was sent home, again via bus, at midnight in bitter cold December weather. In our interview Victorine said, *"I just think people treat people on account of their money and influence."* Victorine's point describes a health care system that callously dismisses the needs of patients and shows little regard for those who are economically disadvantaged.

Donna, who was untreated at the time of our interview, felt that she was ignored by health personnel and left to fend for herself. Beyond the doctor who gave her the diagnosis of breast cancer, Donna received virtually no help in understanding, coping with, and making decisions about what to do once she was diagnosed with breast cancer. She faulted her doctor who continued to press her for a mastectomy and she feared that medical students would operate on her. Talking about her doctor who, at the time of diagnosis, showed her pictures of women whose breasts had been removed, she said, *"First thing you want to do is chop off their damn titty."* Although Donna was terrified of losing her breast, her doctor did not offer her breast reconstruction with a mastectomy, leaving her with no options other than breast amputation, which she refused. When Donna was asked in our interview whether she would have agreed to an earlier mastectomy if reconstruction had been available, she replied, *"Yeah, I probably would have. I just didn't want to go around looking like that."* While Donna understood well the difficult decisions she faced following diagnosis, no one else seemed to—neither the doctors nor the clinic personnel. She said, *"I had found out I had breast cancer, and I wanted to talk to somebody. I think they could have told me how to deal with it without getting it amputated."* No one came forward to help her at a time she was unable to help herself. In sum, Donna found herself completely abandoned by the health care system.

Another barrier to care faced by the women in the study was ethnic discrimination. Several of the Latinas felt that they received inadequate care because their physicians failed to give them sufficient information about their diagnoses, spoke to them as if they were ignorant or not capable of understanding their circumstances, and did not treat them as partners in determining their courses of treatment. While language was a barrier for six of the eight Latinas in the study, many were still able to understand English to varying degrees. Combined with lack of insurance, and with few financial and social resources, several of the Latinas felt their quality of care was compromised.

For instance, Elena felt that she was treated poorly because health personnel kept information from her, were rude, and did not provide translation services. She said that she learned little from them about her medical tests, medications, her diagnosis, and prognosis. She reported that lymph nodes under her arm were surgically removed without her prior knowledge or her consent— an illegal and outrageous act. One doctor said to her directly that her English was *"just so bad."* She said forthrightly, *"Because I don't speak the language, I don't get good treatment."* Although she was the only woman in the study whose health insurance paid for all her care, this fact could not guarantee her appropriate breast cancer treatment.

Aurelia, a woman from Cuba, who was also insured, was told not to worry when the results of a mammogram were lost and she was not informed of the findings indicating she had a malignancy. She later found out that a previous mammogram also had been lost and she was never notified of the results. Josefina, a woman from Mexico, reported that the nurses in the hospital where she was treated were often *"inhuman"* and that they chastised her for crying and being *"weak,"* calling her *"a coward."* Insensitivities, cruelties, negligence, and medical malpractice were all a part of the inferior quality of care these women received.

Few of the Latinas in the study spoke openly of frank ethnic discrimination. And, in a few cases, these women were grateful for the care they received—even though when asked directly about the quality of their care, they acknowledged that it was far less than satisfactory. However, it was clear from the study data that the Latinas, in particular, were treated with disrespect and carelessness, resulting in inferior quality of care.

BURDENS TO CARRY

Under normal life circumstances the 24 women in the study struggled to pay their bills, find and hold on to jobs, raise families, and maintain households, on very limited incomes. When they were diagnosed with breast cancer and while they were pursuing treatment, all the women encountered additional problems that compounded their already difficult lives and the burden of coping with breast cancer.

FEARING LOSS OF HOME OR JOB

Living on limited incomes, several women feared losing their homes or their jobs when they were sick. Sarah, uninsured, was threatened with the loss of her home when she did not have the money to pay for radiation treatments. She said, *"For a week I thought that I would die because I just thought that everything that I had worked so hard for to get* [her own home] *was going to be gone. I did not want to lose everything just because I was sick."* At one point, Sarah was unable to pay an installment on her property tax and, once again, she was threatened with the loss of her home. Just to get by, she borrowed money from friends, which she remains unable to repay. Living on earnings of $8,000 a year as a waitress, without health insurance, and the mother of a dependent child, she was forced to continue working despite doctors' warnings that such heavy physical work was ill advised. She reported that if she had had health insurance or savings she would have taken time off as needed: *"I would love to be able just not to go to work the day after chemo. I never could."*

Like Sarah, Victorine feared losing her home when the collection agencies threatened her for nonpayment of medical bills that Medicare would not cover in full. The fear and anger still fresh she said, *"I did not want them to take my house. Because I don't want to be homeless."* Victorine's limited income had restricted her access to breast and other health care, even though at age 69 she was Medicare eligible. She affirmed that *"This is why people get sick because if you don't have the money you don't want to go. I don't go when the doctor say come. I go when I have the money. And that may be three months later."* Discussing how she paid for some mammograms and other health services out of pocket because Medicare and her supplemental policy did not cover them, she replied, *"You cut back on food. You eat soup seven days a week. You cut back on things you need like pantyhose. You wear socks and slacks so that you do not have to buy those things."* Referring to Medicare coverage and her supplemental Blue Cross/Blue Shield policy, she said, *"Paying all this money to insurance. They don't give you medication. No coverage for your eyes. No dental. It is not doing me no good."* Both Victorine and Sarah confronted the pernicious economic discrimination that accompanies poverty. Their troubles illustrate the consequences of income inequality: Those with few economic resources may face financial ruin as well as threats to their health that the economically privileged rarely encounter.

Jean was threatened with the loss of her job as a legal secretary when she was diagnosed with breast cancer. She feared losing the only income and health insurance she had for herself and her family during a critical time. With the fear of job loss, she was unable to take time off from work to rest during six weeks of daily radiation treatments and four cycles of chemotherapy. In addition, she had a two-hour commute each day. She slept during her lunch breaks in order to make it through the day. Jean feared not only the loss of her job but also discrimination if she tried to find another job with health insurance. She felt certain that, because she is a woman with breast cancer, many employers would not want to hire her. Although her health insurance policy paid 80 percent of her breast cancer care, she was left with close to $4,000 in remaining bills. She said, "*With the insurance bills I felt that I had to keep this job. I think that is what mostly kept me going.*" Of her attempts to pay these over time out of her $19,000 salary, she says, "*It is really hard making ends meet.*" Although Jean was employed and insured, her circumstances illustrate another form of economic discrimination encountered by those who are economically disadvantaged: Health insurance that leaves them in debt. She also confronted the discrimination of job lock, or the inability to leave one workplace for another because of the overt bias against hiring individuals with serious illness.

NOT ENOUGH TO LIVE OR GO ON

The women in the study faced other burdens during the breast cancer crisis. Many of them simply did not have enough money to live on, given the added costs of being sick. Others were so distraught by both the breast cancer and the strain on their already arduous lives that they were not sure they had enough emotional strength to keep going. While half the women received various forms of public assistance or social insurance, one of the chief complaints for many was the lack of income support during the breast cancer crisis. The dual burden of no health insurance and not enough money to pay for needed health services or to maintain their already frugal and fragile standards of living left many of the women at wit's end.

Sarah's perspective on her need for some form of temporary assistance speaks for many of the women. She applied to Social Security and for public aid but was refused both. Still angry, she said, *"I had not abused society. I had not gone to jail. I was not asking for long term help. I was asking to get through these few months while I was sick. Help me out. I have paid you for thirty years."* Sarah appealed the denial, but the stress of pursuing the appeal, coping with breast cancer, raising her son, working daily, and finding a way to pay her bills left her with little strength. Resignation in her voice, she said, *"I was sick as it was and I was doing all I could to work every day and convince myself that I was going to be cancer free. Keep my home in order. Keep the people that I love from worrying too much."*

Marva, too, was barely getting by. She was diagnosed with breast cancer shortly after losing her health insurance and her job. She has a master's degree and had been an educator, but multiple health conditions prevented her from being able to work. She was treated for breast cancer at a public hospital through medical assistance. However, her only income is $100 a month limited public aid and $122 a month in food stamps. She lives with her mother in a very small one-bedroom apartment and relies on her mother and daughter to pay her bills. She said, *"I am not getting by. If my mother or daughter buys me something every blue moon, then that is all I have."* Marva is angry that she does not qualify for full public assistance, which would give her about $500 a month, because she does not meet the qualifications for disability under Social Security. She says she feels entitled to this help. *"I don't want this the rest of my life. But I am entitled to it now. And I intend to get it now until I can do better. I should not have to suffer. I have worked since I was fifteen years old."* Both Marva and Sarah were calling for temporary aid from social programs into which they had already paid. These were not women who were attempting to malinger or take unfair advantage of public monies. However, the mismatch between their distressing circumstances and the empty hand extended to them by society illustrates the inequities faced by those who are already poor.

Carrie, too, had no health insurance, although her husband had worked for the metropolitan transit service for many years. When her husband died and Carrie was coping with breast cancer, she was forced to leave the home where they had lived for many years and had raised their children, because she could not afford to stay there. Although she had been a homemaker for most of her adult years, she began to work part-time in a family-owned business and moved into a small apartment loaned to her to help make ends meet. Carrie said that she did not apply for public aid because she would have had to spend down to $1,200 to qualify and wanted to hold on to a small amount of savings *"for an emergency one day."* She added, *"My husband and I, we have been tax-paying citizens all these years. We got married as teenagers and never been on public aid, not a day in our life, never received food stamps. We took care of ourselves. But then when you get in a hard place, you think well maybe you're gonna get something from them, but, it's too hard. I would rather dig ditches than fool with public aid."* Carrie also tried to qualify for disability but was told that she was able to work. She agreed with that assessment but was simply hoping that she could have temporary disability *"until I get myself on my feet in a little bit."* Carrie says of her financial situation, *"I'm barely making it. The little money I make, I can't sneeze."* Carrie, like Marva and Sarah, confronted society's empty hand when she was most in need, despite her family's pride in lifelong independence.

Donna, who was untreated a year after being diagnosed, had long been without health insurance although she had worked for many years as a hotel housekeeper and as a housekeeping supervisor. She had a bad back and, as a result, she was unemployed at the time she was diagnosed with breast cancer. Donna was angry that she had not previously qualified for such forms of assistance as Medicaid because, although she is poor and single, she does not have children. She lived under difficult circumstances in an area with a thriving drug market, often without a telephone and even gas and electricity, and no transportation to the clinic. By the time of our interview she had begun to receive temporary state medical assistance (which also qualified her for Supplemental Security Income and food stamps), after a neighbor told her how to apply. She was scheduled for a mastectomy and breast reconstruction, after which she would lose all these benefits (which amounted to about $6,000 a year), at that time her only source of income. If prior to surgery she found a job, she also would lose the benefits because she would be employed and ineligible for assistance. As a result, Donna had stopped her job search and was waiting to enter the hospital. Donna had reached a virtual and contorted dead end. A diagnosis of breast cancer entitled her to the benefits of several social programs she otherwise would not have received even though she was desperately poor and temporarily disabled. Had health insurance, temporary income support, or disability been available to her prior to the breast cancer diagnosis, she might have never found herself in the desperate circumstances she described.

Sue, like Donna, had lost her job and accompanying health insurance. This situation occurred one month after she found a breast lump, at the time the company she worked for fired all the pro-union employees. She could not afford the $400 a month insurance premium on her own and sought care at a local low-cost clinic. When the cancer was diagnosed, the clinic was unable to provide further care and she was forced to travel almost two hours each way to a public hospital. She found terrible irony in the fact that her home was right across the street from the hospital where she was born but to which she could not go for breast cancer treatment. She said, *"Every day I just stared at that place when I would pull out of the driveway. It is like why can't I just be walking across the street?"* She was obliged to drive almost four hours a day, five days a week, for five weeks of radiation treatments, and also had additional travel time for six cycles of chemotherapy. After two and a half weeks of radiation treatment, Sue's daily fatigue was considerable and she struggled to complete her daily trips, saying, *"And mostly you try to stay awake on the way home."* With so much time given over to travel and treatment she was unable to work more than temporary part-time jobs, and so had little income. She applied for public aid but was refused because she was told that breast cancer does not qualify as a disability—even in her case where her work as a packer means heavy physical labor. Like Donna, Sue was resentful that public aid programs would have helped if she had children but were indifferent to her financial plight. She said their general attitude was, "*Well, we don't care about you. Just your kids.*" In sum, society had made no provisions for Sue and her lack of insurance, job loss, and diagnosis of breast cancer. Like Donna, she had been ignored and was left to fend for herself. She considered herself fortunate to have finally been admitted and treated at a public hospital.

As many of the women's stories illustrate, social institutions designed to help those in need often fail to do so. Moreover, as a number of women in this study recounted, some institutions actively create barriers that preclude the help these women so desperately need. Maria's story is one last ironic, but, revealing note on how difficult it is for these women to manage when so many odds are arrayed against them. Maria is a single mother of two who earns about $19,000 a year as a billing clerk. She is attempting to pay in installments cancer treatment bills that her previous insurer refused to cover. She also is repaying public aid for overpayments they claim to have made to her at an earlier time. In effect, Maria is paying out to two entities, one private and one public, whose purpose is to pay her when she is in need. As an employee and a taxpayer, she has already underwritten both the insurer and public aid. Yet, as Maria copes with breast cancer, she finds herself hounded by them and forced to make payments she can ill afford.

CONCLUSIONS

Americans, used to hearing their country called the most wealthy and the most powerful nation in the world, do not like to hear much about poverty and powerlessness. And, undoubtedly, Americans do not like to think much about these troubling issues. We do, however, make some assumptions about those among us who live in or near poverty and one of these assumptions is that somehow, someway, the poor get by. It may be that many of the poor do get by. But, we should ask the question, at what price?

The poor and underserved women with breast cancer in this study did, for the most part, get by. The study did ask the question— what price did the women pay? The answer is that the women paid heavily with their health and survival. The full spectrum of the health care system, including health insurance, Medicaid, Medicare, state and local medical assistance and hospitalization programs, community-based clinics, private and public hospitals, and health charities, were unable to provide appropriate breast cancer treatment for the majority of the women. Other social institutions, such as public assistance, Social Security, food stamps, welfare, and disability programs were unavailable for many of the women who lived near financial collapse. As a result, their meager resources became even more fragile during the breast cancer crisis. Consequently, in addition to their compromised physical health and survival, the women in this study also paid heavily with their emotional and psychological well-being.

This group of 24 urban women offers a glimpse of what it means to be poor and sick with breast cancer in contemporary American society. Although the majority of the women were relatively well educated and only five of the women were unemployed, three-quarters of the women lived on incomes of $8,000 or less. Thus, being reasonably well educated did not lift them out of poverty, did not provide a living wage, and did not insure them for health care. Less than half the women had health insurance of any kind, public or private, and only three had health insurance in their own right through employment. Clearly the American dream of education leading to better jobs, higher incomes, and better lives was not accessible to these women. Nor were many of the women who had worked and paid taxes for many years able to count on public assistance programs to help them, even temporarily, manage a health crisis.

One of the consequences of being poor and uninsured is the lack of fit within a health care system that organizes itself for those who are insured or can afford to pay for care. This mismatch resulted in many of the women facing unconscionable delays in locating and receiving treatment services. It also resulted in the women paying unaffordable out-of-pocket costs for needed medical care, being denied treatment for lack of funds, or doing without care. The women were often the recipients of inferior and negligent quality of care, and several encountered discrimination because of their low income or ethnic status. These circumstances led, in turn, to a cascade of other effects, such as the threatened or actual loss of their homes, jobs, and health insurance, as well as the harassment of collection agencies because they were unable to pay medical bills. A few women went into debt to pay for medical care or household expenses while being treated for breast cancer. Others were unable to take time off from work while in treatment, even though they desperately needed to and their doctors advised them to do so.

This lack of fit within the health system also left many of the women to fend for themselves when they were diagnosed with breast cancer. Without sufficient information, personal authority, or a sense of entitlement, many of the women were ill equipped to negotiate institutions, systems, programs, and policies that might have improved their chances of access to treatment services they knew they needed. It is not surprising, then, that many of the women reported an underlying and pervasive fear that they simply would not be able to manage financially, physically, and emotionally. Compounding this fear was the fact that the majority of the women were quite isolated and alone, with limited social and emotional support, a situation that echoes the literature on poverty and isolation discussed earlier.

The context of living in poverty prior to diagnosis set the stage for difficulties the women faced when they attempted to enter the health care system to be diagnosed and treated for breast cancer. Their circumstances of poverty included lives made difficult by very limited financial resources, income insecurity, job instability, difficulty making ends meet to care for themselves and their families, single parenthood, violence in relationships, disrupted neighborhoods, housing instability, lack of acculturation, isolation, and lack of social support and social capital. The risk of poorer health outcomes for these women with breast cancer rested on a foundation of poverty and on a society which seemed to care little for their health and well-being.

Many of the women spoke of being unable to see a doctor or get a mammogram when they believed they needed to, either because they were uninsured, underinsured, did not have the money to pay out of their own pockets, or did not know where to go. Several women were so preoccupied with the difficulties of their lives that their health concerns became secondary. While they were all aware that regular health visits and good health care are important, for many of the women these services were dependent on material and psychological resources they often lacked. The women in this study worried about the consequences of these adversities on their health and survival, and rightfully so. Much is made of the importance of timely and high quality diagnostic and treatment services in public education materials, television, newspapers, and magazines, and the women in the study were all aware of these messages.

Several of the women had been diagnosed with later stage disease. The consequences of lives lived in poverty, compounded by the difficulties of gaining access to medical services, treatment delays, and substandard quality of care that many of the women encountered, may well compromise their health and survival from breast cancer. Sadly, many of these 24 women may be candidates for the statistics of later diagnosis and higher mortality cited earlier in this chapter.

In the absence of universal health insurance, full employment at a living wage, readily available public assistance for individuals and families who face serious hardship, and a national commitment to raise all members of society out of poverty, poor women with breast cancer will continue to face near insurmountable barriers and carry wrenching burdens that few who live outside the boundaries of poverty can imagine.

NOTES

AUTHOR'S NOTE: I am grateful to Alice Dan for her support of this study from its inception and to my research assistants Frances Aranda, Rebecca Levin, and Ami Lynch for their hard work and constancy. I offer much gratitude to the 24 women who participated in the study and were willing to share the difficulties of their experiences with breast cancer and their lives so that other women might benefit. The study was initially supported by the Women's Health Policy Research Fellowship of the Center for Research on Women and Gender at the University of Illinois at Chicago. A grant from the U.S. Agency for Health Care Policy and Research (now the Agency for Healthcare Research and Quality) enabled me to substantially complete the study.

1. Participants for the study were recruited from similar sites in both cities. These sites included hospitals, clinics, breast cancer support groups, health departments, community health centers, shelters, charities, church groups, and women's organizations. Pilot interviews were conducted in 1995 and 1996. The majority of the interviews were conducted in 1998. All interviews were conducted by the author as the principal investigator and a research assistant or a bilingual translator (for six of eight interviews with Latinas). Interviews typically lasted from two to three hours, usually in the participants' homes, and were audio tape recorded. The recorded interviews were transcribed verbatim. Transcripts and field notes were coded for analysis and interpreted using a three-stage content analysis (Kasper 1994).
2. All names used here are pseudonyms. All quotes are taken verbatim from the interview transcripts.
3. The National Breast and Cervical Cancer Early Detection Program (NBC-CEDP) is the source of the breast cancer partnership programs that served several women in this study. The 1990 authorizing legislation for this program provided federal dollars to the Centers for Disease Control and Prevention (CDC) to establish breast and cervical cancer screening programs for low income women at the state level. There now are screening programs in all states, territories, tribes, and the District of Columbia. However, in establishing this national program, Congress left to the states the provision of treatment services for women diagnosed with disease. Many of the partnership programs struggle to find willing providers, negotiate reduced fees, and locate charity care since state and local dollars are often

insufficient. This struggle has increased as providers are more resistant to accepting reduced fees, hospitals do not have the charity and bad debt pools they once had, physicians in managed care settings may not be able to participate, and charities and foundations may not help regularly or indefinitely.

REFERENCES

Agency for Health Care Policy and Research. 1998. "Reasons Vary for Lacking a Usual Source of Health Care." *Research Activities* 215:16.

Ayanian, John Z., Betsy A. Kohler, Toshi Abe, and Arnold M. Epstein. 1993. "The Relation Between Health Insurance Coverage and Clinical Outcomes Among Women with Breast Cancer." *New England Journal of Medicine* 329:326-31.

Center on Budget and Policy Priorities. 1998. "Poverty Rates Fall, But Remain High for a Period with Such Low Unemployment." Washington, D.C.: Center on Budget and Policy Priorities.

Hardisty, Jean V., and Ellen Leopold. 1996. "Cancer and Poverty: Double Jeopardy for Women." Pp. 219-36 in *Myths About the Powerless: Contesting Social Inequalities*, ed. by M. Brinton Lykes, Ali Banuazizi, Ramsay Liem, and Michael Morris. Philadelphia, PA: Temple University Press.

Henry J. Kaiser Family Foundation. 1998. "Kaiser Commission on Medicaid and the Uninsured: Uninsured Facts." Washington, D.C.: Henry J. Kaiser Family Foundation.

Karjalainen, S., and E. Pukkala. 1990. "Social Class As a Prognostic Factor in Breast Cancer Survival." *Cancer* 66:819-26.

Kasper, Anne. 1994. "A Feminist, Qualitative Methodology: A Study of Women with Breast Cancer." *Qualitative Sociology* 17:263-281.

Kawachi, Ichiro, Bruce P. Kennedy, Kimberly Lochner, and Deborah Prothrow-Stith. 1997. "Social Capital, Income Inequality, and Mortality." *American Journal of Public Health* 87:1491-98.

Kawachi, Ichiro. 1999. "Social Capital and Community Effects on Population and Individual Health." Presented at the New York Academy of Sciences Conference, Socioeconomic Status and Health in Industrial Nations, May 10-12, Bethesda, MD.

Kogevinas, M., and M. Porta. 1997. "Socioeconomic Differences in Cancer Survival: A Review of the Evidence." *IARC Science Publications* 138:177-206.

Rawlings, Lynette. 1998. "Poverty and Income Trends." Washington, D.C.: Center on Budget and Policy Priorities.

Reisinger, Anne Lenhard. 1996. "Health Insurance and Women's Access to Health Care." Pp. 324-44 in *Women's Health: The Commonwealth Fund Survey*, ed. by Marilyn N. Falik and Karen Scott Collins. Baltimore: Johns Hopkins University Press.

U.S. Bureau of the Census. 1998. *Current Population Reports*. Washington, D.C.
———. 1999. *Current Population Survey*. Washington, D.C.

U.S. Department of Health and Human Services. 1998. *Health, United States, 1998: With Socioeconomic Status and Health Chartbook*. Washington, D.C.: U.S. Government Printing Office.

Vistnes, J., and A. Monheit. 1998. "Health Insurance Status of the U.S. Civilian Noninstitutionalized Population." *Medical Expenditure Panel Survey, Research Findings No. 1*. Rockville, Md: Agency for Health Care Policy and Research.

Zambrana, Ruth E. 1988. "A Research Agenda on Issues Affecting Poor and Minority Women: A Model for Understanding Their Health Needs." Pp. 137-60 in *Too Little, Too Late: Dealing with the Health Needs of Women in Poverty*, ed. by Cesar A. Perales and Lauren S. Young. New York: Harrington Park Press.

Breast Cancer Policymaking

Carol S. Weisman, Ph.D.

Breast cancer policy can be defined as the set of decisions made by society to allocate resources to research, programs, and services to prevent and treat breast cancer. The fact that we now recognize the existence of national breast cancer policymaking means that there has been a process of constructing breast cancer as a social problem, of formulating alternative approaches to addressing the problem through public policy, and of making social choices among policy options. Various groups have participated in this process, including legislators and government agencies, professional associations, private industry, and citizen interest groups organized to advocate for breast cancer causes. Furthermore, because breast cancer is primarily an illness of women, gender issues have been central to its politics.

The definition of breast cancer as a social problem in the United States might be dated to the 1970s, when mammography screening was first debated and tested nationwide, when consumers first raised concerns about mastectomy as standard treatment, and when celebrity breast cancer cases were first publicized in the media to raise breast cancer awareness. The 1990s, however, witnessed an unprecedented spate of consumer advocacy and governmental action on breast cancer, and it is this episode that most observers associate with breast cancer policymaking. Policy responses during the early 1990s focused on improving women's financial access to mammography screening and clinical procedures for breast cancer, ensuring the quality of mammography, revising mammography screening guidelines, and, perhaps most dramatically, increasing government investment in breast cancer research.

This chapter discusses how breast cancer policy is made, what accounts for the timing of the 1990s policymaking episode, and some implications and unintended consequences for women's health. Several recent accounts of the politics of breast cancer have emphasized the role of breast cancer advocacy organizations in bringing the issue to public attention and spurring government action (Altman 1996; Batt 1994; Ferraro 1993; Kaufert 1998; Soffa 1994; Stabiner 1997). While the policy initiatives of the 1990s could not have happened without these organizations, it is also important to recognize that they operated in a policy context in which health care issues were salient and women's health was a popular bipartisan political issue.

The argument will be made here that the political opportunities for breast cancer policy in the 1990s were expanding and that breast cancer advocacy organizations were well positioned to both shape and exploit these opportunities. In so doing, they helped define the breast cancer policy agenda, craft the policy options, and transform how breast cancer policy is made. They did not, however, always control the agenda. Policymaking has been motivated not only by consumer perspectives, but also by political and economic interests that do not necessarily coincide with those of the advocacy community. In this context, single-issue policymaking may not always benefit women's health.

THE CONTEXT OF BREAST CANCER POLICYMAKING

WOMEN'S HEALTH MOVEMENT ACTIVITY

Breast cancer policymaking in the 1990s benefited from the political opportunities opened by a confluence of health and gender politics. Attention to breast cancer coincided with a larger wave of social movement activity related to a range of women's health issues that emerged around 1990 and built on the base of the Women's Health Movement of the 1960s and 1970s.[1] A nexus of empowered women—including Congresswomen and their staffs, women in the biomedical community (including officials at the National Institutes of Health [NIH], academic researchers, and practicing physicians), and women's professionalized health interest and advocacy groups—focused public attention on gender inequities in biomedical research and medical care and proposed specific governmental remedies. In 1989, the bipartisan Congressional Caucus for Women's Issues, which previously had focused on legal and economic equity for women, began to work collaboratively with other groups on a women's health agenda. They crafted legislation on a number of women's health issues and sought to pressure government agencies, such as the NIH and the Food and Drug Administration (FDA), to change their policies and practices on women's health research. A 1990 report by the General Accounting Office, which had been requested by the Caucus, found that NIH had done little to implement its 1986 policy to encourage researchers to include women as subjects in clinical studies. Impending NIH reauthorization opened a "policy window" for legislators to ensure changes at the NIH, and the Caucus took advantage of this opportunity.[2]

Ironically, the political climate in which these events occurred was not particularly friendly to women's issues, yet women's health would soon emerge as a popular bipartisan issue. The 1980s have been described as a decade of cultural backlash against women's recent social and economic gains (Faludi 1991). In the health arena, the abortion politics of the Reagan and Bush administrations had produced a chilling effect on biomedical research related to some aspects of women's health, including the development and testing of new contraceptives, infertility research, and studies of sexual behaviors related to prevention of sexually transmitted diseases (including HIV/AIDS) and unintended pregnancy.

Two focusing events helped draw public attention to women's issues and concerns between 1989 and 1991. The first was the 1989 U.S. Supreme Court decision in *Webster v. Reproductive Health Services,* which upheld the state of Missouri's restrictive abortion law and was viewed as a major victory for the anti-abortion movement. This ruling helped spur a massive mobilization of abortion rights supporters, as evidenced by increased memberships and donations to such groups as the National Abortion Rights Action League and Planned Parenthood (Staggenborg 1991). The second focusing event was the October 1991 televised confirmation hearings on the appointment of Judge Clarence Thomas to the U.S. Supreme Court, in which law professor Anita Hill, who had accused Thomas of sexual harassment, was treated unsympathetically by the all-male Senate Judiciary Committee. The gender dynamics of the hearings have been credited with activating women voters and candidates for the 1992 election and with increasing the currency of women's issues in Congress and among candidates for political office (Witt, Paget, and Matthews 1994). The 1992 elections nearly doubled the number of women in Congress, and women's votes helped elect President Clinton, who supported many women's issues as well as a national health care reform agenda. In this context, women's health became a good issue for lawmakers seeking to win favor with female constituents.

Furthermore, those promoting women's health issues in and around the federal government cleverly framed the issues so as to deflect the impact of abortion politics. Patricia Schroeder and Olympia Snowe, the co-chairs of the Congressional Caucus for Women's Issues at the time, acknowledged their early strategy of defining a women's health agenda with broad appeal: "We, as Caucus co-chairs, began to look for a new middle ground that could be embraced by Congresswomen on both sides of the abortion divide" (Schroeder and Snowe 1994.92). (The caucus took no official position on abortion until 1993.) By framing women's health in this way, they focused attention on women's health problems that had been under-researched, such as heart disease and breast cancer, and they provided anti-abortion legislators with an opportunity to support women's health initiatives.

BREAST CANCER'S ROOTS AS A SOCIAL ISSUE

Breast cancer became the quintessential women's health issue in the 1990s that appealed to legislators regardless of their position on abortion. This change did not happen by chance; instead, it built on a foundation of media attention and the resources of a growing and increasingly organized breast cancer advocacy community poised to take full advantage of the changing climate for women's health issues.

Once a taboo topic, breast cancer had begun to emerge in public discourse in the 1970s. During that decade, mammography screening was first subjected to nationwide debate; several research studies and personal accounts by breast cancer patients questioned the appropriateness of radical mastectomy as standard treatment for breast cancer, and prominent women—notably, Shirley Temple Black, Happy Rockefeller, and Betty Ford—acknowledged their breast cancer in the national media. The publicity surrounding celebrity cases helped raise women's awareness of the disease. However, many Women's Health Movement participants of this time were members of the post–World War II baby-boom generation and were more concerned about abortion and other reproductive health issues than about conditions such as breast cancer that affect primarily midlife and older women.

By 1990, women of the baby-boom generation were entering midlife and had been exposed to information about mammography screening, which had begun to be actively promoted during the 1980s in media campaigns sponsored by the American Cancer Society (ACS).[3] Screening rates improved as a result of these campaigns and, partly in consequence, breast cancer incidence rates increased by more than 30 percent during the 1980s (Ries et al. 1994). One implication of the trend in incidence was the growing likelihood that a given individual would have contact with a woman with breast cancer. Breast cancer awareness also was heightened by increasing coverage in popular magazines in the late 1980s (Lantz and Booth 1998). Thus, even though breast cancer was not the leading cause of death among U.S. women— or, after 1986, even the leading *cancer* cause of death[4]—the conditions existed in the 1980s to frame breast cancer as an important women's health problem.

THE BREAST CANCER ADVOCACY COMMUNITY

Breast cancer advocacy evolved from local support groups into highly professionalized national interest organizations in little more than a decade. Grass-roots breast cancer groups had begun to appear in many U.S. communities in the late 1970s and early 1980s, often organized by women with breast cancer or their survivors as a means of coping with the illness, providing social support, or drawing attention to the need for information, research, or services. Examples include Y-ME, founded in 1979 by women with breast cancer in Chicago to provide support and information for women with breast cancer; the Susan G. Komen Breast Cancer Foundation, founded in Texas in 1982 by the sister of a breast cancer victim to raise funds for research and services; and Kendall Lakes Women against Cancer, formed in a Florida community in 1985 to investigate a breast cancer cluster thought to be associated with environmental contamination. The Massachusetts-based Women's Community Cancer Project (WCCP), founded in 1989 as a feminist advocacy group, also took up breast cancer as a major issue. Many of the leaders of these groups report that AIDS activists were their models for organizing, publicizing the disease, identifying strategies to influence politicians, and developing policy options such as increased federal funding earmarked for disease-specific research (Ferraro 1993; Kaufert 1998).[5] (For more discussion of breast cancer advocacy groups, see chapter 11 of this volume.)

By the early 1990s, organizational networks were forming to share information and resources and to influence public policy. Most notably, the National Breast Cancer Coalition (NBCC) was founded in 1991 with three major goals: promoting research on the causes, treatments, and cure for breast cancer; improving access to services for all women, including the underserved; and increasing the involvement of women with breast cancer in policy and research (Langer 1992). A planning group consisting of eight organizations soon expanded to a 20-member working board, and, by 1994, the coalition had members in all states and nearly 300 affiliated organizations (Love 1995). Participating groups were quite diverse, including local breast cancer support groups, such as Arm-in-Arm in Baltimore; cancer groups for special populations, such as the Mary Helen Mautner Project for Lesbians with Cancer; and professional and other not-for-profit associations, such as the National Alliance of Breast Cancer Organizations (NABCO) and the American Cancer Society (ACS). Among its first projects, the NBCC spearheaded the 1991 collection of over 600,000 letters demanding increased funding for breast cancer research, of which over 100,000 were delivered to the Bush White House, coincident with the Clarence Thomas hearings. Participants have described the juxtaposition of the hearings and the lukewarm reception from President George Bush as a transforming experience that inspired their activism (Kaufert 1998).

The NBCC is an example of a professionalized health advocacy organization. Although it describes itself as "a grass-roots advocacy effort" and has members in local communities, it is a national organization with a Washington, D.C., office and a hired lobbyist. Its President, Fran Visco, is an attorney as well as a woman with breast cancer, and its board of directors includes breast cancer researchers as well as other professionals. The NBCC organizes regular briefings for Congressional staff and is adept at public relations, media campaigns, and fund-raising efforts targeting the public as well as corporate donors.

The NBCC also reflects an interesting transformation in breast cancer activism. The early support and advocacy groups had been organized largely around women's collective identity as breast cancer patients. By the time the NBCC formed, however, breast cancer had been reframed as a problem for *all* women. The illness was labeled an epidemic by activists and journalists, whose rhetoric emphasized that most women (including younger women) were at risk, that access to screening and treatment services therefore should concern all women, and, resonating with the larger Women's Health Movement of the 1990s, that the failure of public policy to address breast cancer was an issue of gender equity. The advocacy community succeeded in expanding its constituency by defining a generalized gender-based risk to which many women and lawmakers could relate.

KEY POLICY INITIATIVES IN THE 1990S

THE FEDERAL LEVEL: EXPANDING RESEARCH AND SERVICES

Key breast cancer legislation was enacted by Congress between 1990 and 1997, including appropriations for breast cancer research (see figure 7.1). Not surprisingly, breast cancer was among the first health topics addressed by the Congressional Caucus for Women's Issues, when Representative Mary Rose Oakar, whose sister had breast cancer, introduced legislation requiring states to adopt informed consent procedures for breast cancer surgery. Although that legislation was not successful, other breast cancer bills have been a consistent component of the Women's Health Equity Act (WHEA), a series of omnibus legislative packages on women's health research and services first introduced by the Caucus in the 101st Congress (1989-90) and reintroduced in subsequent sessions.

The first bill associated with the WHEA to become law was the Breast and Cervical Cancer Mortality Prevention Act of 1990, which established mammography and Pap test screening programs to be administered by the Centers for Disease Control and Prevention (CDC) for low-income, medically underserved women. Funding

FIGURE 7.1

KEY BREAST CANCER LEGISLATION ENACTED BY CONGRESS AND SELECTED BILLS INTRODUCED, 1990-JULY 1998

	ENACTED	INTRODUCED
101st CONGRESS (1989-90)	Breast and Cervical Cancer Mortality Prevention Act of 1990 (P.L 101-354) Omnibus Budget Reconciliation Act of 1991 (Mammography reimbursement) (P.L. 101-508)	WHEA of 1990 (20 bills, including provisions for breast cancer research funding)
102nd CONGRESS (1991-92)	Mammography Quality Standards Act of 1992 (P.L. 102-539)	Breast Cancer Basic Research Act (H.R. 381/S.512) Breast Cancer Informed Decision Act (H.R. 382) Medicaid Women's Basic Coverage Act (H.R. 1129)
103rd CONGRESS (1993-94)	NIH Revitalization Act of 1993 (Breast cancer research funding) (P.L. 103-62) DOD Authorization Act (Breast cancer research funding) (P.L. 103-160) Breast and Cervical Cancer Mortality Prevention Act Reauthorization (P.L. 103-183)	Medicaid Mammography Coverage Act (H.R. 425) National Breast Cancer Strategy Act (S. 1454)
104th CONGRESS (1995-96)	DOD Authorization Act (Breast cancer research, treatment, and prevention programs) (P.L. 104-61)	Department of Veterans Affairs Mammography Quality Standards Act (H.R. 882) Breast Cancer Research Extension Act (H.R. 3443)
105th CONGRESS (1997-98)	Balanced Budget Act of 1997 (Expanded Medicare mammography coverage) (P.L. 105-33) Stamp Out Breast Cancer Act (Stamp sales to raise research revenue) (P.L. 105-41)	Breast Cancer Patient Protection Act (H.R. 135/S. 143) Reconstructive Breast Surgery Benefits Act (H.R. 164/S. 609) Mammography Quality Standards Act Reauthorization (S. 537) Consumer Involvement in Breast Cancer Research Act (H.R. 1352/S. 86) Mammography Standards for Veterans (S. 999) Breast Cancer Research Extension Act (H.R. 1070/S. 67)

WHEA: Women's Health Equity Act (first introduced in 1990)
NIH: National Institutes of Health
DOD: Department of Defense

Source: Women's Policy, Inc.

for this initiative, the National Breast and Cervical Cancer Early Detection Program, increased from $30 million in fiscal year 1991 to $145 million in 1998. By March 1997, nearly 600,000 mammograms had been provided and over 3,000 women had been diagnosed with breast cancer through the program (Centers for Disease Control and Prevention 1998).

Other policy initiatives also addressed breast cancer screening. As part of the 1991 Omnibus Budget Reconciliation Act, a WHEA provision restored Medicare coverage for biennial screening mammograms for women ages 65 and over after the mammography benefit had been struck from the bill (Schroeder and Snowe 1994). Medicare coverage of mammography was later expanded, and as of 1997 includes annual mammograms for women over the age of 39 (Women's Policy, Inc. 1997). The Mammography Quality Standards Act of 1992 established federal standards and accreditation procedures for mammography facilities to be effective in late 1994.

Beginning in 1990, bills in the WHEA have provided for increased funding for breast cancer research. Between 1990 and 1997, federal funding for breast cancer research increased more than fivefold, from $81 million to $521 million (Women's Policy, Inc. 1997). This included allocations to the NIH, where the National Cancer Institute (NCI) is the main funder of breast cancer research, and to the Department of Defense (DOD). In 1992, at the urging of the NBCC and with the help of Senator Tom Harkin, whose family had experienced breast cancer, Congress appropriated $210 million for breast cancer research in the DOD budget, making DOD the second largest source of support for breast cancer research after the NCI. Researcher Patricia Kaufert points out the powerful symbolism of this event: "The defense budget, the ultimate expression in economic and political terms of male power, had been coopted by and for women" (1998:301). Despite widespread initial skepticism, the DOD breast cancer program has become a model for innovation and consumer participation in research review panels (Cordes 1997).

In 1993, the NBCC delivered 2.6 million petition signatures to the Clinton White House, demanding a national strategic plan to eradicate breast cancer. After a planning conference chaired by Donna Shalala, Secretary of Health and Human Services, President Clinton established the National Action Plan on Breast Cancer in 1994 to craft a national strategy for research, health care, policy, and the education of consumers, providers, and scientists. The National Action Plan was designed as a public-private partnership, co-directed by the Deputy Assistant Secretary of Health for women's health in the Department of Health and Human Services and the President of the NBCC. Its steering committee includes government and nongovernment members from research, policy, health care, breast cancer advocacy, and industry organizations. The National Action Plan's activities have included awarding nearly 100 grants for research and outreach projects, with consumers participating on panels reviewing research grant proposals. In addition, the Plan has monitored insurance coverage of clinical trials and informed consent issues in breast cancer research, published a position paper on genetic testing, provided testimony before Congress, and conducted conferences and workshops.

THE STATE LEVEL: REGULATING MANAGED CARE

Breast cancer policy also was made at the state level, where the major responsibility for regulating insurance resides. In the 1990s, the rapid growth of managed care attracted public scrutiny of its cost containment strategies and benefits structures, and attempts to regulate managed care at the state level often addressed women's health. Examples include state legislation to ensure women's access to obstetrician-gynecologists and to mandate coverage of minimum lengths of hospital stays for deliveries (Hellinger 1996). A reasonable hypothesis is that this legislative initiative occurred because both lawmakers and the groups promoting regulation—usually segments of the medical profession and some consumer groups—

viewed women's health as a popular cause among the public and as a difficult one for politicians to ignore.[6]

Breast cancer issues also figured in state legislation. By the end of 1992, 42 states plus the District of Columbia had legislation mandating insurance coverage of mammograms (Kaufert 1996). In addition, by 1995, at least 14 states had enacted or had legislation pending that required insurers to cover, under some circumstances, autologous bone marrow transplantation (ABMT) for breast cancer treatment (U.S. General Accounting Office 1996). Although ABMT was widely regarded as an unproven, experimental procedure and cost between $80,000 to over $150,000 per patient, some patients had successfully sued insurers who had denied coverage of the treatment. Ironically, an unintended consequence of wider insurance coverage of ABMT was increased difficulty recruiting women to NCI-sponsored clinical trials to determine ABMT's efficacy (Dickersin and Schnaper 1996). The case of ABMT is a poignant illustration of the dilemmas inherent in mandating insurance coverage for experimental medical procedures.

THE ROLE OF BREAST CANCER
ADVOCACY GROUPS IN THE 1990S

Members and staff of the Congressional Caucus for Women's Issues credit the breast cancer advocacy community with much of the policy successes at the national level (Schroeder and Snowe 1994; Women's Policy, Inc. 1996). As we have seen, single-issue breast cancer advocacy groups were becoming organized for national action at the same time that the women's health advocacy community was beginning to shape a new legislative agenda in Washington, and the groups were well positioned both to stir the waters and to catch the wave for the 1990s episode in women's health policymaking. These organizations did more than help frame breast cancer issues for politicians; they also helped identify policy options, they successfully lobbied for increased research funding and new sources of funding, and they defined a participatory role for consumers (i.e., women with breast cancer) in the breast cancer research agenda.

The NBCC entered a policy context in which previous efforts to address breast cancer had focused largely on mammography screening (its safety, efficacy, use, and insurance coverage) and on treatments for breast cancer. What the NBCC introduced into this mix after 1991 was attention to the overall breast cancer research agenda and how it is set. Advocates redirected attention to the need for research on the causes, primary prevention, and ultimate cure for breast cancer. In addition, distrustful of business as usual in the established cancer research organizations, breast cancer groups sought direct consumer participation in policymaking bodies responsible for setting the research agenda (e.g., the NCI's National Cancer Advisory Board), deciding what research projects are funded (e.g., through the DOD and the National Action Plan on Breast Cancer), designing the way in which projects would be conducted, and disseminating findings (Dickersin and Schnaper 1996).

The research community, however, often resists consumer involvement in scientific advisory councils and grant review panels, because consumers are perceived as relying on anecdotal evidence and lacking the expertise to evaluate scientific data and research proposals. Recognizing this concern, the NBCC developed an innovative training program, Project LEAD (Leadership, Education, and Advocacy Development), to prepare consumers for roles on committees and advisory panels, institutional review boards on human subjects in research, and panels to review research grant applications. The original curriculum for Project LEAD was designed by Kay Dickersin, then a University of Maryland epidemiologist, member of the NCI's National Cancer Advisory Board, and a member of the NBCC.

Instituted in 1995, Project LEAD trained 125 women in intensive four day workshops held in different locations around the country during the project's first year of operation (Dickersin and Schnaper 1996). The workshops were conducted by biomedical researchers and NBCC board members on such topics as the epidemiology of breast cancer, basic science relating to the cell, genetics and breast cancer, and research design and methods. By preparing advocates in this way, the NBCC hoped both to place its trainees in more positions from which they could influence breast cancer policy and to give them a basic vocabulary to have a voice in research agenda-setting.

OTHER STAKEHOLDER INTERESTS

Despite their high visibility and recent policy successes, breast cancer groups are not the only stakeholders in breast cancer policy, nor do they always control the public policy agenda. Although breast cancer is a popular bipartisan political issue, this popularity does not imply that all groups share the same interests or agree on strategies. The interests and goals of the various stakeholders in both the public and private sectors may coincide or conflict, and groups may compete for financial resources (e.g., from government agencies, corporate sponsors, or private donors) or social resources (e.g., recognition as the leading authority on some aspect of breast cancer). These dynamics help illuminate some current controversies and suggest some possible consequences of recent breast cancer policymaking.

In the public sector, stakeholders include Congress and a number of federal agencies, such as the NIH, NCI, CDC, and FDA. In Congress, members' careers may depend in part upon appearing responsive to the various constituencies interested in women's issues. Congress appropriates funds and otherwise influences the federal agencies that have specific mandates related to biomedical research, screening or treatment services, and regulation of medical products. These agencies, in turn, have interests in promoting and controlling these mandates, and they view themselves as the guardians of scientific standards in biomedical research and in its applications in clinical practice and policy.

The NIH, for example, traditionally resists earmarked funding allocated to support research on a particular disease, such as breast cancer. Earmarks, however, have been a key policy option supported by breast cancer advocates, the Congressional Caucus for Women's Issues, and some members of the biomedical community whose programs stand to benefit from the funding. Earmarks typically are viewed by NIH as external political interference in its authority to determine its research priorities, to award funding to the most scientifically meritorious projects, and to support basic (as opposed to clinical or applied) research. Some members of Congress also may resist earmarked funding because they are deluged with multiple demands from diverse advocacy groups—often referred to as the disease of the month—or because they would like to spend money on other things. Earmarking NIH funds for one disease takes away from others, unless the NIH budget is increased or another source of funding (e.g., the DOD) is found. Earmarking DOD funds for breast cancer research, however, has been opposed by some Congressional supporters of the defense budget, who see it as detracting from the mission of the nation's defense.

Public and private organizations that comprise the establishment cancer community—such as the NCI, the American Cancer Society (ACS), and cancer research and treatment centers—have a mutual stake in promoting cancer research, screening, and treatment agendas. Typically dominated by physicians active in cancer research or practice, these organizations tend to view themselves as having particular expertise in breast cancer. The ACS is a leading cancer charity, promoter of screening mammography, and funder of cancer research; however, advocacy groups have criticized it for failing to address the problem of poor women's access to mammography, and they have criticized the ACS, NCI, and CDC for neglecting research on environmental causes and primary prevention of breast cancer and on treatments for women diagnosed with breast cancer (Langer 1992). Advocacy groups also are concerned about the ethics of expanded screening in the absence of universal access to treatment and follow-up care.

Associations of health professionals and of organizations involved in cancer research, screening, or treatment represent the interests of their members as providers of services. Physicians' specialty associations (e.g., the American College of Radiology, American College of Surgeons, American College of Obstetricians and Gynecologists) promulgate practice guidelines that define the standard of practice for screening or treatment services, and they often lobby for health insurance coverage or other favorable market conditions for the services they provide. The American College of Radiology, for example, has been an active proponent of insurance coverage for mammography since the 1980s. Medical specialty groups generally resist what they perceive as interference in their authority to set standards in their professional field of expertise, and they tend to oppose efforts to limit third-party reimbursement for the services they provide. In seeking health insurance coverage for such services as mammography, physicians' associations often find allies in consumer groups seeking expanded benefits.

Health insurance companies and managed care organizations typically resist government regulations of their practices, including mandated benefits for screening or treatments, particularly if the covered procedures have not been proven to be effective. Private employers, who are the principal payers of private health insurance and the architects of health insurance benefits packages, similarly resist mandates because they limit employers' efforts to control their health care costs. Unions or trade groups representing women workers tend to advocate for increased access to health services for women and for broader health insurance benefits.

Private industry also has demonstrated its interests in breast cancer. In addition to pharmaceutical firms and other manufacturers that market products related to breast cancer, companies in a variety of industries see benefits in supporting breast cancer initiatives. Corporate donors in the cosmetics and fashion industries, in particular, are interested in marketing to middle-class women's causes and have provided financial support to breast cancer advocacy groups, researchers, breast care centers, and community service programs. Examples include Revlon's support of breast cancer research and the Revlon-UCLA Breast Center, and Ralph Lauren's support of the Nina Hyde Center for Breast Cancer Research at Georgetown University (Belkin 1996).

Finally, women's health advocacy and interest groups that focus either on single issues other than breast cancer, on a broad range of women's health issues, or on the health interests of special groups of women (e.g., ethnic groups, disabled women, lesbians) comprise an issue network in women's health.[7] Examples of multi-issue organizations with a national scope include the National Women's Health Network and the Boston Women's Health Book Collective. While these groups do not command large budgets and could compete with breast cancer groups for public attention and financial resources, they also may form coalitions with the clout to promote a variety of issues. During the health care reform episode of the early Clinton administration, for example, the Campaign for Women's Health coalesced over 100 diverse organizations—including health-focused organizations, women's rights groups, and trade unions—to promote a broad women's agenda and comprehensive benefits package within national health care reform (Kasper 1996). The NBCC participated in the Campaign, which went on hiatus when health reform failed.

A CASE STUDY IN BREAST CANCER POLICYMAKING

The NIH Consensus Development Conference on Breast Cancer Screening for Women Ages 40-49, which convened in Bethesda, Maryland, on January 21-23, 1997, at the request of the director of the NCI, provides a case study in how multiple interests interact in breast cancer policymaking. The case also illustrates that breast cancer advocacy groups do not always control the breast cancer policy agenda.

NIH consensus development conferences are convened to resolve scientific controversies and to produce an authoritative statement based on an objective review of the existing body of evidence.[8] This particular conference was intended to address the longstanding debate about the efficacy of regular mammography screening for women ages 40 to 49. In addition to resolving the scientific issue, however, the conference's findings were expected to have important policy implications for public and private health insurance coverage of mammography, for standard medical practice, and, potentially, for the public health burden of breast cancer.

The context in which this consensus conference was convened included the heightened activity surrounding breast cancer research and services, as well as a history of organizational disagreements on mammography for women in their forties. Regular mammography screening for women 50 years old and over is endorsed by most organizations, but screening for women in their forties had been a contentious issue since the 1970s. Just as experts differed in their interpretations of the scientific evidence, organizations differed in their recommendations to women and their providers. In 1996, the ACS, American College of Radiology, American Medical Association, American College of Obstetricians and Gynecologists, and other organizations recommended mammography screening for women every one or two years beginning at age 40 and annual screening beginning at age 50. Organizations recommending that regular mammography screening begin at age 50 included the American Academy of Family Physicians, the American College of Physicians, the U.S. Preventive Services Task Force, and the NCI (U.S. Preventive Services Task Force 1996).

The positions that organizations took, furthermore, were not immune from partisan politics. In 1993, the NCI had reversed its earlier endorsement of screening for women in their forties, arguing that there was insufficient scientific evidence to justify it. The ACS and 20 other cancer organizations disagreed, however. Both NCI and President Bill Clinton took much criticism for NCI's change of view. For example, in a 1993 article in the *Wall Street Journal,* Dr. Bernadine Healy, who had been Director of the NIH in the Bush administration, accused the Clinton administration of using the reversed NCI recommendations as a rationale for denying mammography coverage to women in their forties under its health care reform plan, which she opposed. She also called for an NCI-funded trial of mammography for women in their forties to resolve the scientific questions (Healy 1993). Clinton administration officials, including Donna Shalala, defended the NCI decision and the health reform package.

Thus, it could be argued that the 1997 NIH Consensus Development Panel was expected to resolve both a scientific and a political controversy. Convened as an impartial panel, it originally consisted of 13 members (one later resigned), including medical and scientific experts (radiologists, obstetrician-gynecologists, surgeons, epidemiologists, and statisticians) and consumer representatives. The latter were Julia Scott, President and CEO of the National Black Women's Health Project, and Constance Rufenbarger, a woman with breast cancer and consumer advocate. The panel held a preconference review of the research literature and an intense, contentious three-day conference in which it reviewed scientific studies and heard presentations and testimony. Radiologists addressing the meeting were particularly strong supporters of mammography for women in their forties, based on recent Swedish data suggesting that such screening could reduce the breast cancer death rate by between 15 and 23 percent (Taubes 1997).

At the end of the conference, the panel issued a preliminary report in which it concluded:

> At the present time, the available data do not warrant a single recommendation for mammography for all women in their forties. Each woman should decide for herself whether to undergo

mammography. Given both the importance and complexity of the issues involved in assessing the evidence, a woman should have access to the best possible information in an understandable and usable form. Her health care provider must be equipped with sufficient information to facilitate her decision-making process. (NIH Consensus Development Panel 1997a:7)

The panel's report referred to this as a "recommendation for informed decision-making" and also recommended that for women in their forties who choose to have mammography, "costs of the mammograms should be reimbursed by third-party payors [sic] or covered by health maintenance organizations" (NIH Consensus Development Panel 1997a:7).

The panel's conclusion on screening was a reasonable one based on the state of the scientific evidence. The language in the preliminary report, however, was perfunctory and did not elaborate the concept of informed decision making nor the key phrase "decide for herself." This language left the panel open to the accusation that it had merely passed the buck to women consumers.

The reaction to the preliminary report was swift and mixed. Although some individuals and organizations not associated with the panel praised the report, on the day of its release (January 23, 1997), NCI Director Richard Klausner stated that he was "shocked" by the panel's recommendations and announced that the National Cancer Advisory Board would soon review the report (Kolata 1997a:A1). This public statement undercut his own consensus panel and probably contributed to some members' reconsideration of the recommendations and to the panel's subsequent publication of both a majority and minority report.[9] In an editorial on January 28, 1997, the *New York Times* called the preliminary report a "muddled message," and Bernadine Healy referred to it as a "panel of Babel" (1997:1). Rather than interpreting the report as supporting women's informed decision making, many commentators interpreted it as a recommendation that women in their forties should *not* get mammograms. Radiologists were particularly strong critics of the report, and Harvard radiologist Daniel Kopans declared the panel's conclusion "fraudulent" (Taubes 1997:1057).

Congress then entered the action. The panel chairman, Johns Hopkins epidemiologist Leon Gordis, was summoned to defend the panel's recommendation before a special hearing of Senator Arlen Specter's Senate Subcommittee on Labor, Health and Human Services, and Education Appropriations, which authorizes spending for NIH and NCI. In statements for the *Congressional Record,* Specter made it clear that he urgently wanted a recommendation endorsing screening for all women in their forties, and he was in a position to pressure NCI for this result because of his power to endorse or oppose budget increases for the agency. His motives were interpreted, at least in part, as a fallout of gender politics: He was thought to have embraced women's health issues after his aggressive interrogation of Anita Hill during the Clarence Thomas confirmation hearings and his subsequent close race for re-election against a female challenger. He was not the only senator supporting expanded mammography screening, however. On February 4, 1997, at the request of Olympia Snowe, the Senate unanimously supported a nonbinding resolution calling for guidelines on the benefits of screening mammography for women in their forties and urging the NCI's National Cancer Advisory Board (NCAB) to reissue its 1993 guidelines recommending screening for women ages 40 to 49 (Women's Policy, Inc. 1997). The entire Senate apparently perceived the issue as a political winner.

In March 1997, the NCAB voted 17 to 1 that the NCI should recommend mammography screening every one to two years for women in their forties. Agreeing with the consensus panel's recommendations, Kay Dickersin cast the dissenting vote. The ACS weighed in with a new recommendation that women in their forties should be screened *annually.* Quickly adopting the NCAB recommendation, the NCI reversed itself again and issued a recommendation that women in their forties should get screening mammograms every one to two years. Both the chair of the NCAB, behavioral scientist Barbara Rimer of Duke University, and the director of the NCI denied that the decision was the result of political pressure (Kolata 1997b).

Nevertheless, this episode has been widely described as a case of politics trumping science. Several scientific bodies, including the NCI and the NCAB, were pressured to change their positions because of political considerations, thus casting doubt on their institutional integrity. How one feels about politics in this case may depend on one's understanding of science. Some see the scientific process as rational and objective, based on evidence and intendedly divorced from politics. Others believe that science is inherently political and subject to biases and special interests in much the same ways as any human endeavor. Political processes, furthermore, may be understood as a way to integrate diverse points of view, including those of scientists and others, as a basis for policy decisions.

Some, however, have mistakenly interpreted these events as a case of "science versus advocacy." For example, two University of North Carolina physicians argued that the policy debate on mammography screening was "distorted" by single-issue advocacy groups and gender politics "led by female senators" (Ransohoff and Harris 1997). They specifically suggested reducing the influence of emotional single-issue advocacy groups and promoting a rational, physician-led public education effort. They failed to acknowledge that single-issue advocacy did not determine the outcome of the screening debate. In fact, the two consumer representatives on the NIH consensus panel endorsed the panel's majority report; the dissenting vote on the NCAB was by an influential member of the NBCC; and breast cancer advocacy groups generally supported the consensus panel recommendations and were not responsible for the ensuing events that caused the NCI to reverse its own panel.

Among the advocacy and interest groups supporting the consensus panel's recommendations were the National Women's Health Network, the National Breast Cancer Coalition, the Center for Medical Consumers in New York, and the Long Island One in Nine Breast Cancer Group.[10] These groups, as we have seen, typically are more interested in promoting primary prevention and effective treatment for breast cancer than in expanding mammography screening. They also are concerned about younger women's increased risks of false positive mammograms, which carry both psychosocial and financial consequences.[11]

Advocates who supported the consensus panel report drew attention to the paternalistic nature of criticisms of the panel for not making a blanket recommendation for mammography screening. They pointed out that women are capable of understanding complex health information, weighing conflicting evidence, and dealing with uncertainty in decisions about their health. Cindy Pearson, Executive Director of the National Women's Health Network, defended the consensus panel recommendation and pointed out: "It is way past time to stop giving women simplistic information. Women deserve to know everything that researchers know, even if it is not clear cut" (Pearson 1997:1).

In this instance, breast cancer advocacy groups were not the most influential architects of breast cancer screening policy. Instead, special interest groups within the medical community—especially radiologists—and members of Congress were dominant. The case illustrates that the mammography screening debate is inherently political. It is not only about resolving differences in interpretations of scientific data on efficacy or incorporating the findings from the latest studies; it is also about the implications of recommended guidelines for health insurance coverage of mammograms, for reimbursement to providers and facilities that provide mammograms, for breast cancer research funding, for the credibility of individuals and organizations on different sides of the debate, and for women's health.

IMPLICATIONS OF
BREAST CANCER POLICYMAKING FOR WOMEN

Recent breast cancer policymaking was part of a larger episode in women's health policymaking in the 1990s that focused on securing equity for women in health research and services. Breast cancer became a popular women's health issue on the national agenda because of the larger context of women's health activism, because it is less controversial than abortion or other hot-button health issues, and because of the efforts of a highly organized advocacy community. Precisely because of its broad appeal, however, breast cancer became an issue championed by diverse groups motivated not only by the desire to improve women's health but also by political or economic self-interest.

On balance, recent breast cancer policymaking could be viewed as having both positive and negative consequences for women. On the plus side, recent policy has increased women's awareness of breast cancer risks and controversies; improved financial access to mammography screening among traditionally underserved segments of the female population and among Medicare recipients; increased overall utilization of mammography; promoted quality assurance in mammography facilities; increased government's financial investment in breast cancer research; broadened the topics investigated in breast cancer research; and established mechanisms for consumer participation in the research agenda–setting process. On the minus side, recent policymaking has exaggerated the risk of breast cancer relative to other threats to women's health; failed to address the nonfinancial access barriers to mammography, such as not having a regular source of health care; provided conflicting messages about mammography screening, particularly for women in their forties; inadequately addressed women's financial access to effective treatments for breast cancer; and generated controversy about the role of consumer advocates in the policymaking process. It is too early to tell whether the policy initiatives of the 1990s will produce the research breakthroughs or the clinical interventions to substantially reduce mortality and morbidity associated with breast cancer.

The current state of breast cancer policymaking raises two key questions about how policy should be made in order to benefit women's health. First, what is the appropriate role of consumer advocates in policymaking? Breast cancer advocacy and interest groups do not always control the policy agenda, but they deserve major credit for raising the profile of breast cancer as an issue on the public agenda. In addition, it can be argued that these groups provide a needed counterweight to the influence of biomedical experts who too often fail to perceive the ways that scientific inquiry and medical practice can be biased in the identification of research priorities or in the interpretation of findings.

Perhaps most notably, breast cancer activists have transformed the policymaking process and have provided models for other consumer groups seeking to influence health policy. Not satisfied with external influence strategies alone, they have crafted mechanisms to participate in formal policymaking processes and to change the institutions within which breast cancer policy is made. Breast cancer organizations have become partners with government in the National Action Plan on Breast Cancer, have placed their representatives on key advisory committees (e.g., the National Cancer Advisory Board) and grant review panels (e.g., in the DOD and as part of the National Action Plan), and have created an innovative program to train consumers to serve in these capacities. In these new participatory roles, advocates are helping to set research funding priorities, to design breast cancer research projects, and to establish breast cancer screening policy. They also provide a model for health policymaking more generally.

These innovations have not been without controversy. The high visibility and participation of breast cancer advocacy groups probably accounts for their sometimes being blamed for creating tensions between consumers and scientists or medical experts. In the case of the consensus panel on mammography screening for women in their forties, as we have seen, blaming advocacy groups for the tensions was an erroneous framing of the situation and served to deflect attention from heated disagreements and competing interests within the biomedical community. In this climate, the credibility of women's health advocacy groups still has not been established with some segments of the health policymaking community, and advocacy groups may expect to continue to encounter resistance.

The second question raised by recent breast cancer policymaking has to do with the relative advantages and disadvantages of single-issue—that is, disease-specific—policymaking. Although there are important political and strategic reasons why breast cancer policymaking emerged in the 1990s, the wisdom of focusing public attention and resources on a single disease, rather than on a broader women's health agenda, is open to debate. The advantages of single-issue women's health policymaking are that it focuses attention and resources on a problem that may have been neglected in the past and for which targeted policy options can be identified, debated, and implemented. In the case of breast cancer, furthermore, the issue was successfully framed as one relevant to all women and therefore of broad appeal and symbolic importance.

The disadvantages of single-issue policymaking, however, are that it encourages competition among diverse health advocacy and interest groups for limited resources, including public attention and financial support; it can arouse opposition to such policy options as earmarked research funding that are perceived as taking resources away from other important health problems; and it can contribute to the fragmentation of women's health care services by focusing attention on one disease or body part rather than on social conditions or services that promote overall health. An unintended consequence of successful single-issue policymaking in women's health is that it can detract attention and resources from a broader women's health agenda. Knee-jerk responses to breast cancer issues have been evident in Congress, as the case of the debate about mammography screening for women in their forties has shown. The danger exists that lawmakers who support various breast cancer policies—whether these policies are promoted by breast cancer advocacy groups or not—will believe that they have responded to women's health concerns and need not address other issues, such as reproductive rights, women's access to health care, or the environmental conditions that promote women's health.

What are the prospects for U.S. breast cancer policymaking? Scholarship on social problems suggests that no matter how persistent breast cancer advocacy groups or other stakeholders are, it may be difficult to sustain the high visibility and political currency of breast cancer issues for long. Women's health issues, like all issues, compete for attention on the public agenda and cycle through periods of high and low recognition as problems requiring policy responses. On the other hand, breast cancer advocates now participate in the institutions responsible for policy, and ongoing programs—such as the National Action Plan on Breast Cancer and funded activities at the NIH, DOD, and CDC—create constituencies for breast cancer initiatives. Even if substantial improvements in breast cancer mortality were realized, the multiple stakeholders in breast cancer policy are likely to focus on new technologies (such as genetic testing and gene therapy) and on continuing issues having to do with prevention or access to services.

The political opportunities for breast cancer policymaking, therefore, are not likely to disappear. Continued efforts will be needed, however, to ensure that policymaking incorporates the viewpoints of consumers and serves the interests of women's health.

NOTES

AUTHOR'S NOTE: I am grateful to Kay Dickersin, Paula Lantz, Susan Ferguson, and Anne Kasper for their helpful comments on a draft of this chapter. My work on this chapter was supported in part by a Robert Wood Johnson Foundation Investigator Award in Health Policy Research.

1. Although the episode during the 1960s and 1970s is commonly referred to as the Women's Health Movement, waves of Women's Health Movement activity have spanned the nineteenth and twentieth centuries. These waves and their interconnections are discussed by Carol Weisman (1998). The 1960s and 1970s wave set the stage for activism in the 1990s, in part by creating a climate in which many women's health problems, including breast cancer, could become a matter of public discourse. In addition, some key women's health advocacy and interest groups were founded during that era (e.g., the National Women's Health Network and the Boston Women's Health Book Collective).

2. The political scientist John Kingdon defines a policy window as "an opportunity for advocates of proposals to push their pet solutions, or to push attention to their special problems" (1995:165). Examples of policy windows include a change of administration, budget cycles, a scheduled renewal of a program, a crisis or focusing event, or a shift in national mood.

3. The history of mammography screening for breast cancer and its surrounding controversies are described by Patricia Kaufert (1996). Cancer control efforts focusing on mammography screening intensified in the mid-1980s and spawned research to establish the safety and effectiveness of screening, debates about clinical guidelines for screening, efforts to establish quality standards for mammography facilities, legislation in some states on insurance coverage of mammograms, and efforts to obtain Medicare coverage of mammography. All of these activities helped set the stage for policy developments in the 1990s.

4. In 1987, lung cancer surpassed breast cancer as the leading age-adjusted cancer cause of death in U.S. women (Collins et al. 1994). Breast cancer, however, is the most frequently diagnosed cancer in U.S. women.

5. This claim is somewhat ironic, given the long history of Women's Health Movements and cases of women organizing to influence policy on specific health problems. Examples include Progressive Era women's activism on infant and maternal mortality, which succeeded in obtaining the first federal programs to address these problems (Skocpol 1992), and the abortion rights movement of the 1960s and early 1970s (Staggenborg 1991). The recent policy successes of AIDS activists, however, may have been more salient to breast cancer activists than these other examples. The breast cancer advocacy community, furthermore, benefited from comparisons between AIDS and breast cancer with respect to number of lives lost (greater for breast cancer) and the relative amount of public resources devoted to the two diseases (greater for AIDS) (Kaufert 1998).

6. Contrary to conventional wisdom, women's health advocacy and interest groups did not lead these legislative initiatives, which tended to be promoted by special interests within the medical community. Women's health groups rarely publicly opposed the initiatives, however. By the end of 1997, 32 states had legislation providing some form of direct access to obstetrician-gynecologists; besides obstetrician-gynecologists—who were the leading proponents of the legislation—groups supporting it included the National Women's Law Center, the March of Dimes, and the Junior League (National Conference of State Legislatures 1998). Women's health advocacy groups did not uniformly support this legislation, and several opposed it.

In the case of the postpartum hospital stays, obstetrician-gynecologists and pediatricians were leading proponents of state and federal legislation mandating insurance coverage of minimum stays. Both the American College of Obstetricians and Gynecologists and the American Academy of Pediatrics issued guidelines on minimum stays. The American College of Nurse-Midwives opposed the Newborns' and Mothers' Health Protection Act in 1995 on the grounds that the time limits on inpatient care were arbitrary and the legal scope of practice of providers other than physicians was not recognized in the legislation (American College of Nurse-Midwives 1995).

7. Women's health advocacy and interest groups are diverse. They vary on a number of dimensions, including whether they are single- or multiple-issue and the degree to which their scope is local or national, membership is predominantly grass-roots or professional, activities are member-focused or policy-focused, and resources are provided largely by members or include corporate or public contributions. A recent study by Sheryl Ruzek and Julie Becker (1999) identifies 223 U.S. women's health advocacy organizations with a national scope.

8. The assumptions built into the NIH consensus process—that important controversies can be resolved in three-day consensus conferences, that conference participants are impartial, or that expert reports change behavior at the clinical level—can, of course, be disputed. Suzanne Fletcher discusses some of these points (1997).

9. Personal communication with Leon Gordis, chairman of the consensus panel. The final consensus panel report was issued with a minority report, coauthored by a radiologist and an obstetrician-gynecologist, concluding that "we should actively encourage routine screening mammography for women in their forties" (NIH Consensus Development Panel 1997b).

10. A key exception was the National Alliance of Breast Cancer Organizations (NABCO), a network of organizations providing screening and treatment services, which supported screening women in their forties.

11. The risk of false positive mammograms in younger women is nontrivial. The NIH consensus panel estimated that "as many as 3 out of 10 women who begin annual screening at the age of 40-years-old will have an abnormal mammogram during the next decade" (NIH Consensus Development Panel 1997b:1017).

REFERENCES

Altman, Roberta. 1996. *Waking Up, Fighting Back: The Politics of Breast Cancer.* Boston: Little, Brown.

American College of Nurse-Midwives. 1995. "The American College of Nurse-Midwives Statement for the Record on S.969 Newborns' and Mothers' Health Protection Act of 1995 before Senate Committee on Labor and Human Resources." Washington, D.C.: American College of Nurse-Midwives.

Batt, Sharon. 1994. *Patient No More: The Politics of Breast Cancer.* Charlottetown, P. E. I., Canada: Gynergy Books.

Belkin, Lisa. 1996. "Charity Begins at . . . the Marketing Meeting, the Gala Event, the Product Tie-In." *New York Times Magazine* (December 22) 40.

Centers for Disease Control and Prevention (CDC). 1998. "The National Breast and Cervical Cancer Early Detection Program At-A-Glance." Atlanta: Centers for Disease Control and Prevention, National Center for Chronic Disease Prevention and Health Promotion.

Collins, Karen Scott, Diane Rowland, Alina Salganicoff, and Elizabeth Chait. 1994. "Assessing and Improving Women's Health." Pp. 109-53 in *The American Woman 1994-95: Where We Stand—Women and Health*, ed. C. Costello and A. J. Stone. New York: W.W. Norton.

Cordes, Colleen. 1997. "Defense Department Wins Praise for Its Research Program on Breast Cancer." *The Chronicle of Higher Education* (December 19) A29-31.

Dickersin, Kay, and Lauren Schnaper. 1996. "Reinventing Medical Research," Pp. 57-76 in *Man-Made Medicine: Women's Health, Public Policy, and Reform*, ed. Kary L. Moss. Durham, N.C.. Duke University Press.

Faludi, Susan. 1991. *Backlash: The Undeclared War Against American Women*. New York: Crown Publishers.

Ferraro, Susan. 1993. "The Anguished Politics of Breast Cancer." *New York Times Magazine* (August 15).

Fletcher, Suzanne W. 1997. "Whither Scientific Deliberation in Health Policy Recommendations? Alice in the Wonderland of Breast-Cancer Screening." *New England Journal of Medicine* 336:1180-83.

Healy, Bernadine. 1993. "Mammograms—Your Breasts, Your Choice." *Wall Street Journal* (December 28).

———. 1997. "Screening Mammography for Women in Their Forties: The Panel of Babel." *Journal of Women's Health* 6:1-3.

Hellinger, Fred J. 1996. "The Expanding Scope of State Legislation." *Journal of the American Medical Association* 276:1065-70.

Kasper, Anne S. 1996. "The Making of Women's Health Public Policy." Working Paper. Chicago: University of Illinois at Chicago, Center for Research on Women and Gender.

Kaufert, Patricia A. 1996. "Women and the Debate over Mammography: An Economic, Political, and Moral History," Pp. 167-86 in *Gender and Health: An International Perspective*, ed. Carolyn F. Sargent and Caroline B. Brettell. Upper Saddle River, N.J.: Prentice Hall.

———. 1998. "Women, Resistance, and the Breast Cancer Movement." Pp. 287-309 in *Pragmatic Women and Body Politics*, ed. Margaret Lock and Patricia A. Kaufert. Cambridge: Cambridge University Press.

Kingdon, John. 1995. *Agendas, Alternatives, and Public Policies*. 2nd ed. New York: HarperCollins.

Kolata, Gina. 1997a. "Mammogram Talks Prove Indefinite." *New York Times* (January 24) A1, A15.

———. 1997b. "Another Group Switches on Frequency of Mammograms." *New York Times* (March 28) A16.

Langer, Amy S. 1992. "The Politics of Breast Cancer." *Journal of the American Medical Women's Association* 47:207-9.

Lantz, Paula M., and Karen M. Booth. 1998. "The Social Construction of the Breast Cancer Epidemic." *Social Science and Medicine* 46:907-18.

Love, Susan M. 1995. *Dr. Susan Love's Breast Book*. 2nd ed. Reading, Mass: Addison-Wesley.

National Conference of State Legislatures. 1998. "Access to OB/GYN." Health Tracking Service. Washington, D.C.: National Conference of State Legislatures.

National Institutes of Health Consensus Development Panel. 1997a. "National Institutes of Health Consensus Development Statement: Breast Cancer Screening for Women Ages 40-49." Draft Report, January 21-23.

———. 1997b. "National Institutes of Health Consensus Development Conference Statement: Breast Cancer Screening for Women Ages 40-49, January 21-23, 1997." *Journal of the National Cancer Institute* 89:1015-21.

Pearson, Cynthia. 1997. "Mammography Controversy." *Network News* 22(2):1.

Ransohoff, David F., and Russell P. Harris. 1997. "Lessons from the Mammography Screening Controversy: Can We Improve the Debate?" *Annals of Internal Medicine* 127:1029-34.

Ries, L. A. B., B. A. Miller, B. Hankey, C. L. Kosary, A. Harras, and B. K. Edwards (eds.). 1994. *SEER Cancer Statistics Review, 1973-1991: Tables and Graphs.* Bethesda, MD: National Cancer Institute.

Ruzek, Sheryl Burt, and Julie Becker. 1999. "The Women's Health Movement in the United States: From Grass-Roots Activism to Professional Agendas." *Journal of the American Medical Women's Association* 54:4-9.

Schroeder, Patricia, and Olympia Snowe. 1994. "The Politics of Women's Health." Pp. 91-108 in *The American Woman 1994-95: Where We Stand—Women and Health,* ed. C. Costello and A. J. Stone. New York: W.W. Norton.

Skocpol, Theda. 1992. *Protecting Soldiers and Mothers: The Political Origins of Social Policy in the United States.* Cambridge: Harvard University Press.

Soffa, Virginia M. 1994. *The Journey Beyond Breast Cancer: From the Personal to the Political.* Rochester, Vt: Healing Arts Press.

Stabiner, Karen. 1997. *To Dance with the Devil: The New War on Breast Cancer.* New York: Delacorte Press.

Staggenborg, Suzanne. 1991. *The Pro-Choice Movement: Organization and Activism in the Abortion Conflict.* New York: Oxford University Press.

Taubes, Gary. 1997. "The Breast-Screening Brawl." *Science* 275:1056-59.

U.S. General Accounting Office. 1996. *Health Insurance Coverage of Autologous Bone Marrow Transplantation for Breast Cancer.* Washington, D.C.: U.S. General Accounting Office, Health, Education, and Human Services Division.

U.S. Preventive Services Task Force. 1996. *Guide to Clinical Preventive Services.* 2nd ed. Baltimore, MD: Williams & Wilkins.

Weisman, Carol S. 1998. *Women's Health Care: Activist Traditions and Institutional Change.* Baltimore, MD: Johns Hopkins University Press.

Witt, Linda, Karen M. Paget, and Glenna Matthews. 1994. *Running as a Woman: Gender and Power in American Politics.* New York: Free Press.

Women's Policy, Inc. 1996. *The Women's Health Equity Act of 1996: Legislative Summary and Overview.* Washington, D.C.: Women's Policy, Inc.

———. 1997. *Women's Health Legislation in the 105th Congress.* Washington, D.C.: Women's Policy, Inc.

Controversies in Breast Cancer Research

Sue V. Rosser, Ph.D.

The cover article "Advances in Breast Cancer Research" of a recent *Harvard Women's Health Watch* exemplifies why much of breast cancer research remains controversial. Although the article begins, "In the last few months, breast cancer research appears to have undergone a climatic shift," its content becomes restricted to two drugs for prevention (tamoxifen and raloxifene) and two for treatment (paclitaxel and Herceptin) of the disease (Robb-Nicholson 1998a). By reporting on drugs with side effects, such as increased risk of uterine cancer and blood clots, and with relatively small effects in preventing and treating the disease in certain high risk groups, this article typifies the biomedical approach to illness that characterizes breast cancer research.

Not surprisingly, controversies in breast cancer research demonstrate many of the problems that women's health, in general, has suffered at the hands of a male-dominated, hierarchical health system that is based on a biomedical model of medicine. The biomedical model focuses on anatomy and physiology and causes of disease at the cellular, hormonal, and genetic levels rather than behavioral, social, and environmental contributions to disease. Since breast cancer is impacted by behavioral and environmental factors and is not a major health problem for men, it has received low priority, funding, and attention. The selection of diseases for investigation in biomedical research is determined primarily by a national agenda that defines what is worthy of study and of receiving funding. This chapter explores how biases in breast cancer research that result from this system and model translate into problems with risk factor prevention, screening, detection, and treatment. These problems contribute to conflicting policies and messages surrounding mammography screening, autologous bone marrow transplantation (AMBT), tamoxifen, and breast implants.

BIOMEDICAL MODEL

ORIGINS OF SCIENTIFIC METHODS

Most researchers in the behavioral, biomedical, and physical sciences are trained in the scientific method and believe in its power. Few, however, are aware of its historical and philosophical roots in logical positivism and objectivity. Positivism implies that "all knowledge is constructed by inference from immediate sensory experiences" (Jaggar 1983:355-56). It is premised on the assumption that human beings are highly individualistic and obtain knowledge in a rational manner that may be separated from their social conditions. This assumption leads to the belief in the possibilities of obtaining knowledge that is both objective and value-free, the cornerstone of the scientific method.

In *Science as Social Knowledge,* Helen Longino (1990) explores the extent to which methods employed by scientists can be objective and lead to repeatable, verifiable results while contributing to hypotheses or theories that are congruent with subjective institutions and ideologies of the society. "Background assumptions are the means by which contextual values and ideology are incorporated into scientific inquiry," she believes (p. 216). The institutions and beliefs of our society reflect the fact that the society is patriarchal. Even female scientists have only relatively recently become aware of the influence of patriarchal bias in the paradigms of science.

FEMINIST CRITIQUES

In the past two decades, feminist historians, philosophers of science, and feminist scientists[1] have elucidated the bias and absence of value neutrality in science, particularly biology. By excluding females as experimental subjects, focusing on problems of primary interest to males, utilizing faulty experimental designs, and interpreting data based in language or ideas constricted by patriarchal parameters, scientists have introduced bias or flaws into their experimental results in several areas of biology. These flaws and biases were permitted to become part of mainstream scientific thought and were perpetuated in the scientific literature for decades. Because most scientists were men, values held by them as males were not distinguished as biasing. Rather, male values were congruent with the values of all scientists and thus became synonymous with the "objective" view of the world (Keller 1982, 1985) and what aspects of it were studied. Since few men experience breast cancer, the relative low priority of breast cancer research may be a reflection of their world view.

A first step for feminist scientists was recognizing the possibility that androcentric or male bias would result from having virtually all theoretical and decision-making positions in science held by men (Keller 1982). Not until a substantial number of women had entered the profession (Rosser 1986) could this androcentrism be exposed. As long as only a few women were scientists, they had to conform to the male view of the world to be successful and have their research meet the criteria for "objectivity."

Once the possibility of androcentric bias was revealed, feminist scientists set out to explore the extent to which it had distorted science at various levels: the choice and definition of problems to be studied, the exclusion of females as experimental subjects, bias in the methodology used to collect and interpret data, and bias in theories and conclusions drawn from the data. They also began to realize that, since the practice of modern medicine uses a biomedical approach based in positivist research in biology and chemistry and depends heavily on clinical research, any flaws and ethical problems in this research are likely to result in poorer health care and inequity in the medical treatment of disadvantaged groups.

The biomedical model, although too restrictive an approach for most diseases, remains especially inadequate for women's health, particularly for breast cancer. Using only the methods traditional to a particular discipline results in limited approaches that fail to reveal sufficient information about the problem being explored. Narrowly focused disciplinary research may provide particular difficulties for studies exploring medical problems of pregnancy, childbirth, menstruation, and menopause, for which the methods of one discipline are clearly inadequate. Social and behavioral factors, such as diet, exercise, and smoking, as well as physiological, hormonal, and other biological parameters may influence each of these reproductive events. Early in this phase of emphasis upon women's health, Jean Hamilton called for interactive models that draw on both the social and natural sciences to explain complex problems: "Research on heart disease is one example of a field where it is recognized that both psychological stress and behaviors, such as eating and cigarette smoking, influence the onset and natural course of a disease process" (1985:VI-62).

BIOMEDICAL MODEL APPLIED TO BREAST CANCER

As with most women's health issues, the biomedical model remains too restrictive for exploring causes, treatments, and prevention of breast cancer. Many critics of breast cancer research have pointed out that overreliance upon the biomedical model has focused attention on the cellular, hormonal, and genetic causes of the disease at the expense of attention to behavioral, social, and environmental causes (Altman 1996; Love 1990). This model, because it explores cancer cells, leads to an emphasis on treatment rather than on prevention (Batt 1994). Biomedicine has a tradition of researching disease and how to cure it rather than studying health and how to prevent illness (Bailar and Smith 1986). This tradition places responsibility at the level of the individual rather than the society as a whole. Focusing basic research at the level of the cell and below also has consequences for the types of treatments developed. Susan Love's characterization of "slash, burn, and poison" as the treatment methods for breast cancer highlights the cellular approach. The theory of cancer as cells growing out of control leads to treatments that attempt to limit cell growth by surgically removing the cells (slash), killing the cancer cells which divide more rapidly than nonmalignant cells (burn through radiation therapy), or changing the cellular environment to one that is less favorable for the growth of cancer cells (poisoning through chemotherapy). Individuals bear responsibility to undergo these cellular treatments; attention to the cellular level also implies a shift in focus to factors in individuals (genes, hormones, cell physiology) from societal factors (behaviors, environments) as causes and cures for cancer. These treatments encourage resources to be directed to treatment in individuals and away from societal prevention of cancer. They center on individual responsibility rather than overall societal responsibility for addressing environmental pollution, advertising to promote tobacco and alcohol, and attention to food additives, fat content, and preservatives.

HUMAN GENOME ERA

The human genome era has produced a particularly reductionistic version of the biomedical model, in which extreme attention is drawn to genetic causes for diseases. This genetic focus becomes necessary to justify the vast resources that are diverted from epidemiology and public health measures to prevent disease and are directed into the three-billion-dollar Human Genome Project. For breast cancer research, this redirection of resources helps to explain the focus on the isolation of the BRCA1 and BRCA2 genes. The media attention surrounding the isolation and copying of the breast cancer genes fueled the public perception that the overwhelming cause of breast cancer is hereditary and that a cure for the genetic cause will soon be found. The reality is that only 5 to 10 percent of breast cancer is inherited, and that the BRCA1 and BRCA2 genes are responsible for only half of the inherited cases (King, Rowell, and Love 1993). This leaves 90 to 95 percent of breast cancer cases unaccounted for by the BRCA1 and BRCA2 genes and points to the role caused by social, behavioral, and environmental factors.

The Human Genome Project and isolation of the BRCA1 and BRCA2 genes have resulted in more than a public misperception about the genetic cause for most breast cancer cases and a diversion of resources and attention away from prevention. It has led to a rush to apply for patents for actual genes and gene sequences (National Breast Cancer Coalition [NBCC] 1997). If these patents are granted, researchers other than those to whom the patents have been granted would be prohibited from using the genes or gene sequences without obtaining a license from the patent holder. The patent holder is free to charge a fee of any amount or to deny use to anyone for up to 17 years, thus stopping research completely or limiting it to only wealthy corporate or institutional researchers. If granted for genes or gene sequences, such patents may promote secrecy in research because once something is public, it is no longer patentable. Such secrecy may restrict collaborative research. Equally important, it will restrict the peer review of the research by competent professionals in two ways. First, researchers will wait to publish results until they have patents; second, other researchers cannot attempt to replicate experimental results unless they can afford to pay the patent fee. Patenting genes may represent an extreme form of the male, hierarchical, biomedical model where the genes become the property of the researcher, controlled for his interests. It seems difficult to imagine how such an approach would lead basic research in a direction to prevent breast cancer in women.

As a result of the isolation and copying of the BRCA1 and BRCA2 genes, several biotechnology firms and at least one academic medical center now market tests to detect genetic susceptibilities to breast cancer. Ignoring the fact that this move, again, takes attention away from social, behavioral, and environmental factors and prevention to focus on inherited susceptibilities, the test raises numerous other problems and ethical dilemmas. Marketed as laboratory services rather than products, the tests do not fall under regulation by the Food and Drug Administration (FDA). Thus, the tests have not undergone standardization before coming on the market, resulting in variation in the data on the effectiveness, safety, and implications of the tests. For example, two laboratories differed in the age estimates of the chance of getting breast cancer if the test is positive (NBCC 1997). Second, there is no "cure" or definitive treatment for a positive test. When an individual learns she has the BRCA1 or BRCA2 genes, she cannot "remove" the gene to prevent the development of cancer and is left with a terrible dilemma— whether to have her breasts removed prior to the development of cancer or live with the anxiety of knowing that she is likely to develop breast cancer at some point in her life. Third, some indicators suggest that insurance companies might view positive results as a basis for a preexisting medical condition (based on what happened with the gene for sickle cell anemia) and cancel coverage for those with the gene(s) (Lerman et al. 1994).

In short, the BRCA1 and BRCA2 gene sequencing may represent an exciting breakthrough in basic research. Yet, its implications for future collaborative and open research may be problematic because of patenting and its immediate impact upon testing and treatment. An unfortunate fallout from the work is the misperception held by some women that the BRCA1 and BRCA2 genes are the exclusive cause of breast cancer, and that, consequently, they might as well stop doing breast self-examination since cancer will be inevitable if they have the gene, or not occur if they lack the gene.

IMPLICATIONS OF THE BIOMEDICAL MODEL

Another limitation of the biomedical model with its cellular, hormonal, and genetic approaches is its tendency to center on the individual and her body while diverting attention from surrounding social, economic, and political factors that may contribute to the disease and its progress. The incidence of invasive breast cancer has increased one percent per year from 1940 until 1982 and four percent per year from 1982 until 1996 (American Cancer Society 1999). Studies from the 1970s documented a fivefold variation in breast cancer rates around the world (Armstrong and Doll 1975). Moreover, the incidence of breast cancer in Japanese women who migrate from their low-incidence home country to the United States becomes that of U.S. women (Buell 1973). These facts suggest that factors besides genetics are significant for the cause of the disease.

Inclusion of social, psychological, and public health perspectives are needed for a more comprehensive research base to also explore why poor women and women of color have higher death rates from breast cancer. Epidemiological approaches include these perspectives; they reveal factors important for disease prevention. Because the poor, in general, have a 10 to 15 percent lower cancer survival rate regardless of race, research that relies on biology alone and ignores socioeconomic factors will be unlikely to uncover the best way to remove this survival differential (See chapter 6 of this volume). Similarly, the fact that the five-year survival rate is 75 percent in white women compared to 63 percent for African American women (Altman 1996) is likely to be most fully explored when methods from social sciences are coupled with those from biomedicine. Such interdisciplinary approaches may tease apart the relative effects that more exposure to workplace and environmental carcinogens (see chapter 9 of this volume) and less access to high-quality medical care (see chapter 3 of this volume), nutritious food, and decent living conditions have upon the higher incidence and lower survival rates experienced by African Americans with regard to breast cancer. The 1994 National Institutes of Health (NIH) Guidelines for Inclusion of Women and Minorities as Subjects in Clinical Research require that the NIH ensure that women and minorities be included in all human subject research. Additionally, these guidelines require that these same groups be included in Phase III clinical trials in numbers adequate to allow for valid analyses of differences in intervention effects (U.S. Department of Health and Human Services 1994).

Epidemiological studies do attempt to consider or at least control for social, psychological, economic, and environmental factors by using matched cohorts (individuals who are the same for all variables except the risk factor under study) or case studies (individuals who differ only in whether or not they have the disease). Use of epidemiology in breast cancer research has begun to elucidate potential contributions of diet, lifestyle, and environmental factors to breast cancer, such as dietary fat content, smoking, exercise, and environmental contaminants. Due to the complexity of breast cancer, different epidemiological studies often yield conflicting results; sample size, failure to control for all variables, and length of study contribute to these conflicting results. Increased funding of epidemiological studies might not only lead to improved studies but also shift the focus to prevention.

MALE BIAS

Although difficulties with breast cancer research reflect the general problems facing women's health research in the United States at this time, breast cancer research faces some unique problems, partially as a result of the male-dominated hierarchical medical system. The $323.7 million 1995 budget of the National Cancer Institute (NCI) for breast cancer research demonstrates the biases in funding. This budget equals approximately the cost of one B-1 bomber. In fiscal year 1998, the National Institutes of Health received $460 million for breast cancer research funding. The Department of Defense breast cancer research program received an appropriation of $135 million for fiscal year 1998 (NBCC 1997:8) and requested $175 million for 1999 (NBCC 1998). Even compared to other diseases, breast cancer has received relatively little funding. For example, in 1989 the NIH spent far more money on AIDS research than it did on breast cancer research. From 1981 to 1994, 620,000 women died of breast cancer while approximately 270,000 people died of AIDS, a disease that can be prevented (Altman 1996).

In addition to assigning lower priority and directing relatively fewer dollars to women's health research, male domination of Congress and the leadership of the scientific and medical establishment leads to other demonstrated biases in medical research. Cardiovascular diseases (Healy 1991) and AIDS (Norwood 1988; Rosser 1994) stand as classic examples of diseases studied using the male-as-norm approach. Aspects of this approach included research designs that failed to assess gender differences in cardiovascular disease, case definitions that failed to include gynecologic conditions and other symptoms of AIDS in women until 1993, and exclusive use of males as research subjects in clinical trials.[2] This male focus resulted in an accumulation of data and methods that work for exploring health and disease in the male body against which to compare new data from research on cancer; a similar accumulation of data does not exist for the female body against which to assess new research in breast cancer.

LEGACY FROM EXCLUSION
OF WOMEN FROM CLINICAL TRIALS

Menstrual cycles may complicate drug metabolism, leading to increased time and cost in drug testing. Pharmaceutical companies also fear litigation from possible birth defects in fetuses that can result from testing drugs in women of childbearing age. These concerns deterred pharmaceutical companies from including women in clinical trials, despite the fact that, once the drugs came on the market, they often were prescribed more frequently for women than for men. Exclusion of women from clinical drug trials was so pervasive that a meta-analysis, published in September 1992 in the *Journal of the American Medical Association,* surveying the literature from 1960 to 1991 on clinical trials of medications used to treat heart attack, found that women were included in less than 20 percent and the elderly in less than 40 percent of those studies (Gurwitz, Nananda, and Avorn 1992). Thus, individuals most likely to benefit from these medications were excluded from most of the clinical trials. After the 1990 General Accounting Office critique of the NIH for inadequate representation of women and minorities in federally funded research and the passage of the Women's Health Equity Act, women were included more frequently in clinical trials. Unfortunately, including women failed to ensure that research results were analyzed by gender. A 1996 study including all prospective treatment and intervention studies published in the *New England Journal of Medicine,* the *Journal of the American Medical Association,* and the *Annals of Internal Medicine* between January and June in 1990 and 1994 revealed that only 19 percent of the 1990 studies and 24 percent of the 1994 studies reported any data analysis by gender, despite the fact that 40 percent of the subjects were female (Charney and Morgan 1996).

IMPACT ON BREAST CANCER

The research bias that excludes women from clinical trials and uses a male-as-norm approach has had negative effects for women when scientists study diseases that occur in both sexes. How has this bias affected a disease such as breast cancer? Since more than 90 percent of cases of breast cancer occur in women, the male has not usually been perceived as the norm for the disease in the way that he often is in other diseases such as AIDS and cardiovascular diseases.

Biomedical researchers used significant biological reasons, including estrus cycles in nonhuman females, menstrual cycles in women, and life span changes correlated with changes in the reproductive cycle, such as pregnancy and menopause, to justify their male focus. Only now, as a result of the Women's Health Initiative and other forces for change, are data comparable to that for the male body being collected on the effects of these female cycles to fill this dearth of information. For breast cancer research, this missing information would appear critical to understand causes and treatments of a disease where hormone levels and reproductive history have documented, critical roles. Differing estrogen levels among women and changing levels associated with pregnancy, breast-feeding, and menopause have been correlated with different risks, treatment successes, and mortality outcomes in breast cancer. A long history of understanding changes in hormone levels over the life cycle of women from diverse races, ages, and social classes, with differing reproductive backgrounds, would appear crucial for breast cancer research. The very cyclical nature of the female body and interactions between estrogen and other drugs may serve as keys to breast cancer breakthroughs. For example, the differential survival rate of women receiving surgery for tumor removal in the follicular compared to the luteal phase of the menstrual cycle (Hrushesky 1996; Hrushesky et al. 1989; Senie et al. 1991) suggests that stage of the ovulation cycle—i.e., hormone levels—significantly influence disease progression. Surgery in the early luteal stage of the cycle, which occurs just after ovulation, results in better survival rates. The substitution of a history of female-as-norm approaches, in which phases of the menstrual cycle and hormone levels and their interactions with drugs and surgery had been well studied, might have led to this discovery before 1989. Some of the current controversies in screening and treatment, such as mammography for premenopausal women and use of tamoxifen for prevention, might be better understood if decades of research had focused on pre- and postmenopausal women, their cycles, and hormonal interactions.

In a similar fashion, the history of general exclusion of women from clinical trials of drugs also has distorted clinical trials of medications to treat breast cancer. Some clinical trials for drugs, such as the early testing of estrogen treatments to prevent miscarriage (e.g., diethylstilbestrol [DES]), used male subjects only (Seaman and Seaman 1977). Although exclusive testing in male subjects was rare, failure to test on the individuals most likely to benefit from the medications was not. Through the 1980s less than five percent of American women with breast cancer participated in clinical trials; older women and African American women—those most at risk of dying from breast cancer—had even lower participation rates in clinical trial research,[3] often due to lack of knowledge about clinical trial research and access to participation (Paskett et al. 1996). Restricted eligibility criteria and low participation may limit the applicability of the data gleaned from such trials to all breast cancer patients and particularly to those at highest mortality risk. Physician bias in selection of patients (Begg 1988) and failure of physicians to offer trial participation (Paskett et al. 1996) become significant deterrents to participation for breast cancer patients.

HIERARCHY

The hierarchical nature of both the politics and funding of medical and scientific research in this country suggests why research on women's health issues has received relatively little attention and support, despite women being the majority of the population and health care consumers. As Marxist, African American, and feminist critics[4] of scientific research have pointed out, the research that is undertaken reflects the societal bias toward the powerful, who are overwhelmingly white, middle- to upper-class, and male. Significantly, the majority of the members of the U.S. Congress, who appropriate funds for the NIH and other federal agencies, fit this description, as do the individuals in the theoretical and decision-making positions within the medical hierarchy and scientific establishment. As a result, the relatively small amount of money directed toward research in women's health goes to the agencies controlled by the white male hierarchy and certainly little or none toward women's health groups. The lion's share of funding for breast cancer research has gone for years to the NIH; since 1993, the Department of Defense (DOD) has received approximately $1 billion directed toward breast cancer research (Department of Defense 2000:II-1).

Pressure from the contemporary women's movement provided the impetus to put women's health on the national agenda. The Women's Health Movement dismantled many of the underpinnings that support sexist treatment of women in research and medical practice (Altekruse and Rosser 1992). The feminist analyses of physicians' portrayal of women in textbooks (Scully and Bart 1973), the audacity of the Boston Women's Health Book Collective members to claim their bodies as their own (1973), and the founding of organizations, such as the National Women's Health Network in 1975, affected every aspect of reproductive and other women's health issues. Eventually, the pressure resulted in institutional and legal changes. For example, women began to use legal means, including class action suits, to gain admittance to medical schools. Moreover, medical malpractice actions (such as the case of the Dalkon Shield contraceptive) were initiated against physicians and pharmaceutical houses (Dowie and Johnston 1977). In 1973, the U.S. Supreme Court ruled abortion legal.

After the 1985 U.S. Public Health Service survey recommended that the definition of women's health be expanded beyond reproductive health, the General Accounting Office (GAO) reported that the NIH expended only 13 percent of its budget on women's health issues. In 1990, the GAO criticized the NIH for inadequate representation of women and minorities in federally funded studies (Taylor 1994). The same year the Congressional Caucus for Women's Issues introduced the Women's Health Equity Act. In 1991, Bernadine Healy, the first female director of the NIH, established the Office of Research on Women's Health and announced plans for the Women's Health Initiative (Healy 1991). The Women's Health Initiative was designed to collect baseline data and look at interventions to prevent cardiovascular disease, breast and colorectal cancer, and osteoporosis. This study and breast cancer funding within the NCI have been monitored carefully by women in Congress and others in an attempt to change the funding priorities and bias against women's health in general and breast cancer in particular.

Another aspect of hierarchy appears in the organization of medical subspecialties that may contribute to the dearth of research and lack of focus on breast cancer. The primary issue is that the breast does not fit into the territory of any particular specialty. The breast fails to fit the traditional location of obstetrics and gynecology, usually considered to be a woman's reproductive system below the waist—ovaries, oviduct, uterus, vagina, urethra, and associated glands. Even its involvement in sexual activity has not resulted in the breast being claimed as the province of obstetrics and gynecology. After birth, during lactation, the breast may briefly fit under pediatrics. For palpation to detect changes or lumps, it may fall into the territory of the obstetrician/gynecologist, general practitioner, or the internist during the course of a physical examination. Radiologists claim the breast for mammography screening.

Only after the breast becomes cancerous does it intersect with the territory of other specialists—the surgeon for lumpectomy or mastectomy, the pathologist for determination of malignancy, the oncologist to oversee chemotherapy, and the radiologist who delivers radiation to kill cancerous cells. Eventually, a plastic surgeon may undertake breast reconstruction. In brief, the breast is the territory of virtually all specialists and of none. Although the notion of a team of specialists now enjoys recognition as the favored approach for patient treatment, the typical breast cancer research project does not routinely use such a large, interdisciplinary team of researchers. Since the organization of the NIH correlates with the medical specialties, it is not remarkable that breast cancer research fell through the cracks until fairly recently.

TRANSLATION OF RESEARCH BIASES INTO PRACTICE

Not surprisingly, the biases of male-dominance, hierarchy, and overreliance on the biomedical model that distort basic research have led to problems with breast cancer risk factor determination, prevention, screening, detection, and treatment. Conflicting policies and messages surrounding mammography screening, autologous bone marrow transplantation for advanced breast cancer, tamoxifen as a preventive agent, and the FDA breast implants decision result from biases in research and policy.

MAMMOGRAPHY

The most recent outrage in the continuing controversy over the advisability of routine mammography screening for women in their forties exemplifies the legacy of these biases. This controversy came to a head over the NIH Consensus Development Conference on Breast Cancer Screening for Women Ages 40-49 in early 1997. (See chapter 7 of this volume.) The conference panel's report of January 23, 1997 found insufficient evidence to make a recommendation regarding efficacy of screening to reduce breast cancer mortality for women in this age group (Fletcher 1997).

Although many interpretations can be made from these continuing debates over mammography screening, one interpretation is that they are a consequence of the impact of a male-dominated, hierarchical health system that is based on a biomedical model of medicine. The influence of Congress and the Director of the National Cancer Institute (NCI) reveal the hierarchical nature of the system where funding priorities drive the research. More than a decade of disagreements over interpretations of mammography research between prestigious biomedical professional groups led to the NIH Consensus Development Conference. The American Cancer Society, the NCI, the American Medical Association, and the American College of Radiology ultimately recommended routine screening beginning at age 40. The U.S. Preventive Services Task Force, the American College of Physicians, and the Canadian Task Force on the Periodic Health Examination recommended beginning at 50 years old (Fletcher 1997). As the major federal medical research institute, the NIH was at the top of the hierarchy to settle this discrepancy.

Consumer advocates and women in Congress have come up against male-dominated medicine in the mammography controversy in particular and in attempts to increase women's health research and funding in general. Prior women's health examples should have increased the understanding of the importance of including women in research. Instead, failure to come to consensus on policy implications resulting from medical research sounds suspiciously similar to earlier arguments that women should be excluded from clinical trials.

The biomedical model contributed to the outrage of the scientists when Congress and the public questioned their failure to make decisions on the basis of the scientific experiments. Richard Klausner, Director of the NCI, noted honest disagreements, saying, "The data are complex and the evidence is not transparent. Different groups come to different conclusions because they have different standards of evidence" (Marwick 1997:1181). Other scientists suggested this controversy raised the issue of whether scientific debates should be approached by examining facts deliberately and carefully with the aid of unbiased, independent, scientific experts representing multiple disciplines, or within Congress and the *New York Times* (Fletcher 1997). In her *New England Journal of Medicine* article, Suzanne Fletcher suggests that questions about health care are increasingly being distorted by emotional, political, financial, and legal issues.

Unfortunately, she does not note that these same issues, especially political and financial ones, appear to have a direct impact on breast cancer research and survival rates. She also does not mention that the resources poured into research on genetic and cellular levels divert money from more and better designed epidemiological studies that might provide results to make consensus possible.

SILICONE IMPLANTS

The FDA decision to remove silicone implants from the market again demonstrated the biases that permeate issues in women's health and breast cancer research. Marcia Angell, Executive Editor of the *New England Journal of Medicine*, supported the Consensus Conference in its decision not to recommend a decision on mammography. She cited a lack of evidence and questioned the pressure from Congress and the NCI Director on the NCI Advisory Board to make a recommendation. Angell also wrote *Science on Trial: The Clash of Medical Evidence and the Law in the Breast Implant Case* (1997). In this book, she contends that the legal system and scientists use different criteria to judge the results of medical research. Angell argues that David Kessler, former Commissioner of the FDA, decided prematurely to ban silicone breast implants because of pressure from the legal system, breast cancer advocates, politicians, and the media. As in the case with mammography, the epidemiological results from studies on the effects of implants conflicted. Angell believes that the FDA ban occurred because of large financial settlements awarded to women by juries, based on anecdotal evidence of illness in individual women not supported by epidemiological studies. Angell contends that the scientific evidence from new studies that became available after the ban proves that the implants are not unsafe. Therefore, she casts the FDA ban as a horrifying trend where the anti-science, anti-medical American public, using the media and legal system, has taken over judgment of scientific and medical evidence.

Critical of feminists, lawyers, politicians, and health care consumers, Angell denounces them as anti-science, money seeking, and hypochondriacal. She fails to understand how the biased history of funding research may have contributed to the push for the ban. Although she mentions diethylstilbestrol (DES), the Dalkon Shield contraceptive, and the exclusion of women from clinical trials in passing, she does not seem to link the politicians, women's health advocates, and the legal system, which revealed the cover-up or disregard of scientific evidence in these earlier cases, to why these groups may have mobilized in the implants case. She demonstrates little sympathy for time pressures faced by women who have breast cancer and want guidelines upon which they can base decisions for reconstructive surgery and their health care.

Angell's critique appears to reflect a hierarchical approach in which the physicians and scientists make decisions with little consensus or interchange with other affected parties, such as women with breast cancer, Congress, and health consumer advocates. The critique accepts a restricted biomedical approach that gives limited attention to the psychological, social, and economic aspects of breast cancer's impact on women's lives. Her criticism does not appear to be woman-centered, despite her claim that she is a feminist (Angell 1997:13). She directly attacks feminists, as well as humanists, multiculturalists, and others who have criticized science as it is currently practiced. Angell interprets Sandra Harding's feminist critiques of science as not recognizing the reliability and verifiability of the scientific method, failing to understand Harding's "strong objectivity," which calls for the recognition of the cultural, social, and historical forces that shape the questions asked by scientists, their approaches, and the theories and conclusions drawn from their data (Harding 1993:17). This strong objectivity might correct a science that is too narrow. For the case of breast implants, strong objectivity provides a mechanism to include the data reported by women with implants, which Angell's more narrow view of science appears to overlook. In addition to the issues addressed by Angell in *Science on Trial*, the implant controversy raises other questions, such as the uses of science to make products that turn out to be harmful, the lack of rigorous testing, and the denial by the manufacturers of any responsibility for the science they have supported. Because implants remained on the market for almost 30 years without regulation, the implant controversy also raises questions about the role of the FDA in product testing, marketing, and regulation (see chapter 2 of this volume). Similar questions surrounding the FDA's role in testing and timing of product release arise in the tamoxifen trials.

TAMOXIFEN

The Breast Cancer Prevention Trial is a randomized, placebo-controlled clinical trial to evaluate the ability of tamoxifen to prevent breast cancer development in women at increased risk for the disease (Fisher et al. 1992). The suggested reason for the initial trial was that in three of eight studies of women with breast cancer, tamoxifen appeared to cause a statistically significant reduction in tumors in the other breast (Fugh-Berman and Epstein 1992). Problems arose, however, that included the extrapolation of data on reduction of additional tumors in women who already have cancer to women who are healthy and cancer-free. There was also evidence that tamoxifen might increase the risk of uterine cancer, blood clots, damage to the retina, and hepatitis. Nevertheless, the trial was initiated.

Before its initiation and throughout the trial, debate raged over giving a potentially carcinogenic drug to healthy women (Herman 1994). Two years into the study, data revealed that women taking tamoxifen tripled their risk for uterine cancer. This finding, plus emerging evidence of increased risk of blood clots, led the National Women's Health Network to describe the study as "an exercise in disease substitution rather than disease prevention," based on the argument of Adriane Fugh-Berman and Samuel Epstein (1992:1596). From March until the summer of 1994, recruitment of new women for the trial was suspended while investigation of research fraud and mismanagement were investigated in another NCI study also managed at the University of Pittsburgh by the National Surgical Adjuvant Breast and Bowel Project (NSABP). Almost simultaneously, Canada's Hamilton (Ontario) Regional Cancer Centre unanimously withdrew from the NCI Breast Cancer Prevention Trial because of informed consent issues arising from whether data on deaths and side effects of tamoxifen had been passed on to volunteers in the trial in a timely manner. They viewed this issue as particularly salient because the trial participants were healthy women, so that ethics of informed consent should include "medicine's special obligations to healthy volunteers" (Raloff 1994:6).

Throughout the trial, volunteers and the public continued to receive confusing messages. On September 3, 1998, the FDA panel recommended approval of tamoxifen for healthy women at high risk for breast cancer; high risk was defined for this study as women over 60 years old or younger women with a strong family history or a previous abnormal biopsy. The study of 13,388 high-risk, healthy women showed that after four and one-half years of therapy, those on tamoxifen were 45 percent less likely to get breast cancer than those on a placebo. The same report announced that tamoxifen more than doubled the risk of uterine cancer, tripled the risk of blood clots and cataracts, and may cause fetal abnormalities in pregnant women (Robb-Nicholson 1998b).

Almost simultaneously, two European studies, the Italian Tamoxifen Prevention Study of 5,408 women and the United Kingdom study of 2,494 women were released, showing no protective effect for the drugs. Although the differences between the findings from the two European studies and the results of the U.S. trial may be partially due to variation in the studies' composition, the U.S. study had a shorter follow-up period. The European studies suggest that tamoxifen may only delay, rather than prevent, breast cancer (Robb-Nicholson 1998b).

Once again, women at risk for breast cancer face confusing messages about how to address their risk. Should they take tamoxifen and possibly delay their chances of getting breast cancer but increase their risk of uterine cancer, blood clots, cataracts, and perhaps other diseases? Will the FDA's approval of this drug after a shorter period of testing than undertaken in European studies lead to healthy women developing disease in the United States?

The confusing messages sent to the public over implants and the use of tamoxifen for breast cancer prevention appear again in the debate over the use of autologous bone marrow transplantation (AMBT) for breast cancer therapy, revealing similar biases of hierarchy, male dominance, and overreliance on the biomedical model. (For a discussion of AMBT see chapter 4 of this volume.)

CONCLUSION

As researchers announce new climatic shifts in breast cancer studies (Robb-Nicholson 1998a), behavioral, social, and environmental factors should become part of the climate for this research. Continuing to focus on the cellular, hormonal, and genetic causes represents a reductionistic approach to the problem. These approaches lead to drugs, radiation, and surgery as logical treatments for cancer. Reliance on these approaches will likely produce more drugs as the major treatments.

Feminist scholars have revealed the biases of male-dominance, hierarchy, and overreliance on the biomedical model that distort basic scientific research. These biases in research have led to failures to properly assess breast cancer risk factors, prevention, screening, detection, and treatment. Conflicting policies and messages surrounding mammography screening, ABMT for advanced breast cancer, tamoxifen as a preventive agent, and the FDA breast implants decision result from biases in research and policy. This research backdrop has permitted a steady increase in the incidence of breast cancer during the last 30 years, with relatively stable mortality and little progress in decreasing the death rate. Recently developed women-focused research agendas, as exemplified by the Women's Health Initiative, provide models to begin to eliminate research bias. Increased research and funding directed toward social, behavioral, and environmental causes of breast cancer initiate the steps needed to correct overreliance on the biomedical model.

NOTES

1. For feminist critiques of science, see Fee 1981, 1982; Haraway 1978, 1989, 1997; Harding 1986, 1993, 1998; Longino 1990; and Birke 1986; Bleier 1984, 1986; Fausto-Sterling 1992; Keller 1983, 1985, 1992; Rosser, 1988, 1994, 1997; Spanier 1995.
2. For more on the male-as-norm approach, see Grobbee et al. 1990; Multiple Risk Factor Intervention Trial Research Group (MRFIT) 1990; Steering Committee of the Physician's Health Study Group 1989; and Rosser 1994.
3. For more on women in clinical trials, see Lippman and Chabner 1986; Goodwin et al. 1988; Yancik, Ries, and Yates 1989; Hunter 1989.
4. See Zimmerman et al. 1980; McLeod 1987; Hubbard 1990.

REFERENCES

Altekruse, Joan M., and Sue V. Rosser. 1992. "Feminism and Medicine: Cooptation or Cooperation?" Pp. 27-40 in *The Knowledge Explosion,* ed. Cheris Kramarae and Dale Spender. New York: Teachers College Press.

Altman, Roberta. 1996. *Waking Up/Fighting Back: The Politics of Breast Cancer.* Boston: Little, Brown.

American Cancer Society 1999. "Breast Cancer Facts and Figures." Atlanta, Ga.

Angell, Marcia. 1997. *Science on Trial: The Clash of Medical Evidence and the Law in the Breast Implant Case.* New York: W.W. Norton.

Armstrong, B., and Richard Doll. 1975. "Environmental Factors and Cancer Incidence and Mortality in Different Countries, with Special Reference to Dietary Practice." *International Journal of Cancer* 15:617-31.

Bailar, John C., and Elaine Smith. 1986. "Progress Against Cancer?" *New England Journal of Medicine* 8:1226-32.

Batt, Sharon. 1994. *The Politics of Breast Cancer.* Charlottetown, P. E. I, Canada: Gynergy Books.

Begg, C. B. 1988. "Selection of Patients for Clinical Trials." *Seminars in Oncology* 15:434.

Birke, Lynda. 1986. *Women, Feminism, and Biology.* New York: Methuen.

Bleier, Ruth. 1984. *Science and Gender: A Critique of Biology and its Theories on Women.* New York: Pergamon Press.

———. 1986. "Sex Differences Research: Science or Belief?" Pp. 147-64 in *Feminist Approaches to Science,* ed. Ruth Bleier. New York: Pergamon Press.

Boston Women's Health Book Collective. 1973. *Our Bodies, Ourselves.* New York: Simon & Schuster.

Buell, P. 1973. "Changing Incidence of Breast Cancer in Japanese-American Women." *Journal of the National Cancer Institute* 51:1479-1783.

Charney, Pamela, and Carole Morgan. 1996. "Do Treatment Recommendations Reported in the Research Literature Consider Differences Between Women and Men?" *Journal of Women's Health* 5(6):579-84.

Department of Defense. 2000. Breast Cancer Research Program, Program Announcement. U.S. Army Medical Research and Materiel Command. Fort Detrick, Md.

Dowie, Mark, and Tracy Johnston. 1977. "A Case of Corporate Malpractice and the Dalkon Shield." Pp. 89-104 in *Seizing Our Bodies,* ed. Claudia Dreifus. New York: Vintage Books.

Fausto-Sterling, Anne. 1992. *Myths of Gender.* New York: Basic Books.

Fee, Elizabeth. 1981. "Is Feminism a Threat to Scientific Objectivity?" *International Journal of Women's Studies* 4:213-33.

———. 1982. "A Feminist Critique of Scientific Objectivity." *Science for the People* 14(4):8.

Fisher, Bernard, Carol Redmond, Leslie Ford, and Susan Nayfield. 1992. "Investigators of the Breast Cancer Prevention Trial Reply." *New England Journal of Medicine* 327(22):1596-97.

Fletcher, Suzanne. 1997. "Whither Scientific Deliberation in Health Policy Recommendations: Alice in the Wonderland of Breast-Cancer Screening." *New England Journal of Medicine* 336(16):1180-83.

Fugh-Berman, Adriane, and Samuel Epstein. 1992. "Should Healthy Women Take Tamoxifen?" *New England Journal of Medicine* 327(22):1596.

Goodwin, J. S., W. C. Hunt, C. R. Key, and J. M. Samet. 1988. "Cancer Treatment Protocols: Who Gets Chosen?" *Archives of Internal Medicine* 148:2258.

Grobbee, D. E., E. B. Rimm, E. Giovannucci, G. Colditz, M. Stampfer, and W. Willett. 1990. "Coffee, Caffeine, and Cardiovascular Disease in Men." *New England Journal of Medicine* 321:1026-32.

Gurwitz, J. H., F. C. Nananda, and J. Avorn. 1992. "The Exclusion of the Elderly and Women from Clinical Trials in Acute Myocardial Infarction." *Journal of the American Medical Association* 268(2):1417-22.

Hamilton, Jean. 1985. "Avoiding Methodological Biases in Gender-Related Research." In *Women's Health Report of the Public Health Task Force on Women's Health Issues.* Washington, D.C.: U.S. Department of Health and Human Services.

Haraway, Donna. 1978. "Animal Sociology and a Natural Economy of the Body Politic, Part I: A Political Physiology of Dominance;" and "Animal Sociology and a Natural Economy of the Body Politic, Part II: The Past is the Contested Zone: Human Nature and Theories of Production and Reproduction in Primate Behavior Studies." *Signs: Journal of Women in Culture and Society* 4(1):21-60.

———. 1989. "Monkeys, Aliens, and Women: Love, Science, and Politics at the Intersection of Feminist Theory and Colonial Discourse." *Women's Studies International Forum* 12(3):295-312.

————. 1997. *Modest_Witness@Second_Millenium: Femaleman⊕Meets Oncomouse:™ Feminism and Technoscience*. New York: Routledge.

Harding, Sandra. 1986. *The Science Question in Feminism*. Ithaca: Cornell University Press.

————. 1993. *The "Racial" Economy of Science: Toward a Democratic Future*. Bloomington: Indiana University Press.

————. 1998. *Is Science Multicultural?* Bloomington: Indiana University Press.

Healy, Bernadine. 1991. "Women's Health, Public Welfare." *Journal of the American Medical Association* 264(4):566-68.

Herman, Robin. 1994. "Tamoxifen on Trial." *Washington Post* (September 23) 9-10.

Hrushesky, William. 1996. "Breast Cancer, Timing of Surgery, and the Menstrual Cycle: Call for Prospective Trial." *Journal of Women's Health* 5(6):555-66.

Hrushesky, William, A. Z. Bluming, S. A. Gruber, and R. B. Sothern. 1989. "Menstrual Influence on Surgical Cure of Breast Cancer." *Lancet* 2:949.

Hubbard, Ruth. 1990. *Politics of Women's Biology*. New Brunswick: Rutgers University Press.

Hunter, C. P. 1989. "Cancer Control and the Community Oncology Programs: Minority Participation in the National Cancer Institute Clinical Trials Network." P. 94 in *Minorities and Cancer*, ed. L. A. Jones. New York: Springer-Verlag.

Jaggar, Alison M. 1983. *Feminist Politics and Human Nature*. Totowa, N.J.: Rowman and Allanheld.

Keller, Evelyn Fox. 1982. "Feminism and Science." *Signs* 7(3):589-602.

————. 1983. *A Feeling for the Organism: The Life and Work of Barbara McClintock*. New York: W. H. Freeman.

————. 1985. *Reflections on Gender and Science*. New Haven: Yale University Press.

————. 1992. *Secrets of Life, Secrets of Death*. New York: Routledge.

King, Mary-Claire, Sara Rowell, and Susan M. Love. 1993. "Inherited Breast and Ovarian Cancer: What Are the Risks? What Are the Choices?" *Journal of the American Medical Association* 269(15):1975-80.

Kuhn, Thomas S. 1970. *The Structure of Scientific Revolutions*. 2d ed. Chicago: University of Chicago Press.

Lerman, C., M. Daly, A. Masny, and A. Balshem. 1994. "Attitudes about Genetic Testing for Breast-Ovarian Cancer Susceptibility." *Journal of Clinical Oncology* 12:843-50.

Lippman, Mark, and Bruce Chabner. 1986. "Editorial Overview of NIH Consensus Development Conference on Adjuvant Chemotherapy and Endocrine Therapy for Breast Cancer." *National Cancer Institute Monograph 1*. Bethesda, MD: National Institutes of Health.

Longino, Helen. 1990. *Science as Social Knowledge: Values and Objectivity in Scientific Inquiry*. Princeton: Princeton University Press.

Love, Susan M. 1990. *Dr. Susan Love's Breast Book*. New York: Addison-Wesley.

Marwick, Charles. 1997. "Final Mammography Recommendation." *Journal of the American Medical Association* 277(15):1181.

McLeod, S. 1987. *Scientific Colonialism: A Cross-Cultural Comparison*. Washington, D.C.: Smithsonian Institution Press.

Multiple Risk Factor Intervention Trial Research Group. 1990. "Mortality Rates After 10.5 Years for Participants in the Multiple Risk Factor Intervention Trial: Findings Related to a Prior Hypothesis of the Trial." *Journal of the American Medical Association* 263:1795.

National Breast Cancer Coalition (NBCC). 1997. "Legislative Update." *Call to Action* 4(3-4):6-8.

———. 1998. "Campaign: Vote Breast Cancer." *1998 Voting Record* 2 5(1):2.

Norwood, Chris. 1988. "Alarming Rise in Deaths." *Ms.* (July) 65-67.

Paskett, Electra D., Hyman B. Muss, L. Douglas Case, and M. Robert Cooper. 1996. "Participation in Clinical Treatment Trials: Factors Affecting Participation for Women with Breast Cancer." *Journal of Women's Health* 5(6):585-92.

Raloff, Janet. 1994. "Tamoxifen Turmoil: New Issues Emerge as Healthy Women Volunteer to Take Potent Drug." *Science News* 146(17):268-69.

Robb-Nicholson, Celeste. 1998a. "Advances in Breast Cancer Research." *Harvard Women's Health Watch* V(11):1-2.

———. 1998b. "New Studies Question Tamoxifen's Benefits." *Harvard Women's Health Watch* VI(1):7.

Rosser, Sue V. 1986. *Teaching Science and Health from a Feminist Perspective: A Practical Guide.* Elmsford, N.Y.: Pergamon Press.

———. 1988. "Women in Science and Health Care: A Gender at Risk." Pp. 3-15 in *Feminism Within the Science of Health Care Professions: Overcoming Resistance,* ed. Sue V. Rosser. Elmsford, N.Y.: Pergamon Press.

———. 1994. *Women's Health: Missing from U.S. Medicine.* Bloomington: Indiana University Press.

———. 1997. "The Next Millennium is Here Now: Women's Studies Perspectives on Biotechnics and Reproductive Technologies." *Transformations* 8(1):1-27.

Rubin, Rita. 1998. "FDA Panel Oks Two Breast Cancer Drugs." *USA Today* (September 3) 1D, 5D.

Scully, Diana, and Pauline Bart. 1973. "A Funny Thing Happened on the Way to the Orifice: Women in Gynecology Textbooks." *American Journal of Sociology* 78:1045.

Seaman, Barbara, and Gideon Seaman. 1977. *Women and the Crisis in Sex Hormones.* New York: Rawson.

Senie, R., P. Rosen, P. Rhondes, and M. Lesser. 1991. "Timing of Breast Cancer Excision During the Menstrual Cycle Influences Duration of Disease-Free Survival." *Annals of Internal Medicine* 115:337.

Spanier, Bonnie. 1995. *Impartial Science: Gender Ideology in Molecular Biology.* Bloomington: Indiana University Press.

Steering Committee of the Physician's Health Study Group. 1989. "Final Report on the Aspirin Component of the Ongoing Physician's Health Study." *New England Journal of Medicine* 321:129-35.

Taylor, C. 1994. "Gender Equity in Research." *Journal of Women's Health* 3:143-53.

U.S. Department of Health and Human Services. National Institutes of Health. 1994. "NIH Guidelines on the Inclusion of Women and Minorities as Subjects in Clinical Research; Notice." *Federal Register* 59:14508-15413.

Yancik, R., S. G. Ries, and J. W. Yates. 1989. "Breast Cancer in Aging Women: A Population-Based Study of Contrasts in Stage, Surgery, and Survival." *Cancer* 63:976.

Zimmerman, B., et al. 1980. "People's Science." Pp. 299-319 in *Science and Liberation,* ed. Rita Arditti, Pat Brennan, and Steve Cavrak. Boston: South End Press.

The Environmental Link to Breast Cancer

Sandra Steingraber, Ph.D.

> The possible contribution to recent cancer trends of the substantial worldwide increases in chemical production that have occurred since World War II (and the resulting increases in human exposure to toxic chemicals in the environment) has not been adequately assessed. It needs to be systematically evaluated.
>
> —Philip Landrigan, M.D.,
> Mount Sinai School of Medicine, 1992

When I first read these words, they prompted me to think about writing a book that would address the gap between knowledge about cancer trends and knowledge about environmental carcinogens. Five years later, I published *Living Downstream: A Scientist's Personal Investigation of Cancer and the Environment,* which represents my best attempt as both a biologist and a former cancer patient to examine the evidence—however preliminary—that we do have for an environmental link to human cancers. How much evidence is there? How should we take action in light of it?

Apparently, these questions are now on the minds of many people because I spent the next year traveling to different community groups, universities, hospitals, churches, and Congressional offices to talk about this link, often at the invitation or insistence of breast cancer activists. In June 1998, driving home from one of these speaking engagements in upstate New York, I thought about Landrigan's words again after an unexpected encounter on the highway.

The sun had just broken through the clouds. Cows grazed on the hills. Rain-wet roses bloomed in farmhouse yards. No traffic. Far ahead, a silver truck crawled slowly up the interstate's long upgrade, flanked front and rear by two red cars moving at an identical pace. It was a puzzling procession. As I approached, I could begin to make out the black letters stenciled onto the back of the truck: CAUTION: CHEMOTHERAPEUTIC WASTE. Around these words were other stencils: the red and yellow flowers that are the universally recognized symbols for radioactivity.

The possible contribution to recent cancer trends . . . increases in human exposure . . . needs to be systematically evaluated . . .

I was six months pregnant with my first child. Only two months earlier, I had held in my hands a vial of amniotic fluid that had just been withdrawn from my uterus for genetic evaluation. In that moment, I had felt once again the exquisite communion between body and earth: The water I drink—brought to me by rain and rivers and underground springs—fills the aquifer inhabited by the body of my unborn daughter. Now I could feel her turn and lurch within me as the words written on the back of the truck sank into my consciousness, and my hands gripped the steering wheel harder.

Whatever the specific contents inside that silver truck, I felt intimately familiar with them. A cancer patient by the age of 20, I have walked through plenty of doors marked with the same atomic flowers. I have held out my arm to receive injections of radioactive isotopes for CAT scans, bone scans, and intravenous pyelograms. I have dutifully drunk the chalky barium for GI series x-rays. I have placed my breasts between glass plates for mammograms. I have watched (through a video monitor) my best friend receive proton beam therapy at the Harvard University cyclotron. Always in the back of my ecologist's mind I have wondered what happened to the waste created by such activities. Where does the old radiation equipment end up when it is retired? Where do the contaminated gloves and syringes, the expired chemotherapy drugs, and all those radioactive implants go? In whose community are they laid to rest? In their toxic graveyards, do they threaten as many lives as they once claimed to have saved?

I have also tailed a few hazardous-waste hauling trucks in my day—mostly those hauling incinerator ashes to landfills. But I was not doing this kind of environmental detective work now that I was pregnant. I took my foot off the gas pedal and let my car drop back. In fact, I was frightened enough by the surreal parade in front of me that I took the first exit and found an alternative route home. However, I could not shake from my mind the quote that had started me thinking six years earlier about the necessity of addressing the historical and ecological contexts of human cancer.

Perhaps there is no more urgent need to do so than with breast cancer, a disease whose public conversation seems firmly focused on detection, treatment, and cure, and whose causes remain officially shrouded in mystery and silence. I believe we do have the beginnings of an ecological understanding of breast cancer. The evidence comes from several sources: studies of cancer registry data, studies of the geographic distribution of breast cancer, occupational studies, radiation studies, studies of the chemical contamination of the breast itself, and endocrinological studies of estrogen-mimicking chemicals. Altogether, these lines of evidence are beginning to tell a consistent story.

TIME TRENDS IN
BREAST CANCER INCIDENCE AND MORTALITY

Breast cancer is one of several cancers that have risen in incidence rate since the end of World War II, an event that marked the beginning of an exponential rise in the production and use of toxic chemicals. In general, U.S. European-American women born in the 1940s have had 30 percent more non-smoking-related cancers than did women of their grandmother's generation. Researchers estimate that women born in the United States between 1947 and 1958 have three times the rate of breast cancer than their great-grandmothers did when they were the same age. The most reliable data, however, come from the national cancer registry, which was only initiated in 1973. In the two decades since then, breast cancer incidence rose by nearly 24 percent in the United States.

During that time, of course, the introduction of mammography changed the way many U.S. women were diagnosed with the disease, presumably because malignancies could be identified before being felt as a lump. How much of the apparent rise in breast cancers, since the 1970s, can be explained by better and earlier detection? To answer this question, statisticians first look to see whether breast cancer incidence began to rise at the same time mammography became widely available. An internal audit of the data also can show whether groups of women with the highest rates of cancer are those receiving the most mammograms. Additionally, since mammograms purportedly detect cancer earlier, statisticians can check whether the diagnosis of small breast tumors has been increasing faster than the diagnosis of large advanced ones.

While still a matter of some debate, the most widely accepted estimate is that between 24 and 40 percent of the recent upsurge in breast cancer is attributable to earlier detection (Liff 1991; Proctor 1995:251). Underlying this acceleration still exists a gradual, steady, and long-term increase in breast cancer incidence. This slow rise—between one and two percent each year since 1940—predates the introduction of mammograms as a common diagnostic tool. Moreover, the groups of women in whom breast cancer incidence is ascending most swiftly—African Americans and the elderly—are among those least served by mammography.

Between 1973 and 1991, the incidence of breast cancer in females age 65 and older in the United States rose nearly 40 percent, while the incidence of breast cancer in African American females of all ages rose more than 30 percent (Feuer and Wun 1992; Harris 1992). Therefore, the majority of the increase in breast cancer cannot be explained by mammograms.

Since 1993, breast cancer incidence has begun to level off and even shows signs of declining. At this writing, this downward trend is neither strong enough (the decrease is very slight) nor stable enough (has not occurred long enough) to interpret. Some activists have pointed out that the leveling off of new breast cancer cases is coincident with a significant rise in the incidence of ductal cell carcinoma *in situ* (DCIS; a type of breast cancer that is confined within the breast ducts and which has not yet invaded surrounding tissue). DCIS is most often found by mammography rather than by self-examination and, because it is not invasive, is not counted in cancer registry data. If mammograms are indeed discovering breast cancers at earlier, more treatable stages, then perhaps the apparent decline in new breast cancer cases can be accounted for by this rise in DCIS cases. Not enough information is available to answer this question yet.

SPATIAL TRENDS IN
BREAST CANCER INCIDENCE AND MORTALITY

Several large studies have detected elevated breast cancer rates around hazardous waste sites. In 21 different New Jersey counties, breast cancer mortality among European American women rose as the distance from residence to dump site shrank (Najem et al. 1983; Najem et al. 1985a; Najem et al. 1985b). However, many of the clusters of excess breast cancer occurred in heavily industrialized counties so that air pollution from these sources confounded the results. Thus, a woman with breast cancer in northeastern New Jersey cannot know with certainty whether she is dying because of the air wafting down from the factory stacks or because of the water contaminated by the dump site.

In another large study, researchers scoured the United States for counties that met two criteria: First, their hazardous waste sites had contaminated the groundwater, and, second, this groundwater served as the sole source of drinking water for the residents. Meeting these qualifications were 593 waste sites in 339 counties in 49 states. Next, researchers obtained for each of these 339 counties 10 years' worth of cancer mortality data and compared them to cancer mortality data from counties without hazardous waste sites. Women living in hazardous waste counties turned out to suffer significantly higher mortality from breast cancer as well as lung, bladder, colon, and stomach cancers. In fact, counties with hazardous waste sites were 6.5 times more likely to have elevated breast cancer rates than counties without such sites (Griffith and Riggan 1989; Hoover and Fraumeni 1975).

A third large-scale study later corroborated these results. Looking specifically at breast cancer, researchers found that mortality rates at the county level were significantly correlated with hazardous waste sites slated for clean up on the National Priorities List (the so-called Superfund roster). Counties with the highest breast cancer mortality had four times as many facilities that treated and stored hazardous waste than the national average (Goldman 1991:116).

Studies, such as these three, are considered preliminary rather than definitive because possible confounding factors could not be eliminated. These include the possibility that residents living in counties with hazardous waste facilities are getting more cancers not because of the dumps but because they work for the companies that create the wastes or because they smoke or drink more.

Recent studies have attempted to control for these so-called lifestyle factors. In 1994, the New York State Department of Health released the results of a carefully controlled study of Long Island women that showed a significant association between residence near chemical plants and risk of contracting breast cancer. In other words, women with breast cancer were more likely to live near a chemical facility than women without the disease. Moreover, breast cancer risk rose with the number of facilities: The more chemical plants in the community, the higher the incidence of breast cancer. Risk also was related to distance. The closer a woman lived to one of these plants, the greater her chance of developing breast cancer. These associations were most pronounced from women who had lived near these industries between 1965 and 1975, as compared with 1975 to 1985, when state air standards had become stricter (Lewis-Michl et al. 1996; Melius et al. 1994; Schemo 1994). Although such links had already been established in animal studies, this study was the first to indicate that breast cancer in humans may be associated with air pollution. The Long Island Breast Cancer Study Project is still ongoing.

Similar studies are now underway on Cape Cod, Massachusetts. By 1993, the Massachusetts Department of Public Health had established that breast cancer in almost all the towns on the Cape exceeded the statewide average. Of the 10 towns with the highest breast cancer incidence in the state, seven are located on the Cape. These elevated rates cannot be explained by differences in screening practices. U.S. census data show that the women of Cape Cod are similar to the state's women in ethnicity and income. Out on Cape Cod, the Silent Spring Institute has not yet solved the puzzle of why breast cancer rates are 20 percent higher than elsewhere in Massachusetts (Steingraber 1998:80-84). By 1998, researchers had ruled out the possibility that the rate is skewed by a high retirement-age population; the most significant elevations in breast cancer are occurring among women younger than 65 years old. They also have ruled out most factors of lifestyle and inheritance: Smoking, alcohol consumption, early detection, reproductive history, and family history of breast cancer are not significantly different on the Cape (Rudel et al. 1998; Saltus 1997; Silent Spring Institute et al. 1997). Initial analysis of public drinking water supplies found few detections of cancer-causing or hormone-disrupting chemicals, although ground water analysis in areas near septic tanks show troubling signs of contamination with detergent surfactants that are known to mimic estrogens. A complete analysis of private wells remains to be done. In addition, research teams are now poised to collect environmental samples—dust, soil, and air—directly from women's homes. Having created an information system that combines environmental factors about the Cape—including pesticide use back to the 1940s and historic patterns of land use—the institute's team of scientists now has the ability to estimate exposures for every house lot on the Cape. These estimations will be the focus of the next phase of their research. Solvent-leaching water pipes that appear to be responsible for the clusters of bladder cancer on the Cape are also being investigated for their possible role in creating breast cancer risk.

Investigators in Kentucky have found a connection between breast cancer incidence and a class of pesticides called triazine herbicides. With demographics and reproductive histories corrected for, the highest breast cancer rates in Kentucky occur in the counties with the highest use of triazines (Kettles et al. 1997). The triazine herbicides are the most frequently used pesticides in the United States, primarily because they are used as weed-killers in corn fields. They are notorious ground water leachers, which means that many of us in the Midwest and Great Plains regions drink high levels of these farm chemicals in our tap water, especially in the spring months during the planting season. All of us are exposed through diet: Oranges and apples, for example, can bear residues of triazines as do meat, milk, poultry, and eggs, resulting from the ubiquitous use of corn in animal feed. Atrazine, the most popular of the triazines, has been shown to cause breast cancer in one strain of laboratory rat. Exposure to trace levels of atrazine also causes changes in the pituitary hormones that govern ovulation. In Italy, researchers have shown a correlation between exposure to triazine herbicides and ovarian cancer among women farmers (Donna et al. 1984; 1989). In spite of their enormous popularity in the United States, the triazines are heavily restricted for use in much of Europe precisely because of studies linking them to breast and ovarian cancers.

OCCUPATIONAL EXPOSURES AND BREAST CANCER

Links between breast cancer and workplace exposures to carcinogens are not well understood because, historically, women workers have not been the objects of study in occupational health investigations (Infante, personal communication).

Consider vinyl chloride, which is used in the manufacture of a substance familiar to us all—polyvinyl chloride, otherwise known as PVC or simply vinyl. Credit cards are made of PVC, as are garden hoses, lawn furniture, floor coverings, children's toys, and food packaging materials. PVC, in turn, is made up of many vinyl chloride molecules all bonded together. Vinyl chloride, a sweet-smelling gas at room temperature, has long been classified as a known human carcinogen. Its cancer-causing properties were discovered when high numbers of male vinyl chloride workers began contracting angiosarcoma, a rare cancer that causes tumors to grow inside the liver's blood vessels. The incidence among vinyl chloride workers was found to be 3,000 times higher than among the general population (Chiazze et al. 1977; Infante and Pesak 1994). Animal studies as well as further studies of male workers, also revealed the ability of vinyl chloride to contribute to lung and brain cancers. In response to these results, allowable workplace air levels of vinyl chloride were drastically reduced. However, it was not until researchers also studied female workers that vinyl chloride's potential as a breast carcinogen was uncovered. Subsequent laboratory studies showed that atmospheric vinyl chloride triggers breast tumors in female rats, even at the lowest dosages; so does ingestion of PVC dust. Such an association is certainly biologically plausible since vinyl chloride has an affinity for fat tissue.

Evidence for a link between vinyl chloride and breast cancer in women workers has broad implications for the rest of us. While vinyl chloride levels are very much lower outside the factory, significant exposures can occur among residents living near vinyl chloride and PVC facilities. The air currents that blow across hazardous waste sites also contain elevated levels of vinyl chloride. Vinyl chloride is a frequent contaminant of ground water, where it can remain for months or years because there is no pathway to the atmosphere. The flesh of fresh water fish also contains vinyl chloride.

According to the U.S. Agency for Toxic Substances and Disease Registry (ATSDR), each of these pathways exposes the general public to "negligible amounts" of this known carcinogen. However, no one knows the cumulative lifetime risk from all of these negligible exposures. The ATSDR also stated that "exposure to vinyl chloride either in the prenatal period or during early childhood years may result in an increased risk of cancer" later in life (U.S. Agency for Toxic Substances and Disease Registry 1990:4). If vinyl chloride caused only a very rare form of liver cancer, perhaps these multiple routes of tiny exposures would be less cause for alarm. However, as of 1994, breast cancer was the leading cause of death of American women age 35 to 50, and we are the first generation of women born after World War II when chlorinated chemicals, such as vinyl chloride, were first widely dispersed in the general environment (Women's Cancer Resource Center 1994).

In spite of all this preliminary evidence, no comprehensive study has ever been undertaken to examine vinyl chloride's contribution to breast cancer. In fact, the 1977 study of women PVC fabricators has never been followed up, even though cohorts of men exposed to vinyl chloride, and who demonstrate excesses of brain, liver, and lung cancer, have been periodically updated. This omission is especially frustrating to Peter Infante, the Director of the Health Standards Program at the Occupational Safety and Health Administration, whose job it is to set limits on vinyl chloride levels in workplace air. Lack of interest in investigating a possible vinyl chloride–breast cancer link, says Infante, serves as an example of indifference to the plight of women in the workplace—indeed, to the plight of women everywhere (Infante and Pesak 1994).

LINKS BETWEEN
CHEMICAL EXPOSURE AND BREAST CANCER

We know with certainty that trace amounts of chemicals linked to breast cancer in laboratory animals are found within the breast tissue of most U.S. and European women as well as in human breast milk. We do not know with certainty, however, what role these chemicals play in causing or contributing to the rise in human breast cancer over the past half century. Some studies show a direct connection and others do not.

In the mid-1970s, researchers reported that women with breast cancer had significantly higher levels of DDE (a metabolic break-down product of the pesticide DDT) and PCBs (a chlorinated organic chemical used in industry) in their tumors than in the surrounding healthy tissues of their breasts. Similar but weaker trends held for the pesticides lindane, heptachlor, and dieldrin. The study was small—involving only 14 women—but the findings were provocative because DDT and PCBs were already linked to breast cancer in rodents.

Other small studies followed. Some showed an association between breast cancer and residues of pesticides or PCBs; some did not. In 1990, Finnish researchers reported that women with breast cancer had higher concentrations of a lindane residue in their breasts than women without breast cancer. Indeed, women whose breasts sequestered the highest levels were ten times more likely to have breast cancer than women with lower levels. Moreover, the pooled blood from women with breast cancer contained 50 percent more of this pesticide residue than the blood from women without breast cancer (Mussalo-Rauhamaa et al. 1990). Similarly, in 1992, a study of 40 Connecticut women revealed that levels of PCB, DDE, and DDT in the breasts of women with breast cancer were 50 to 60 percent higher than in women who did not have breast cancer (Falck et al. 1992).

In 1993—17 years after the first pilot study—biochemist Mary Wolff and her colleagues conducted the first carefully designed major study on this issue. They analyzed DDE and PCB levels in the stored blood specimens of 14,290 New York City women who had attended a mammography screening clinic. Within six months, 58 of these women were diagnosed with breast cancer. Wolff matched each of these 58 women to control subjects—women without breast cancer but of the same age, same menstrual status, and so on—who also had visited the clinic. The blood samples of the women with breast cancer were then compared to their cancer-free counterparts.

On average, the blood of breast cancer patients contained 35 percent more DDE than that of healthy women. (PCB levels were only slightly higher.) The most stunning discovery was that the women with the highest DDE levels in their blood were four times more likely to have breast cancer than the women with the lowest levels. The authors concluded that residues of DDE "are strongly associated with breast cancer risk" (Wolff et al. 1993; Hunter and Kelsey 1993; Longnecker and London 1993).

On the heels of the Wolff study came another by the Canadian researchers Eric Dewailly and colleagues in Quebec. Dewailly obtained breast tissue from women who had undergone biopsies for breast lumps. He chose 20 women whose lumps turned out to be cancerous and 17 women whose lumps were benign. The removed lumps were then analyzed for chemical residues. Consistent with the findings of previous studies, the concentrations of several pesticides and industrial chemicals were moderately higher in the tissues of women with cancer than women without. When Dewailly restricted his comparison to estrogen receptor-positive tumors (that is, tumors sensitive to the presence of estrogen), the difference became more striking: DDE levels were substantially higher in women with estrogen receptor positive cancers than in the women of the control group (Dewailly et al. 1994).

Following Wolff's and Dewailly's work came the Krieger study (1994), which yielded a more complex picture. Harvard University epidemiologist Nancy Krieger, then at the Kaiser Foundation in Oakland, California, examined DDE and PCB levels in blood drawn from women in the 1960s and then frozen and stored for nearly 30 years. She compared the blood from 150 women who went on to get breast cancer sometime during those intervening three decades to blood from 150 women who remained cancer free. The central question: Can exposure to DDT and PCBs many years earlier predict whether a woman will contract breast cancer? Previous studies looked at DDE and PCB levels at the time of diagnosis. Her study would be the first study to take into account the lag time between exposure and onset of disease. Three racial-ethnic groups were represented—African Americans, Asian Americans, and European Americans. When the three groups were combined, no significant differences were found. However, when each racial group was considered separately, the results changed. European Americans and especially Asian American women with breast cancer had significantly higher levels of DDE than women without breast cancer, even as Asian American women continued to reflect the overall pattern of no difference. More mysteriously, while African American women with breast cancer showed more past exposure to PCBs than their counterparts without breast cancer, the trend for European American women went in the opposite direction: The highest levels of blood PCBs tended to occur in women *without* the disease.

The interpretation of these results—which are not inconsistent with earlier studies but which do not actually confirm them either—has sparked considerable debate. Do DDE and PCB levels in blood serum accurately mirror their levels in women's breasts? (Evidence from other studies indicates they do (MacMahon 1994; Savitz 1994; Sternberg 1994.) Do we know whether DDE and PCB molecules remain stable when stored for thirty years? (Persistence is certainly a well-known trait of both chemicals.) What about the red rubber tops that capped the test tubes? Could chemical contaminants have migrated into the blood and marred the chemical analysis? (A speculative concern.)

The evidence that PCBs may be contributing to breast cancer, on the other hand, has not been supported in the past year. Nor has the evidence for DDT and breast cancer. A large, well-designed study published in the *New England Journal of Medicine* found no link between blood levels of certain PCB and DDT metabolites and risk of breast cancer (Hunter et al. 1997). Researchers analyzed blood samples from thousands of subjects, and those who went on to get breast cancer were matched with those who did not. No differences in median levels of these two contaminants were identified. However, as one of the authors of the study cautioned, abandoning the PCB/DDT hypothesis on the basis of these data alone is premature. Exposure to these two chemical species may be important for some groups of women and not others, or for some types of breast cancer and not others. (No distinction was made in this study between pre- and postmenopausal breast cancers, for example, or between estrogen receptor-positive and estrogen receptor-negative cancers.) Timing of exposure, rather than absolute amount of exposure, also may be critical. Furthermore, the particular metabolites chosen for measurement may not be the actual agents of harm. Remember, there are 209 different PCBs; they have wildly differing metabolic fates and wildly differing effects on the body.

Such considerations have not prevented detractors from declaring, on the basis of this single study, the exoneration of not just DDT and PCBs—but of *all* pesticides and industrial contaminants—from accusations of breast carcinogenicity. The irresponsibility of such statements is revealed in the results of other papers recently published. For example, a new study by Canadian researcher Eric Dewailly found that the concentration of estrogen receptors in breast tumors correlates closely with the concentration of DDT metabolites in surrounding breast fat (Dewailly et al. 1997). Although small in scale, this study is particularly intriguing because organochlorine compounds like DDT are known to stimulate estrogen receptor levels in breast tumor cells growing in laboratory cultures and because, collectively, women's breast tumors have become increasingly rich in estrogen receptors over the past two decades.

In short, we have even more reason than ever to pursue an environmental investigation of breast cancer.

THE XENOESTROGEN HYPOTHESIS

The first clue that estrogen might play a role in breast cancer came in 1896, when a British surgeon reported that removal of the ovaries sometimes caused breast tumors to shrink. Many exhaustive studies conducted since then have clearly indicated that a woman's chances of developing breast cancer are related in some way to her lifetime exposure to estrogen. Early first menstruation, late menopause, and late or no childbirths all raise a woman's lifetime exposure to estrogen; all are considered established risk factors for breast cancer, as is having a mother or sister with the disease. Even so, taken together, such factors still account for only a minority of breast cancer cases.

Since the origin of most breast cancers remains unexplained and since there exists an apparent connection between breast cancer and naturally occurring estrogen, scientific attention has begun to turn to the possible role of xenoestrogens—chemicals foreign to the body that, directly or indirectly, act like estrogens.

Estrogen is manufactured from cholesterol by a woman's ovaries each month and circulates in the blood, passing freely in and out of all organs and tissues. Eventually, the hormone is metabolized by specific enzymes and, with the help of the liver, is eliminated from the body through the gut. Most cells are completely unaffected by all this activity. The cells of certain tissues, however, contain receptors that latch onto estrogen molecules as they float through. The estrogen receptor complex then goes to work inside the nucleus. Certain genes are activated while others are switched off. Different messages are sent out from the nucleus and, hence, different proteins are manufactured. For tissues possessing estrogen receptors, the net effect of these various alterations is an increase in cell proliferation. The cells of the vagina, uterus, and breast all contain large numbers of estrogen receptors. In the presence of estrogen, they divide. Ovulation, breast development, menstruation, and pregnancy are all made possible by estrogen's actions (Davis and Bradlow 1995; Toniolo et al. 1994).

Estrogen comes in several chemical configurations, each with its own name. By far, the most potent one is estradiol. Its particular structure allows it easy passage from blood into surrounding cells. To regulate this movement, estradiol molecules are attached to serum proteins that slow down their entry into target tissues and thereby blunt their dramatic effects.

Like estradiol, xenoestrogens slip from blood serum into the interior of cells, attach themselves to estrogen receptors, and, by tinkering with particular genes, elicit growth-promoting changes within target tissues. The ability of certain synthetic chemicals to mimic estrogen in this way has been known for some time, but until recently, many researchers had assumed that any breast cancer risk created by this sort of mischief paled in comparison to the sovereign power of a woman's own hormones (Houghton and Ritter 1995). This assumption was based on several observations. First, few synthetic chemicals closely resemble the ornately designed estrogen molecule, and estrogen is the key that must fit into the receptor's lock in order to ignite the whole process. Second, assays show that foreign estrogens are much less potent than naturally occurring estradiol. Indeed, most are thousands, even millions of times weaker. Third, xenoestrogens exist in much lower concentrations in the body than naturally occurring estrogens, which surge to impressive levels during the first half of a woman's menstrual cycle. Also, many of the plants we eat, such as soy, contain naturally occurring plant estrogens, which are far more commonly encountered by our cells than their synthetic counterparts, such as pesticide residues. In short, xenoestrogens have been presumed rare, ineffective, and dilute.

Several recent findings have cast doubt on such reassuring suppositions. It turns out, for example, that close physical resemblance is not required for successful estrogen impersonation. As a lock, the estrogen receptor accepts many keys, some widely divergent in shape and size. Organic compounds that look nothing like estradiol—from pesticides to plastics to detergents—can possess estrogenic properties. Moreover, xenoestrogens are far more common than anyone had imagined (Common 1994).

Additionally, xenoestrogens appear able to compensate for their lack of individual potency through remarkable interactions: Together, they can exert estrogenic effects many times higher than any one working alone (Howard 1997). Many artificial estrogens further compensate for their low numbers through longevity and enhanced availability. Synthetic estrogens are not easily metabolized and excreted. They linger in the body, sometimes for decades. Also, they are often not as tightly bound to blood proteins as estradiol. They can, therefore, enter target cells more quickly and at lower concentrations; they are more available (Arnold et al. 1996).

Medical researchers Ana Soto and Carlos Sonnenschein at Tufts University are two of the leading researchers investigating the phenomenon of xenoestrogens and their relevance to breast cancer. Using tumor cultures growing in petri dishes, they have documented increased rates of growth in estrogen-sensitive breast cancer cells exposed to low levels of several kinds of estrogen-mimicking chemicals (Soto et al. 1991). One is the pesticide endosulfan, introduced to the market in 1954, and now widely used on salad crops. Others include plastics additives (which are known to leach from plastic food containers onto food stuffs), and the fat-soluble pesticides dieldrin and toxaphene. Not only does toxaphene cause breast cancer cells to divide more rapidly, Soto and Sonnenschein discovered, it does so at levels well within the range of concentrations now found in the flesh of some salmon (Soto et al. 1994). Other researchers have observed similar effects with red dye number 3 (Dees et al. 1997).

Xenoestrogens not only mimic natural estrogens directly but also can indirectly enhance their effects. For example, some xenoestrogens appear to stimulate the manufacture of more estrogen receptors. More receptors means an amplified response to estradiol. Still other xenoestrogens influence how estradiol is metabolized and eliminated from the body. This second effect has been the subject of several recent studies led by biochemical endocrinologist Leon Bradlow and his collaborator Devra Davis (Davis 1993; Davis and Bradlow 1995).

As explained by Bradlow and Davis, estradiol molecules can be broken apart by metabolic enzymes in one of two ways. The first one alters carbon atom number 2; the second alters carbon atom number 16. Which of these two pathways estradiol takes turns out to be critical. The 16-metabolite is still estrogenic; it is easily reabsorbed across the gut and is capable of binding to the estrogen receptors just like its parent, estradiol. More menacingly, the 16-metabolite can directly damage DNA. It is believed capable of both initiating and promoting breast cancer. Indeed, many researchers consider the level of this metabolite a potential marker for breast cancer risk. In contrast, the 2-metabolite is minimally estrogenic and nontoxic to DNA, and it may even protect the breast against cancerous changes. According to Bradlow and his colleagues, a low 16-to-2 ratio is desirable (Bradlow et al. 1995; Davis and Bradlow 1995; Telang et al. 1992).

Unfortunately, many contaminants push the ratio in the other direction. In cultured cells, the pesticides DDT, atrazine, and endosulfan—as well as benzene and certain PCBs—all skew the balance away from 2 toward the 16 pathway. In essence, these environmental contaminants turn the natural hormone estrogen into a weapon that is aimed at the breasts it caused to grow in the first place.

LINKS BETWEEN MEDICAL
IONIZING RADIATION AND BREAST CANCER

In November 1997, the National Action Plan on Breast Cancer, administered by the U.S. Department of Health and Human Services, hosted a two-day workshop to review the state of knowledge on medical ionizing radiation (x-ray exposure) and breast cancer risk. The scientists who gathered there reported the following results.

First, exposure to ionizing radiation is a known cause of breast cancer, and medicine is the largest contributor to man-made radiation exposure. In fact, ionizing radiation is the only environmental agent that is *proven* to induce breast cancer. Animal studies, studies of women who were atomic bomb survivors, and studies of women who were medically exposed to radiation are all in complete agreement with each other on this issue. Moreover, radiation-related breast cancer risk rises proportionally with the lifetime dose of radiation received by the breast. The timing of exposure also is crucial. Women exposed to x-rays before age 20 have a much higher chance of developing breast cancer in response to this exposure than women exposed after age 40.

Second, a woman's reproductive status influences her risk of developing breast cancer in response to radiation exposure. Women who have never experienced a full-term pregnancy and women who gave birth to their first child at a late age are more susceptible to radiation-induced breast cancers than women who had children while they were young. Interestingly, the protective effect of an early first full-term pregnancy appears to be retroactive because it mitigates the risk associated with radiation exposure during childhood or early adolescence as well as at older ages. The explanation provided by experimental studies on animals is that the final development of the breast for lactation (which occurs late in pregnancy) inhibits the ability of breast cells to develop into cancer, whether or not they are exposed to radiation.

Genetic factors also influence the breast's susceptibility to damage from x-rays. About 1.4 percent of the population are carriers of a gene called ataxia-telangiectasia (AT), which bestows an elevated sensitivity to radiation. Women carriers of AT are not able to detect and repair chromosomal damage caused by radiation exposure as effectively as noncarriers and are, therefore, far more likely to develop breast cancer as a result of medical x-ray exposure (Breast Cancer Etiology Working Group 1997).

Medical procedures associated with breast cancer risk are numerous. Women who underwent frequent fluoroscopies (real-time x-ray images) for tuberculosis and those who received x-ray therapy for enlarged thymuses when they were newborns have substantially higher breast cancer rates. Pediatric films also have high potential for increasing the risk of radiation-related breast cancer, especially fluoroscopic images of the heart. Amazingly enough, in most states, no training is required to administer fluoroscopies, which generate the highest dosages of radiation, and no certification is required beyond being a licensed health care practitioner (Breast Cancer Etiology Working Group 1997).

Also amazing is the fact that there are established dose limits for radiology technicians but not for patients (Breast Cancer Etiology Working Group 1997). Because there are no records kept on an individual patient's lifetime exposure to radiation, there is currently no way of estimating what cancer risk future x-rays may pose. Establishing dosages, however, is not an easy task: Dose depends on the body size of the patient and, in the case of mammograms, on the density of the breast itself.

In response to these presentations, breast cancer activists who attended the 1997 workshop entitled the Breast Cancer Etiology Working Group, issued the following consensus statement:

Ionizing radiation is an immediately preventable known cause of breast cancer and other cancers, and the breast is particularly susceptible to damage from ionizing radiation. The earlier the age at exposure, the greater the risk; the lower the dose, the less risk there is, but the accumulation of low doses may put a person at high risk. No "acceptable" levels of exposure have been determined. People are exposed to ionizing radiation from many sources. While many of these sources cannot be modified at this time, the medical use of ionizing radiation can be identified as a universal problem that is modifiable. It has been estimated that a threefold reduction of dose from diagnostic radiology is technologically feasible. *Reducing the quantity and improving the quality of medical x-rays and other radiologic procedures is a step that can be taken in the fight against breast cancer* [emphasis added].

THE MASQUERADE OF LIFESTYLE

In 1832, at the height of an epidemic, the New York City medical council announced that cholera's usual victims were those who were imprudent, intemperate, or prone to injury by the consumption of improper medicines (Rosenberg 1962). Lists of cholera prevention tips were posted publicly. Their advice ranged from avoiding drafts and crude vegetables to abstaining from alcohol. Maintaining regular habits also was said to be protective. Decades later, improvements in public sanitation finally brought cholera under control, and the pathogen responsible for the disease was finally isolated by Robert Koch in 1883. Of course, the behavioral changes urged by the 1832 handbills were not all without merit: Uncooked produce, as it turned out, was an important route of exposure, but it was a fecal-borne bacteria—and not a salad-eating lifestyle—that was the cause.

The orthodoxy of lifestyle today finds its full expression in the public educational literature on breast cancer. In scores of cheerful pamphlets, women are exhorted to exercise, lower the fat in their diets, perform breast self-examinations, ponder their family history, and receive regular mammograms. "Delayed childbirth" (after age 20) is frequently mentioned as a risk factor—although I have never seen "prompt childbirth" mentioned in the accompanying list of cancer prevention tips, undoubtedly because such advice would be tantamount to advocating teenage pregnancy. In short, public education on the topic of breast cancer emphasizes personal habits rather than chemical carcinogens as the underlying cause of the disease. As such, breast cancer, like cholera before it, has been framed as a problem of *behavior* rather than as a problem of *exposure* to disease-causing agents.

All by itself, a lifestyle approach to breast cancer is inadequate. First, the majority of breast cancers cannot be explained by lifestyle factors, including reproductive history. Second, mammography and breast self-examinations are tools of cancer detection, not acts of prevention. Detecting a tumor, however early in its development, precludes its prevention. Third, the adage that high-fat Western diets are the cause of breast cancer has not yet been supported by data. Dietary fat has long been a centerpiece of study in the investigation of breast cancer risk, and yet, several long-term, heavily funded studies have indicated that dietary fat is unlikely to play a major role by itself (Giovannucci et al. 1993; Hunter et al. 1996; Hunter and Willett 1993). Rather than continuing to focus single-mindedly on the absolute quantity of fat consumed, several researchers have called for a more refined, ecological approach to diet. Two obvious starting points would be to assess the link between breast cancer and diets high in animal fat and to launch a definitive investigation into the extent to which various kinds of fats are contaminated by carcinogens. We already know with certainty that animal-based foods are our main route of exposure to organochlorine pesticides, PCBs, and other contaminants that bioaccumulate as they move up the food chain (Willett 1996).

Even reproductive choices have environmental implications. Breasts do not complete their development until the last months of a woman's first full-term pregnancy. During this time, the lattice-work of mammary ducts and milk-producing lobules differentiate into fully functioning secretory cells. This process of specialization permanently slows the rate of mitosis, dampens the response to growth-promoting estrogens, and renders breast DNA less vulnerable to damage (Krieger 1989; Korenman 1980). In other words, a full-term pregnancy early in life protects against breast cancer precisely because its reduces a woman's vulnerability to carcinogens and other cancer promoters. Hence, childless women and women who have their babies later in life actually need *more* protection from breast carcinogens because they spend a longer number of years walking around with undifferentiated, vulnerable breasts.

Harvard epidemiologist Nancy Krieger has urged a redirection of breast cancer research toward environmental questions. Noting that researchers have repeatedly confirmed that reproductive history contributes to breast cancer risk, Krieger argues that we now need to know whether women with similar reproductive histories but divergent exposure to carcinogens have marked differences in breast cancer incidence. This need is made urgent by the results of animal studies showing that exposure to certain synthetic chemicals hastens the onset of puberty. Early menstruation—along with late parenthood—is considered a classic risk factor for breast cancer in women.

HEAR NO EVIL, SEE NO EVIL, BLAME THE VICTIM

Late in the summer of 1997, a series of articles appeared in the *Toronto Globe and Mail* that made me wonder if the collective neglect around the topic of breast cancer and the environment is not sometimes backed by outright aversion and hostility—at least at the level of the media.

In August of that year, the University of Buffalo sent out a press release reporting the results of a breast cancer investigation conducted by several of their researchers. The study found that women with breast cancer who had never breast-fed had significantly higher levels of organochlorine chemicals in their breasts than women without breast cancer who also had never breast-fed. These contaminants included the pesticides DDT, HCB, and mirex, as well as PCBs. However, no such difference in levels of toxic chemicals was seen for women who had nursed an infant at some point during their lives. According to the principle investigator, Dr. Kirsten Moysich, "These results suggest that higher blood levels of organochlorines were a risk factor for breast cancer only for women with no history of breast-feeding." The explanation for this difference, she believed, had to do with cleansing effects of lactation. "These chemicals are stored in fatty tissue, including breast tissue. The chief mechanism for eliminating them from the breast tissue is lactation, which flushes them from the system" (University of Buffalo 1997). By this statement, she meant that a woman can rid her breasts of toxic chemicals—presumably lowering her subsequent risk of breast cancer—by transferring these contaminants into her infant. An astonishing admission.

Oddly enough, however, the press release subordinated the positive findings to the negative ones in its headline by defining women who had never breast-fed as existing outside the "general population" and relegating them to lower-case subtitle status: "UB STUDY FINDS NO LINK BETWEEN BREAST CANCER RISK AND PESTICIDES OR PCB EXPOSURE FOR GENERAL POPULATION. Increased risk shown for women who have never breast-fed."

A few days later, the *Toronto Globe and Mail* magnified the bias by running the story under a headline that made no mention of the positive findings at all: "NO LINK BETWEEN CANCER, PESTI-CIDE. Breast cancer target of study." Only deep into the story—many paragraphs after the lead, does the reader find the following mention of the results for non-lactating women, "Women who had not breast fed had significantly higher levels of DDE, a residue of DDT, in their blood and twice the rate of breast cancers as women of similar age and habits who breast fed" (Immen 1997:A12). Two days later, the *Toronto Globe and Mail* ran an editorial entitled, "Science, Belief and Breast Cancer," which repeated only the negative findings and made no mention at all of the doubling rate of breast cancer among women who had never nursed. At this point, nonlactating women were not just defined as outside the norm but were dropped from existence altogether. The editorial then concluded that those who cling to the belief that environmental chemicals play a role in breast cancer in spite of the lack of evidence (I was named directly as one such person) are engaging in "voodooism which faithfully treads the old and fearful pathways of a disease-fearing heart" ("Science, Belief and Breast Cancer" 1997).

The classification of nonlactating women as existing outside the general population (or not existing at all) may come as a surprise to the one of every six couples struggling with infertility, mothers who bottle-fed their infants (especially since formula-feeding was practiced by the majority of mothers throughout the 1950s and 1960s), adoptive mothers, and all those who, for whatever reason, have chosen not to give birth. It certainly surprised my own mother, a biologist and breast cancer survivor who adopted her two daughters more than three decades ago. But for all of us women—lactating mothers and all others, alike—the implicit message that women should alter their own reproductive and child-rearing choices rather than question the practices of industry and agriculture should give us pause. Such an argument rests on the twin assumptions that women can do nothing but passively collect toxic wastes in their breasts and that their infants are a reasonable repository for this pollution. The idea that all women—whatever their lactational status—deserve protection from breast carcinogens is not even within the frame of the debate (Steingraber and O'Brien 1998). These misplaced emphases and unspoken premises are not only antifeminist, they make for bad science and bad public health policy. As I await the birth of my own daughter, I believe more than ever that the feminist cancer activist community must speak loudly and clearly about the science addressing the causes of breast cancer and about its public reportage.

REFERENCES

Arnold, S. F., et al. 1996. "A Yeast Estrogen Screen for Examining the Relative Exposure of Cells to Natural and Xenoestrogens." *Environmental Health Perspectives* 104:544-48.

Bradlow, H. L., et al. 1995. "Effects of Pesticides on the Ratio of 16 alpha/2-Hydroxyestrone: A Biologic Marker of Breast Cancer Risk." *Environmental Health Perspectives* 103(supp. 7):147-50.

Breast Cancer Etiology Working Group. 1997. "Workshop on Medical Ionizing Radiation and Human Breast Cancer, Summary of Presentations." U.S. Department of Health and Human Services, National Action Plan on Breast Cancer, Washington, D.C. (November 17-18) 35.

———. 1997. "Workshop on Medical Ionizing Radiation and Human Breast Cancer, Advocates' Conclusions and Recommendations to the NAPBC Steering Committee." U.S. Department of Health and Human Services, National Action Plan on Breast Cancer, Washington, D.C. (November 17-18) 10.

Chiazze, L., et al. 1977. "Mortality Among Employees of PVC Fabricators." *Journal of Occupational Medicine* 19:623-28.

Common, P. 1994. "Environmental Estrogenic Agents Area of Concern." *Journal of the American Medical Association* 271:414-16.

Davis, D. L. 1993. "Medical Hypothesis: Xenoestrogens as Preventable Causes of Breast Cancer." *Environmental Health Perspectives* 101:372-77.

Davis, D. L., and H. L. Bradlow. 1995. "Can Environmental Estrogens Cause Breast Cancer?" *Scientific American* (October) 166-72.

Dees, C., et al. 1997. "Estrogenic and DNA-damaging Activity of Red No. 3 in Human Breast Cancer Cells." *Environmental Health Perspectives* 105:625-32.

Dewailly, Eric, et al. 1994. "High Organochlorine Body Burden in Women with Estrogen Receptor-Positive Breast Cancer." *Journal of the National Cancer Institute* 86:232-34.

Dewailly, Eric, et al. 1997. "Could the Rising Levels of Estrogen Receptor in Breast Cancer Be Due to Estrogenic Pollutants?" *Journal of the National Cancer Institute* 89:888.

Donna, A., et al. 1984. "Ovarian Mesothelial Tumors and Herbicides: A Case-Control Study." *Carcinogenesis* 5:941-42.

Donna, A., et al. 1989. "Triazine Herbicides and Ovarian Epithelial Neoplasms." *Scandinavian Journal of Work Environment and Health* 15:47-53.

Falck, F., et al. 1992. "Pesticides and Polychlorinated Biphenyl Residues in Human Breast Lipids and Their Relation to Breast Cancer." *Archives of Environmental Health* 47:143-46.

Feuer, E. J., and L. M. Wun. 1992. "How Much of the Recent Rise in Breast Cancer Incidence Can Be Explained by Increases in Mammography Utilization?" *American Journal of Epidemiology* 136:1423-36.

Giovannucci, E., et al. 1993. "A Comparison of Prospective and Retrospective Assessments of Diet in the Study of Breast Cancer." *American Journal of Epidemiology* 137:502-11.

Goldman, B. A. 1991. *The Truth about Where You Live: An Atlas for Action on Toxins and Mortality*. New York: Random House.

Griffith, J., and W. B. Riggan. 1989. "Cancer Mortality in U.S. Counties with Hazardous Waste Sites and Ground Water Pollution." *Archives of Environmental Health* 44:69-74.

Harris, J. R. 1992. "Breast Cancer." *New England Journal of Medicine* 327:319-28.

Hoover, R., and J. F. Fraumeni, Jr. 1975. "Cancer Mortality in U.S. Counties with Chemical Industries." *Environmental Research* 9:196-207.

Houghton, D. L., and L. Ritter. 1995. "Organochlorine Residues and Risk of Breast Cancer." *Journal of the American College of Toxicology* 14:71-89.

Howard, V. 1997. "Synergistic Effects of Chemical Mixtures—Can We Rely on Traditional Toxicology?" *The Ecologist* 27:192-95.

Hunter, D. J., et al. 1996. "Cohort Studies of Fat Intake and the Risk of Breast Cancer—A Pooled Analysis." *New England Journal of Medicine* 334:356-61.

Hunter, D. J., et al. 1997. "Plasma Organochlorine Levels and the Risk of Breast Cancer." *New England Journal of Medicine* 337:1253-58.

Hunter, D. J., and K. T. Kelsey. 1993. "Pesticide Residues and Breast Cancer: The Harvest of a Silent Spring?" *Journal of the National Cancer Institute* 85:598-99.

Hunter, D. J., and W. C. Willett. 1993. "Diet, Body Size, and Breast Cancer." *Epidemiology Reviews* 15:110-32.

Immen, W. 1997. "No Link Between Cancer, Pesticide. Breast Cancer Target of Study." *Toronto Globe and Mail* (August 21) A12.

Infante, P. F., and J. Pesak. 1994. "A Historical Perspective of Some Occupationally Related Diseases of Women." *Journal of Occupational Medicine* 36:826-31.

Infante, Peter F. Health Standards Program, Occupational Safety and Health Administration, personal communication.

Kettles, M. A., et al. 1997. "Triazine Herbicide Exposure and Breast Cancer Incidence: An Ecologic Study of Kentucky Counties." *Environmental Health Perspectives* 105:1222-27.

Korenman, S. G. 1980. "Oestrogen Window Hypothesis of the Aetiology of Breast Cancer." *Lancet* 700-701.

Krieger, N. 1989. "Exposure, Susceptibility, and Breast Cancer Risk." *Breast Cancer Research and Treatment* 13:205-23.

Krieger, N., et al. 1994. "Breast Cancer and Serum Organochlorines: A Prospective Study Among White, Black, and Asian Women." *Journal of the National Cancer Institute* 86:589-99.

Lewis-Michl, E. L., et al. 1996. "Breast Cancer Risk and Residence Near Industry or Traffic in Nassau and Suffolk Counties, Long Island, New York." *Archives of Environmental Health* 51:255-65.

Liff, J. M. 1991. "Does Increased Detection Account for the Rising Incidence of Breast Cancer?" *American Journal of Public Health* 81:462-65.

Longnecker, M. P., and S. J. London. 1993. "Re: Blood Levels of Organochlorine Residues and Risk of Breast Cancer." *Journal of the National Cancer Institute* 85:1696-97.

MacMahon, B. 1994. "Pesticide Residues and Breast Cancer?" *Journal of the National Cancer Institute* 86:572-73.

Melius J., et al. 1994. "Residence Near Industries and High Traffic Areas and the Risk of Breast Cancer on Long Island." Albany: New York State Department of Health.

Mussalo-Rauhamaa, H., et al. 1990. "Occurrence of beta-Hexachlorocyclohexane in Breast Cancer Patients." *Cancer* 66:2124-28.

Najem, G. R., I. S. Thind, M. A. Lavenhar, and D. B. Louria. 1983. "Gastrointestinal Cancer Mortality in New Jersey Counties and the Relationship to Environmental Variables." *International Journal of Epidemiology* 12:276-89.

Najem, G. R., et al. 1985a. "Female Reproductive Organs and Breast Cancer Mortality in New Jersey Counties and the Relationship with Certain Environmental Variables." *Preventive Medicine* 14:620-35.

Najem G. R., D. B. Louria, M. A. Lavenhar, M. Feuerman. 1985b. "Clusters of Cancer Mortality in New Jersey Municipalities, with Special Reference to Chemical Toxic Waste Disposal Sites and Per Capita Income." *International Journal of Epidemiology* 14:528-37.

Proctor, R. N. 1995. *Cancer Wars: How Politics Shape What We Know and Don't Know about Cancer.* New York: Basic Books.

Rosenberg, C. E. 1962. *The Cholera Years: The United States in 1832, 1849, and 1866.* Chicago: University of Chicago Press.

Rudel, R. A., et al. 1998. "Identification of Alkylphenols and Other Estrogenic Phenolic Compounds in Waste Water, Sewage, and Groundwater on Cape Cod, Massachusetts." *Environmental Science and Technology* 32:861-69.

Safe, S. H. 1997. "Xenoestrogens and Breast Cancer." *New England Journal of Medicine* 337:1303-4.

Saltus, R. 1997. "Study Narrows Causes of Cape Breast Cancers." *Boston Globe* (December 12).

Savitz, D. A. 1994. "Re: Breast Cancer and Serum Organochlorines: A Prospective Study Among White, Black, and Asian Women." *Journal of the National Cancer Institute* 86:1255.

Schemo, D. J. 1994. "Long Island Breast Cancer Is Possibly Linked to Chemical Sites." *New York Times* (April 13) A1, B6.

"Science, Belief and Breast Cancer." 1997. *Toronto Globe and Mail* (August 23).

Silent Spring Institute, et al. 1997. "Cape Cod Breast Cancer and Environmental Study, Final Report." Newton, Mass.: Silent Spring Institute.

Soto, A. M., et al. 1991. "*p*-Nonylphenol: An Estrogenic Xenobiotic Released from 'Modified' Polystyrene." *Environmental Health Perspectives* 92:167-73.

Soto, A. M., et al. 1994. "The Pesticides Endosulfan, Toxaphene, and Dieldrin Have Estrogenic Effects on Human Estrogen-Sensitive Cells." *Environmental Health Perspectives* 102:380-83.

Steingraber, S. 1998. *Living Downstream: A Scientist's Personal Investigation of Cancer and the Environment.* New York: Vintage Books.

Steingraber, S., and M. O'Brien. 1998. "All Women Deserve Protection from Cancer-Causing Chemicals." *Toronto Globe and Mail* (Sept. 1).

Sternberg, S. S. 1994. "Re: DDT and Breast Cancer." *Journal of the National Cancer Institute* 86:1094-96.

Telang, N. T., et al. 1992. "Induction by Estrogen Metabolite 16 alpha-Hydroxyestrone of Genotoxic Damage and Aberrant Proliferation in Mouse Mammary Epithelial Cells." *Journal of the National Cancer Institute* 84:634-38.

Toniolo, P., et al. 1994. "Reliability of Measurements of Total, Protein-Bound, and Unbound Estradiol in Serum." *Cancer Epidemiology, Biomarkers, and Prevention* 3:47-50.

University of Buffalo. 1997. "UB Study Finds No Link Between Breast-Cancer Risk and Pesticides or PCB Exposure for General Population." Buffalo: University of Buffalo. Press release.

U.S. Agency for Toxic Substances and Disease Registry (ATSDR). 1990. "Case Studies in Environmental Medicine: Vinyl Chloride Toxicity." Atlanta: U.S. Agency for Toxic Substances and Disease Registry (ATSDR).

Willett, W. C. 1996. "Diet and Nutrition." Pp. 438-61 in *Cancer Epidemiology and Prevention*, 2nd ed., ed. D. Schottenfeld and J. F. Fraumeni Jr. Oxford: Oxford University Press.

Wolff, M. S., et al. 1993. "Blood Levels of Organochlorine Residues and Risk of Breast Cancer." *Journal of the National Cancer Institute* 85:648-52.

Women's Cancer Resource Center. 1994. Berkeley, CA.

PART THREE

BREAST CANCER
AND SOCIAL CHANGE

CHAPTER TEN

Breast Cancer in Popular Women's Magazines from 1913 to 1996

Jennifer R. Fosket, Angela Karran, and Christine LaFia, Ph.D.

In her writing about cancer in 1977, Susan Sontag illuminated the ways that cultural accounts of cancer represent not merely facts and information but transmit larger metaphorical and ideological ideas about illnesses and the people who live with them. Her work profoundly asserts that dominant ideologies are embedded in accounts of illness and fundamentally shape what are often mistaken to be neutral narratives. In this chapter we argue, in agreement with Sontag, that dominant ideologies infiltrate representations of cancer and blame people for being sick. Taking up the challenge implied by her work, we explore representations of breast cancer in popular media not merely as sources of medical knowledge and information but as sources of cultural messages and ideologies about women, their bodies, and disease and illness.

Specifically, we examine meanings and messages transmitted about breast cancer in popular women's magazines from 1913—when the first article on breast cancer appeared in the *Ladies' Home Journal*—to 1996. Our research explores how popular discussions about breast cancer continue to offer shifting, and at times, contradictory speculations about what breast cancer is, how it can be treated, and how women experience the illness. Specifically, we investigate the continuities and changes in messages about early detection, breast cancer risk and causation, and experiences of breast cancer over time. Here, we highlight a dominant, recurring pattern in representations of breast cancer: personal responsibility. Women are depicted as responsible for detecting, preventing, and surviving breast cancer. We argue that by focusing responsibility on women, media messages effectively shift our focus away from larger social, environmental, political, and economic issues surrounding breast cancer and, instead, blame individual women for their illness.

THE MEDIA

In the United States, mass media play a key role in providing information on health issues. News media are such significant channels for the transmission of scientific and medical information that they are often mentioned as second to the doctor as the primary source of such information (Bratic and Greenberg, as cited by Clarke 1992). In particular, magazines serve as an important source of health information, especially information regarding breast cancer (Johnson 1997; Kessler 1989). The accessibility of magazines and other popular media partly explains their importance as health information sources. For many individuals, it is often much easier to locate and to understand information in a magazine than to access a doctor or other health care provider. For all of these reasons, magazines represent an important site of health information and are worthy of sociological investigation.

In addition to providing health information, the media also produce cultural ideologies. Stuart Hall defines cultural ideologies as "those images, concepts and premises which provide the frameworks through which we represent, interpret, understand and 'make sense' of some aspect of social existence" (1995:18). The media are precisely in the business of producing those images, concepts, and premises—those frameworks—through which we come to understand and make sense of the world. A number of journalism analysts have observed that women's magazines, in particular, produce cultural ideologies about womanhood and femininity that shape the way we understand the supposed best and most appropriate ways to be a woman.[1] In the magazines that we examined, the model of womanhood most often depicted was white, middle class, heterosexual, slender, young, and happy.

Media representations of breast cancer emerge out of and reinforce dominant ideologies of femininity, individuality, and personal responsibility.[2] For example, Paula Lantz and Karen Booth (1998) argue not only that popular media articles emphasize dominant ideologies of femininity and personal responsibility, but that in these articles breast cancer is attributed to women's nonconformity to dominant gender identities (i.e., heterosexual marriage and reproduction). Breast cancer poses a challenge to women's magazines' depictions of femininity, which idealize femininity as nonconflicted, carefree, youthful, and healthy, among other things. The resulting magazine representations erase much of the pain, suffering, and politics of breast cancer. Scores of media stories on breast cancer report instead on women who triumphantly emerge from the trenches of treatment to tell their tales.

In order to understand breast cancer representations in popular media, it is important to understand the context in which mass media are produced. In the United States, a few large corporations own most major media outlets (Bagdikian 1997). Magazines operate with the often conflicting goals of disseminating health information and maximizing profit, goals that often result in advertising products that may be dangerous to health (Johnson 1997) or in self-censoring health information so as not to contradict the interests of large advertisers (Kessler 1989). Women's magazines are particularly prosperous advertising vehicles and ensure their existence and profitability by actively selling women consumers to advertisers

(Goldman 1992). Further, what is unique about today's corporate ownership is that corporations own not just one type of media but multiple types including television stations, magazines, book publishing companies, radio stations, and a wide variety of other products and services. Thus, magazine editors need to worry about producing stories that may conflict with the interests not just of advertisers but also of the corporations that own their magazines and sign their paychecks. With this background of corporate politics and conflicting interests, we examine how the topic of breast cancer is represented in the mass media.

THE STUDY

Our analysis consists of 255 articles that were found in 11 of the most popular U.S. women's magazines published since 1913: *Good Housekeeping, Ladies' Home Journal, Woman's Home Companion, Cosmopolitan, Vogue, Redbook, Ms., Mademoiselle, Glamour, Harper's Bazaar,* and *Working Woman.* We identified the articles through the *Reader's Guide to Periodical Literature,* using the category "cancer" until the subject "breast cancer" was included as a separate listing in the guide in the 1940s. All articles that focused on breast cancer during the 1913 to 1996 time period are included in the sample.

We organized the articles by sorting them into three main categories: *etiology*—articles that explored breast cancer causes and risk factors; *detection and treatments*—articles focused on detection practices, technologies, and breast cancer treatment issues; and *personal experiences*—articles focused on women's personal experiences with breast cancer. Within these three main categories, we then sorted the articles into subcategories based on the main topics covered by the articles. We also sorted them according to the "voice" (expert, journalist, or woman with breast cancer) by which the information was transmitted. The expert voice included those articles either written by or relying heavily on quotes from health professionals, usually doctors or scientists; 110 articles were written in the voice of the expert. The 69 articles written by journalists are distinct for their attempts to appear nonbiased and neutral. This neutrality is often accomplished through the absence of authorship so that the information appears uninterpreted and purely factual. Finally, 76 articles were either written by or relied on quotes from women with breast cancer, a distinct voice because it is presented as speaking about the authentic breast cancer experience. Since many of the articles span all three categories, skim the surface of a number of topics, or contain more than one voice, we identified and ranked each article by the top three categories, topics, and voices. In so doing, we were able to unravel the most dominant categories, topics, and voices in U.S. popular women's magazines.

Finally, we summarized the main messages that repeatedly occurred throughout the articles. These messages are especially important because they represent the principal ideas and expectations generated about breast cancer over time. This analysis reveals the most apparent ideologies about women, their bodies, and diseases. The most dominant message and the one most frequently occurring in these articles—that of personal responsibility—forms the basis for discussion in this chapter. Other common messages included the implication that medical science and technology can conquer cancer and that doctors know best. In some ways, these messages contradict the personal responsibility message by emphasizing the role of medicine and medical professionals instead of individual women. Despite this apparent contradiction, it was not uncommon for these messages to appear side by side in the same article. In this chapter, we discuss the ways that personal responsibility emerges within the realms of detection, prevention, and survival.

PERSONAL RESPONSIBILITY FOR DETECTION
"HOW TO EXAMINE YOUR BREASTS AND SAVE YOUR LIFE"[3]

Personal responsibility for detection first appears as a major topic in a 1953 *Woman's Home Companion* article entitled "You Can Fight

Cancer in Your Own Home." This headline symbolically links personal health practices of early detection to the home. In the text of the article, women are implored to practice early detection strategies that take "less time than it takes to darn a pair of socks" (Ratcliff 1953:44). The analogy between breast self-examination and darning socks links this practice to popular models of domesticity. Implicit is the idea that taking care of oneself through breast self-examination is part of a woman's responsibility to her family and home along with the other activities of domestic work. In the 1950s, women's responsibility for domestic work was taken for granted. Whether or not she worked outside the home, widespread cultural messages reinforced the notion that maintaining the domestic sphere was fundamentally a woman's responsibility (Stacey 1990). Thus, by creating this association between domestic work and health and by integrating breast self-examination into the requirements of caring for family and home, the message of personal responsibility is articulated loudly and clearly.

Early though it was, the 1953 *Woman's Home Companion* article is one of the few to appear before the 1970s with this message of personal responsibility for detection. For instance, in the same 1953 article women are told that, "In no other disease is the layman's burden of responsibility so large. In no other disease must the patient and the patient alone exercise so large a measure of alertness, suspicion and critical apprehension of cancer's early presence." Simultaneously, however, this article continues to assert a clear-cut distinction between women's roles in their health and that of the experts: Women are told that self-exam is "by no means as effective as an examination by a competent physician" (Ratcliff 1953:44). This sentiment is echoed in other early articles, such as a 1969 *Ladies' Home Journal* piece that states that their "candid guide" to breast self-exam is "intended to help you know more about your breasts, but not to help you make judgments about your health. Leave that to your doctor" (Ramsey 1969:82). However, this emphasis on doctors as the only experts of breast health profoundly shifted in the 1970s. Beginning in the 1970s and continuing today, personal responsibility for detection became a pervasive message. The emergence of this shift can be linked to the Women's Health Movement and the subsequent co-optation of certain ideas and strategies from this movement by dominant biomedicine. Analyses of the Women's Health Movement highlight the adoption of many of its strategies and institutions (Ruzek 1980; Whatley and Worcester 1989; Zimmerman 1987).

The prospect of women taking control of their own health and bodies was crucial to the Women's Health Movement of the 1970s, which resulted in a fundamental change in the ways women were thought about and treated in the medical encounter (Ruzek 1978). The ideas of empowerment and self-help brought about by this movement are reflected in the emphasis on women as competent surveyors of the health of their breasts. However, the ways that the practice of breast self-examination became less a tool of empowerment and self-help and more a way to make women personally responsible for breast cancer detection reflects medicine's co-optation of the Women's Health Movement. This co-optation shifted the idea of women having a *crucial role* in their own health care to women being *held responsible* for their health care, and then being blamed when things go wrong. Self-help taken out of the context of feminist empowerment has become individualized and victim blaming. It also has succeeded in taking health issues out of their social contexts and transformed them into individual problems (Whatley and Worcester 1989).

This history is reflected in the magazine articles on breast self-examination that began in the 1970s by emphasizing women's *knowledge* and *expertise* of their own bodies and quickly shifted during the 1980s and 1990s to emphasize women's *responsibility* for breast cancer detection. By the mid-1970s, the statistic that 95 percent of all breast cancers are found by women themselves is a prevalent message in the magazines. This statistic continues to be propagated in various forms and marks a shift from doctors as the only competent surveyors of the health of women's breasts to women themselves. This shift was firmly in place by the late 1980s. A 1987 *Glamour* article describes why breast self-examination is the best method of detection: "Though professionally trained, a doctor is at a disadvantage because she often has only a once-a-year exposure to your breasts and can't become as familiar with the unique characteristics and geography of your breasts as you can by monthly examination" ("Breast Update: Why Women Don't Do Self-Examination" 1987:182). This statement asserts women as experts of their own bodies by virtue of intimate knowledge, while diminishing the responsibility of doctors in the detection process.

Aside from changes in the relative expertise attributed to women over time, the general thrust of self-examination articles is remarkably consistent. Women are told that examining their breasts is their best protection against breast cancer. The language of cure and prevention is used to highlight the importance of early detection practices. A 1973 *Good Housekeeping* article states, "Nearly 1/3 of the 350,000 Americans who will die of cancer this year could have been cured if the disease had been diagnosed and treated in its early stages" ("The Better Way: Cancer Tests that Can Save Your Life" 1973:73). Here, cure is practically synonymous with early detection. This statement is problematic because it sends the false message that breast cancer is curable, and it rhetorically blames those women whose breast cancer is not cured for not detecting it soon enough.

Many of the articles that emphasize individual responsibility for detection provide a step-by-step guide to breast examinations accompanied by drawings and, more recently, photographs. These photographs almost always depict young, glamorous, slim, white women in sensuous poses examining their breasts. This deliberately sexy image of the breast-examining woman can be juxtaposed against the earlier articles. Whereas breast self-examination was once linked to domesticity and the care of one's family, now it is linked with sexuality and beauty. As before, breast self-examination is linked to a specific, dominant model of femininity, thereby implying that personal responsibility for health is part of the litany of things one must do in order to become the "right" kind of woman. By depicting the race of breast-examining women overwhelmingly as white, the articles reinforce the false idea that breast cancer primarily impacts white women.

PERSONAL RESPONSIBILITY FOR RISK AND CAUSATION
"PREVENTING BREAST CANCER: WHAT'S A GIRL TO DO?"[4]

Personal responsibility for the risk, causation, and prevention of breast cancer is another pervasive message in women's magazines. Many of the articles on risk and causation promote the idea of personal responsibility by emphasizing diet or exercise, and thus transmit the overly optimistic notion that breast cancer can be prevented if only women ate right and exercised. At the same time, risk factors related to genetics and hormones are often described as innate to a woman's body and thus communicate fear and inevitability. The individual is the focus of the articles; larger social factors such as the environment, lack of access to health care, poverty, educational attainment, employment barriers, social class, racism, or inequality are typically ignored. In this way, the articles focus the microscope on the individual woman as the site at which to locate risk and causation. In this section, we discuss the message of personal responsibility for risk and causation as it has emerged in discussions of risk factors and prevention strategies outlined in the magazine articles.

The most persistent risk factor for breast cancer present across the magazine articles is reproduction. Women are told that it is within their control to protect themselves against breast cancer by fulfilling the culturally prescribed roles of reproduction and motherhood. For example, in a 1982 *Glamour*, readers were told that an important factor in the reduction of risk of breast cancer, "is whether or not you had children, and your age when you gave birth to them. The more children you've had by the time you reach thirty, the more protected you appear to be against developing breast cancer" (Cherry 1982:239). That many women cannot reproduce or do not want to do so is not discussed in the magazine articles. Breast cancer is also linked to reproduction through the birth control pill. Starting in the 1970s, the Pill is cited as a possible risk factor for breast cancer. By focusing on the birth control pill and so-called delayed childbirth, the magazines send the message to women that controlling their reproduction may be hazardous to their health.

Other risk factors for breast cancer are represented more explicitly as within individual women's control. In the early decades of the twentieth century, bras were included as risk factors. The relationship between bras and breast cancer was explicated in a 1936 *Good Housekeeping* article where, under prevention for breast cancer, the only advice is to "avoid tight or chafing brassieres" (Little 1936:79). Another *Good Housekeeping* article, "Care of the Breast" that appeared in 1949 goes into more detail about bras and breast cancer:

> [A] one-piece garment that pulls down the breasts is never desirable . . . she needs a brassiere that raises and gently supports without compressing the breasts. From the point of view of health and beauty, the brassiere is one of the most important items in any woman's wardrobe . . . The main requirements are that the cups are neither too large nor too small, that the bra is not too tight, and that it holds the breasts in a natural position. Otherwise there will be friction, pressure, or stagnation in the milk-secreting glands, all of which seem to favor development of cancer. (Davis 1949:247)

In this article, health and beauty are linked and described as easily achieved through the purchase of the right bra. Thus, not only is personal responsibility reinforced but the method by which women can fulfill their responsibility for reducing breast cancer risk is specified, that is by spending money on gender-specific products.

Psychological and personality factors also emerge at various times in the data and suggest that breast cancer is individually preventable through positive thinking and optimistic attitudes. In 1936, a physician wrote in Good Housekeeping, "In no other physical ailment is psychology so important as it is in cancer" (Little 1936:110). In 1960, almost 25 years later, a Cosmopolitan article informs its readers that, "Dr. Pendergrass went on to relate cases of persons who, while being successfully treated for cancer, underwent some emotional stress, after which the disease flared up again with lethal effect" (James 1960:40). In 1972, Ladies' Home Journal readers were told, again with the authority of an expert, that, "Dr. Dunbar says that only certain types of people succumb to cancer." In this article, "cancer-prone" personalities are described as "hopeless, inadequate and desperate" (Lewis and Lewis 1972:96). Such personalities also are described as repressed, bottling up fear and anger. There are few ways to more directly blame women for causing their own breast cancer than by describing their personalities as cancer-prone as these articles do.

A few decades later, a 1985 Harper's Bazaar article entitled "Can Sex Hang-ups Cause Breast Cancer?" reporting on the research of Dr. Peggy Boyd asserts: "A woman's attitude toward her body, her degree of satisfaction with her first sexual experience and current partner, and confidence in her sex-role identity all have a far greater influence on her likelihood of getting a breast malignancy than does her family medical history or environmental profile" (p. 44). This article never explains how so-called psychological hang-ups and sexual inadequacies from an early age can increase women's susceptibility to breast cancer. By simply linking breast cancer to inadequate feelings about body and sexuality, this article reinforces gendered ideologies about female psychology and sexuality, which emphasize weakness and instability. Women's relationships with sexuality are implied to be so extremely problematic that disease is the result. Without describing why sexuality and sexual experiences are linked to cancer, readers are left to surmise that sex itself must somehow be potentially disease causing.

Throughout the 1970s, and especially in the 1980s and 1990s, magazine articles highlighting the link between women's diets and breast cancer proliferated. Women were and continue to be told that by changing their diets in multiple ways, including avoiding meats and increasing vegetable and fruit intake, eating low-fat diets, drinking less alcohol, and consuming vitamins and supplements, they can protect themselves against breast cancer. Again, the message is that breast cancer is a controllable disease, often through such simple life changes as eating five fruits or vegetables a day.

While current messages admonish women to exercise, change their diets, and avoid alcohol, in the past fear and inevitability were communicated through messages that breast cancer arises as a result of innate aspects of a woman's body such as hormones, cells, and genetics. For example, a 1955 *Woman's Home Companion* article written by a physician relates: "As for the relationship between your sex and cancer, we know that in certain kinds of cancer the abnormal cell growth is stimulated by hormones—particularly those secreted by the sex glands. The ovaries, for instance, seem to play an active role in the spread of breast cancer" (Day 1955:28). This representation and others like it identify women's bodies with disease and construct vivid portrayals of innate and hidden cancer-causing agents such as cells, hormones, and genes. These agents, located inside the body and thus out of the control of the individual, are described in a language that depicts them as hostile forces at war with the body.

Even in one of the earliest articles from 1914, military metaphors prevail in *Good Housekeeping*'s description of the relationship between menopause and cancer: "The reason why the period of greatest liability to cancer in women is some five years before the change of life, is that these rebellious glands or cell-groups require a certain amount of vigor and of blood supply to start their rebellion" (Hutchinson 1914: 534). Here, cells are depicted as an organized rebellion that use a woman's own blood to maintain the vigor of their attack against her body. These articles suggest that not only are women responsible for their cancers, but the disease is somehow inherent in their biological make-up—that through menopause and other processes, a woman's own body mounts attacks on itself from within. These bodily processes are depicted as innate and gender specific, and represent another way to blame women for developing breast cancer. While this message does not imply personal responsibility in the same way as articles that link cancer to diet, nevertheless, it locates cause at the level of the individual and deflects responsibility from social or environmental causes of illness.

In similar fashion, a 1964 *Good Housekeeping* article describes hormonal attacks on women's bodies in an explanation for why breast-feeding seems to reduce breast cancer risk. The article relates, "A woman who nurses two children . . . misses only three or four more menstrual periods . . . but those few respites from attacks of female hormones may account for her slight margin of protection" (Frank 1964:45). In these articles, breast cancer is depicted as emerging out of the "attacks" that a woman's own body mounts against itself. By attacking itself, women's bodies are thus implied to be innately diseased, unstable, and problematic.

Ultimately, the magazines send the message that women can locate the causes of breast cancer in either their lifestyle behaviors or in their bodies. Breast cancer then becomes a personal problem rather than a social issue. By glossing over the social aspects of breast cancer causation, multiple crucial issues are erased. For example, by emphasizing diet as an individual choice, the media ignores such social factors as the production of unhealthy foods, the links between pesticides and other toxins and breast cancer, and socioeconomic inequalities in access to potentially healthier foods and medical care. Similarly, emphasizing exercise as a personal choice ignores a host of social factors that structure one's ability, time, or desire to engage in this health practice. Overall, the emphasis on the individual in representations of breast cancer risk erases political, economic, environmental, and social factors; many of these factors are discussed elsewhere in this volume. This erasure of complex and interconnected social issues also is evident in articles on personal experience, where breast cancer is depicted as a white, middle-class women's disease, and the appropriate ways to experience the illness are formulated to mirror dominant models of femininity in society.

PERSONAL RESPONSIBILITY FOR SURVIVAL
"BACK TO BUSINESS, SURVIVING THE BIGGEST CRISIS OF ALL"[5]

Personal experience articles are particularly important because they are presented as a representation of what breast cancer is really like, what to expect, and how best to deal with the illness. These articles have a tone of authenticity not captured in the other articles because the reader is presented presumably with a true story about a real woman. The articles create a popular discourse based on women's own experiences rather than those of the expert and, as such, bring the reader to a supposedly more realistic understanding of how women experience breast cancer. However, on a deeper level, the articles convey important normative lessons for women about how to deal with illness and disease.

One of the most prominent messages in personal experience articles is that of survival. Personal experience narratives are almost always written by women who describe themselves as having had breast cancer but triumphed over the disease. Further, these women describe themselves as better off as a result of their experiences. The point stressed throughout the articles is that breast cancer is an illness that an individual can conquer. The articles transmit the value of personal actions, lifestyle choices, and positive psychological attitudes as contributors to recovery and survival. In this way, the personal responsibility message maintains a prominent presence in articles on the experience of breast cancer.

For example, a 1947 *Ladies' Home Journal* article describes the cancer experience of Mary Roberts Rinehart, a popular American fiction writer. The story chronicles events in her life that demonstrated hard work, success, personal strength, and courage in overcoming life's obstacles: "Cancer struck at her, cutting across as brilliantly successful a life as has been lived by any American woman of her day . . . She survived it and she let the experience sink in. For here is a woman who knows how to turn every experience to account. That is why she is still teachable today, and why she is worth listening to" (Palmer 1947:145). In this article, personal responsibility and inner strength are noted as key ingredients to overcoming a life-threatening disease.

In 1991, 44 years after Mary Roberts Rinehart's experience, an article entitled, "I Feel Very Lucky!" shares the story of another celebrity. In this article, actress Kate Jackson tells *Redbook* magazine readers, "I could either wallow in misery or accept what has happened . . . I could choose to die, but instead I chose to live, I feel lucky . . . because of early detection I'm fine, I'm cured, I'm well . . . I have the enthusiasm of a twenty-year-old. That's because I'm taking care of myself" (McElwaine 1991:38). In this statement, the message that one can *choose* to live or die is literally stated. Jackson tells readers that by taking care of themselves, women can survive breast cancer and even come out of the experience with "the enthusiasm of a twenty-year-old." Further, both the 1947 and the 1991 articles present their messages with the authority of a famous, successful woman. In this way, they can be seen as role models enacting the "right" and "womanly" way to respond to breast cancer.

The approach to breast cancer represented in the stories about Kate Jackson and Mary Roberts Rinehart reinforces the idea that positive thinking and optimism are far more appropriate responses to illness than are complaint, anger, or fear. Personal experience articles reveal a cultural approach to illness that is characterized by profound optimism, often presented in a Pollyanna-ish tone and style. The womanly response to breast cancer is approved of as transforming it into a positive experience by focusing on the good and de-emphasizing the pain, sadness, or suffering. In 1975, another celebrity, Marvella Bayh, wife of then U.S. Senator Birch Bayh, explains in *Ladies' Home Journal:*

> I remember with what dread I finally looked at myself in the mirror. It wasn't that bad. And I came to realize how lucky I was. If I had to be one out of every four Americans who will get cancer then this was the best kind to have. Losing a breast is so much better than losing an eye or an arm or a leg . . . the only way my life has changed since my surgery is that I enjoy it more now. The sunsets are rosier, the fall leaves are more radiant, and I take time to watch the squirrels play. Although I would not have chosen to have this, I can honestly say that it has changed my life for the better. (p. 102)

This quote reflects the common theme in personal experience stories of looking on the bright side of a breast cancer diagnosis. Repeatedly, women discuss feeling lucky and undergoing a beneficial personal transformation because of breast cancer. The pervasiveness of these kinds of depictions implicitly sends the message that feeling sad, angry, and entirely unlucky to have breast cancer are not appropriate responses.

Further, it is of profound significance that these stories of optimism and survival erase so many women's experiences of death and dying. It is important to give voice to women who are surviving breast cancer and important to transmit the reality that cancer does not necessarily result in death. However, it is also important to critique the absence of articles on death, suffering, anger, and emotional hardship. As it stands, these articles present the idea that women have all of the resources within themselves that they will need to overcome and even benefit from breast cancer. While affirming women's inner strength is positive, it is not so positive to overlook the multiple social resources that women need—and often do not have—to deal with breast cancer. By promoting the idea that women can *choose* to live, the women's magazines do a profound disservice to the more than 40,000 women who die from breast cancer each year in the United States. Clearly, these women would have chosen to live if personal choice was simultaneously an alternative and a means to survival. These are the women whose voices are not heard in the personal experience articles and whose lives also shape the landscape of breast cancer. Their stories and experiences should be represented if we are to understand the true impact of breast cancer.

MEDIA ABSENCES AND SILENCES

This chapter described messages in women's magazine articles about breast cancer that are laced with metaphors falsely associating detection, prevention, and survival with personal responsibility. Women are repeatedly told what breast cancer is and is not, how they can "conquer" the disease, and even how to make it a "gainful experience." The presentation of breast cancer in popular women's magazines creates a distorted sense of knowing about the disease while promoting a blame-the-victim motif.

However, what is equally important about the representations of breast cancer in popular media is what is left out. Two profoundly significant absences in the magazine articles are race and social class. The absence of discussions of race and social class is particularly striking because it is well known in the United States that while white women of high socioeconomic status are statistically more likely to get breast cancer, African American women and poor women are more likely to die from it. While white women's survival rates are improving, the rates for women of color are not (Wells and Horm 1992; Gordon et al. 1992). The absence of discussions about race and social class extends across the articles, notably in the category of personal experience, so that breast cancer is depicted as a disease relevant for only white women of high socioeconomic statuses. One consequence of these absences is that issues of access to care, discrimination, and inequality do not enter the breast cancer discussion.[6]

CONCLUSION

Our research demonstrates that women's magazines are successful at individualizing breast cancer. Just as risk factors that are highlighted in the magazines tend to be located in women's bodies or "in their control," *breast cancer is consistently depicted as a private issue and not as a public problem.* The recurring focus on risk factors as personal in nature coupled with the absence of discussion about breast cancer within the broader societal framework reinforce the media's role as an ideological tool that deflects responsibility from institutions onto the individual. The media representations of breast cancer continually focus attention on individual women who are removed from the communities, institutions, and societies in which their experiences are taking place. Society and social structures are absent from women's magazines and, therefore, the issue of breast cancer is depoliticized and decontextualized.

As we explore what is left out of media representations of breast cancer, it also is important to highlight our own omissions and absences in this analysis. Any cultural product, like a magazine story about breast cancer, will be interpreted within the particular context of the person who is reading it. Thus, there are potentially multiple interpretations of any media representation—differences that are in part structured by race, social class, nationality, sexuality, gender, and other identities, as well as by individual experiences and biographies (Kellner 1995). In particular, future research should explore the ways that women interpret and make sense of media representations of breast cancer.

Representations of breast cancer in women's magazines are shaped by larger ideologies about women, health, and beauty. Situated within the larger capitalist system in the United States, these magazines are motivated by the need to increase profit; this need ultimately shapes the way information is presented. Magazine editors are focused on capturing the widest possible audience and, thus, one rarely reads a story about death, devastation, anger, or political activism. Such stories invoke controversy and unease, which contradicts the "feel-good" genre of women's magazines. Instead, we read about food, beauty, and optimism—subjects that are easy to digest and noncontroversial. The ways that breast cancer is represented in women's magazines are important not just for their reflection of larger ideological ideas, but also because they shape the way breast cancer is thought about and addressed within U.S. society. As a primary source of information about health, magazines are influential in constructing the ideas people have about disease and illness, which, in turn, shape the decisions they make. This construction affects individual women worried about their risk, caretakers for women struggling with breast cancer, policymakers and funders deciding what kinds of research and policies to support, and researchers deciding what kinds of issues are important to pursue. Whether directly or indirectly, the messages conveyed in popular discourse about breast cancer have real and multiple consequences.

NOTES

AUTHOR'S NOTE: After being diagnosed with breast cancer in 1993, Christine LaFia turned her sociological imagination toward the problem of breast cancer and initiated this project with the help of Jennifer Ruth Fosket and Angela Karran. Her critical, sociological perspective, enthusiasm, and inspiration infuse this project, which she was unable to see completed. Christine died of metastatic breast cancer on April 20, 1996.

1. For examples of ways media send messages regarding dominant modes of femininity see Coutts and Berg 1993; Lupton 1994; Ortiz and Ortiz 1989; Winship 1991.

2. See for example, Clarke 1991, 1992; Edwards 1994; Lantz and Booth 1998; Lupton 1994; Yadlon 1997.
3. Title of a January 1975 article in *Harper's Bazaar.*
4. Title of an October 1992 article in *Mademoiselle.*
5. Title of an April 1981 article in *Working Woman.*
6. While these issues may have been present had we sought out magazines aimed explicitly at women of color (e.g., *Jet, Essence, Ebony*), the magazines that we chose are not advertised as being for white women, but rather are identified as women's magazines and thus represent the breast cancer experiences of women in all of our diversity and differences.

REFERENCES

Bagdikian, Ben. 1997. *The Media Monopoly.* 5th ed. Boston: Beacon Press.
Bayh, Marvella. 1975. "Betty, Happy, and Me." *Ladies' Home Journal* (January) 127.
"Better Way: Cancer Tests That Can Save Your Life, The." 1973. *Good Housekeeping* (April) 73-74.
"Breast Update: Why Women Don't Do Self-Examination." 1987. *Glamour* (January) 182.
"Can Sex Hang-ups Cause Breast Cancer?" 1985. *Harper's Bazaar* (April) 44.
Cherry, Laurence. 1982. "The Outlook on Breast Cancer." *Glamour* (November) 238.
Clarke, Juanne N. 1991. "Media Portrayal of Disease from the Medical, Political Economy, and Life-Style Perspectives." *Qualitative Health Research* 1:287-308.
———. 1992. "Cancer, Heart Disease and AIDS: What Do the Media Tell Us About These Diseases?" *Health Communication* 4:105-20.
Coutts, L. Block, and D. H. Berg. 1993. "The Portrayal of the Menstruating Woman in Menstrual Product Advertising." *Health Care for Women International* 14:179-91.
Davis, Maxine. 1949. "Care of the Breast." *Good Housekeeping* (November) 40.
Day, Emerson. 1955. "Cancer and a Woman's Sex." *Woman's Home Companion* (January) 28.
Edwards, Jane. 1994. "Private Cancer, Public Cancer: Guilt and Innocence in Popular Literature." *Australian Journal of Communication* 21:1-13.
Frank, Stanley. 1964. "Reassuring Facts About the Breast Cancer Controversy." *Good Housekeeping* (February) 45-47.
Goldman, Robert. 1992. *Reading Ads Socially.* London: Routledge.
Gordon, Nahida H., Joseph P. Crowe, Jane Brumberg, and Nathan Berger. 1992. "Socioeconomic Factors and Race in Breast Cancer Recurrence and Survival." *American Journal of Epidemiology* 135:609-18.
Hall, Stuart. 1995. "The Whites of Their Eyes: Racist Ideologies and the Media." Pp. 18-22 in *Gender, Race and Class in Media,* ed. G. Dines and J. Humez. London: Sage.
"How to Examine Your Breasts and Save Your Life." 1975. *Harper's Bazaar* (January) 54.
Hutchinson, Woods. 1914. "Nature's Mothers' Pension." *Good Housekeeping* (April) 530-34.
James, T. F. 1960. "Cancer and Your Emotions." *Cosmopolitan* (April) 40-43.
Johnson, J. David. 1997. "Factors Distinguishing Regular Readers of Breast Cancer Information in Magazines." *Women and Health* 26:7-27.

Kellner, Douglas. 1995. "Cultural Studies, Multiculturalism and Media Culture." Pp. 5-17 in *Gender, Race and Class in Media*, ed. G. Dines and J. Humez. London: Sage.

Kessler, L. 1989. "Women's Magazines' Coverage of Smoking Related Health Hazards." *Journalism Quarterly* 66: 316-22.

Lamberg, Lynne. 1981. "Back to Business: Surviving the Biggest Crisis of All." *Working Woman* (October) 85.

Lantz, Paula M., and Karen M. Booth. 1998. "The Social Construction of the Breast Cancer Epidemic." *Social Science and Medicine* 46:907-18.

Lewis, Howard R., and Martha A. Lewis. 1972. "Personality Traits that May Lead to Cancer." *Ladies' Home Journal* (April) 96.

Little, Clarence Cook. 1936. "The Conquest of Cancer." *Good Housekeeping* (May) 78.

Lupton, Deborah. 1994. "Femininity, Responsibility and the Technological Imperative: Discourses on Breast Cancer in the Australian Press." *International Journal of Health Services* 24:73-89.

Menagh, Melanie. 1992. "Preventing Breast Cancer: What's a Girl to Do?" *Mademoiselle* (October) 111-12.

McElwaine, Sandra. 1991. "I Feel Lucky!" *Redbook* (March) 36.

Ortiz, Jeanne A., and Larry P. Ortiz. 1989. "Do Contemporary Women's Magazines Practice What They Preach?" *Free Inquiry in Creative Sociology* 17:51-55.

Palmer, Gretta. 1947. "Face Your Danger." *Ladies' Home Journal* (June) 143.

Patterson, James T. 1987. *The Dread Disease: Cancer and Modern American Culture*. Cambridge: Harvard University Press.

Ramsey, Judith. 1969. "A Healthier Bosom." *Ladies' Home Journal* (April) 82.

Ratcliff, J. D. 1953. "You Can Fight Cancer in Your Own Home." *Woman's Home Companion* (May) 44.

Ruzek, Sheryl Burt. 1978. *The Women's Health Movement: Feminist Alternatives to Medical Control*. New York: Praeger.

———. 1980. "Medical Response to Women's Health Activities: Conflict, Accommodation and Cooptation." *Research in the Sociology of Health Care* 1:335-54.

Sontag, Susan. [1977] 1988. *Illness as Metaphor*. New York: Doubleday.

Stacey, Judith. 1990. *Brave New Families: Stories of Domestic Upheaval in Late Twentieth Century America*. Berkeley: University of California Press.

Wells, Barbara L., and John W. Horm. 1992. "Stage at Diagnosis in Breast Cancer: Race and Socioeconomic Factors." *American Journal of Public Health* 82:1383-85.

Whatley, Mariamne H., and Nancy Worcester. 1989. "The Role of Technology in the Co-optation of the Women's Health Movement: The Cases of Osteoporosis and Breast Cancer Screening." Pp. 199-200 in *Healing Technology: Feminist Perspectives*, ed. Kathryn Strother Ratcliff, Myra Marx Ferree and Gail O. Mellow. Ann Arbor: University of Michigan Press.

Winship, Janice. 1991. "The Impossibility of Best: Enterprise Meets Domesticity in the Practical Women's Magazines of the 1980s." *Cultural Studies* 5:131-56.

Yadlon, Susan. 1997. "Skinny Women and Good Mothers: The Rhetoric of Risk, Control, and Culpability in the Production of Knowledge about Breast Cancer." *Feminist Studies* 23:644-77.

Zimmerman, Mary. 1987. "The Women's Health Movement: A Critique of Medical Enterprise and the Position of Women." Pp. 442-72 in *Analyzing Gender: A Handbook of Social Science Research*, ed. Beth B. Hess and Myra Marx Ferree. London: Sage.

CHAPTER ELEVEN

Sister Support:
Women Create a Breast Cancer Movement

Barbara A. Brenner, J.D.

> When I dare to be powerful, to use my strength in the service of my vision, then it becomes less important whether or not I am unafraid.
>
> —Audre Lorde, *The Cancer Journals*

Writing in 1980, six months after she underwent a modified radical mastectomy at the age of 44, Audre Lorde spoke of the fear experienced by virtually every woman who hears the dreaded words, "You have breast cancer." At the time, almost no one had heard of breast cancer support groups and there was no breast cancer movement.[1] When Lorde died from breast cancer in November 1992, the social and political landscape had changed dramatically. Breast cancer was no longer a personal secret; the breast cancer movement in the United States had grown from support groups to national organizations. Grass-roots groups were scattered across America.

The evolution and the politics of the breast cancer movement reflect the birth and growth of a social movement born out of women's recognition that being forced by social pressures to hide breast cancer meant that none of their needs would be met. Women recognized that support, effective treatments, and real prevention would come about only if they stepped out of their houses and united to satisfy their needs or to demand that others take steps to address them. The seeds of these developments lay in women's personal experiences of the illness and in their willingness to "use their strength in the service of their vision" (Lorde 1980:15). Growing from women's experiences with breast cancer, the breast cancer movement has become an influential force. Millions of dollars have been raised for the cause, and funding for breast cancer research has increased significantly. Moreover, issues of racial and economic diversity and of the links between breast cancer activism and social and political efforts directed at social change have begun to surface.

BREAST CANCER SUPPORT—THE ROOTS OF ACTIVISM

Breast cancer support groups, where women diagnosed with the disease receive psychological and emotional support for the myriad issues that confront a woman with breast cancer, have been critically important to women struggling with the many issues raised by a breast cancer diagnosis. These groups have been the point of origin of the breast cancer movement, arguably one of the most effective health movements in the United States.

The first organized mutual support activity was the Reach to Recovery program, but it took years to materialize. Probably because the program had an intentionally apolitical orientation, it became the background against which the breast cancer support movement was founded and became politicized. Initiated in 1952 by two women who underwent Halsted radical mastectomies and who offered emotional support and practical help to other women hospitalized with the same surgery,[2] the Reach to Recovery program was adopted by the American Cancer Society (ACS) in 1969.

The program involved a woman volunteer visiting a woman hospitalized for breast cancer surgery and delivering a message that was carefully controlled by the ACS. The philosophy of the program was to convince women that they did not have what was then considered a disabling handicap.[3] The support was short term, providing newly treated women with a temporary breast prosthesis and instructing them in exercises to restore freedom of movement. The volunteers were breast cancer survivors who were to serve as walking evidence of medicine's ability to "cure" breast cancer and were forbidden to give any medical advice so as not to contravene anything the patient's doctor might have told her (Batt 1994:218). The formation of mastectomy clubs where women could gather to share their experiences was explicitly rejected by the ACS because of its belief that a mastectomy was not a permanent handicap, and that even the worse scars could be hidden by a well-fitting prosthesis and the right clothes (p. 222). But women knew better.

In 1973, the women's health book *Our Bodies, Ourselves* was published. The book, published by and for women, permitted women for the first time to readily inform themselves about a wide range of women's health issues. It was in the environment of women's self-help efforts characterized by the publication of *Our Bodies, Ourselves* that Rose Kushner was diagnosed in 1974 with breast cancer. Almost immediately, Kushner began demanding that the ACS provide women in the Reach to Recovery program with the opportunity to share with each other their experiences with the long-term physical and emotional consequences of mastectomy surgery.

The ACS, presumably convinced that masking the frightening impact of a breast cancer diagnosis and breast cancer surgery was in the organization's and women's best interest, and unwilling to challenge the established biomedical model that doctors know best, could not be moved. But Kushner, determined to support other women who were struggling with breast cancer, established the Breast Cancer Advisory Center in 1975, a hotline and mail service that provided information about breast cancer to women and men confronted with an illness about which they knew virtually nothing (Altman 1996:295). Kushner made breast cancer a public matter, inspiring support services and access to information that have characterized the world of breast cancer over the last 25 years. Rejecting the ACS's role as gatekeeper to breast cancer information and support, women began to form postmastectomy clubs. A year after Kushner started the Breast Cancer Advisory Center, a Post Mastectomy Discussion Group, organized by a doctor who specialized in breast cancer, began in New York. Though the doctor facilitated the first meeting, a mental health professional quickly took over the role (Altman 1996:298).

In March 1977, the Post Mastectomy Discussion Group turned their personal support into political action. Saks Fifth Avenue, an upscale department store, had offered a job to Jacqueline Bleibert as a sales clerk in the pocketbook department. When Bleibert informed the store's nurse that she had had a mastectomy, the job offer was immediately withdrawn. Members of the Post Mastectomy Discussion Group joined the National Organization for Women (NOW) in a lunchtime demonstration of women in fur coats who chanted "this store discriminates against women" and cut up their Saks credit cards. The store reinstated the job offer (Altman 1996:297).

The impetus for the Saks demonstration came from NOW—an organization focused principally on issues related to women's equality—and the theme of the demonstration was more about employment discrimination than about breast cancer. Apparently not ready to devote itself to political activity, the Post Mastectomy Discussion Group returned its focus to support and evolved into SHARE (Self-Help Action Rap Experience), the first formal organization established for the purpose of giving women an opportunity to support each other through their experiences with breast cancer.

As breast cancer has come out of the closet and as the medical and scientific communities have reported on studies that show extended survival for women in support groups (Spiegel 1993), support groups and organizations have developed throughout the country. Today, SHARE is an agency with a yearly budget in excess of $1.2 million that runs dozens of volunteer-led support and educational groups on a wide variety of breast cancer issues throughout New York City (Fonfa 1998). Significantly, the 1998 Breast Cancer Resource List published by the National Alliance of Breast Cancer Organizations (NABCO) lists 350 breast cancer support organizations. (Because the list does not distinguish between support groups and education and advocacy organizations, the number may be overstated.)

Faced with intransigence from the ACS, the growth of so many formal organizations focused on emotional support for women with breast cancer reflects both the understanding that women can and do benefit from others' experience and the determination to share that experience. Predictably, these organizations exist for the most part in large urban areas, leaving those who live in more rural areas to struggle to find support in less-organized, more one-on-one ways. However, the local support movement also inspired the creation of national organizations focused on supporting people with or at risk of developing breast cancer. Y-ME was the first such organization. Founded in Chicago in 1979 by two women who first started a local support group, Y-ME has grown into a large breast cancer support program, operating a national toll-free information hotline and a telephone counseling service that provides support and tailored packets of information to women with breast cancer (Batt 1994:301).

In the mid- to late-1980s, the prevalence of breast cancer also inspired other kinds of assistance to cancer patients besides breast cancer support groups: organizations providing support to people with all kinds of cancer (Cancer Support Community, San Francisco, 1986), organizations providing practical support services such as home-based assistance and legal services (Women's Cancer Resource Center, Berkeley, 1986), organizations focused on lesbians with cancer (Mary Helen Mautner Project for Lesbians with Cancer [Mautner Project], Washington, D.C., 1985), and organizations that combine a concern for direct support with a feminist political agenda (Women's Community Cancer Project [WCCP], Boston, 1989).

While many of these organizations were started or inspired by women with breast cancer, they broadened the breast cancer support movement by bringing to it an explicitly feminist perspective that included addressing the needs of women with any form of cancer. Unfortunately, the issue of the needs of women with all kinds of cancer remained a matter discussed among small groups of feminists rather than in the board rooms where the national breast cancer movement was taking shape.

THE BIRTH OF BREAST CANCER ACTIVISM

While women throughout the United States were working to guarantee that their sisters with breast cancer received the emotional and practical support they needed, many women in support groups began to see other breast cancer issues—from research funding to access to care—that needed to be addressed. Coming together to support each other emotionally, women with breast cancer made the personal, social, and professional connections that grew into the political breast cancer movement.

For example, a support group at the Cancer Support Community was the birthplace of Breast Cancer Action (BCA). One of the first breast cancer organizations with a decidedly political agenda, San Francisco-based BCA held its first meetings in 1990 at the Cancer Support Community, where many of the original members were in a support group together. Elenore Pred, one of the founders of BCA, stressed the importance of moving beyond emotional support to organizing politically to demand a true cure and effective prevention. Her passion came from her own experience of having been told that she was cured, only to be diagnosed several years later with metastatic breast cancer. BCA's founding mission statement—to serve as a catalyst for the prevention and cure of breast cancer through education and advocacy—reflected a new direction for the breast cancer movement .

At the same time that BCA was forming, other organizations with similar agendas were emerging in many places. Organizations that had been focused on support began to develop political strategies. In northern California, Save Our Selves (Sacramento) and Bay Area Breast Cancer Network (San Jose), a Y-ME affiliate, joined together to demonstrate at the California capitol in the first Mother's Day March for Breast Cancer Awareness in May 1991. At that demonstration, which received heavy media coverage, Ellen Hobbs, founder of Save Our Selves, gave a speech in which she waved both her breast prosthesis and her wig above her head and told the crowd that she had been told these things would make her feel better. She then told the assembly, "But I don't feel better and I won't feel better until more research is done into this horrible disease" (Batt 1994:233).

Hobbs' reference to feeling better was an explicit rejection of the ACS's "Look Good, Feel Better" program which evolved out of the Reach to Recovery program as breast cancer treatments extended beyond hospitals and surgery to outpatient radiation and chemotherapy. "Look Good, Feel Better" encouraged women to take advantage of wig and make-up programs, "learning to disguise the physical evidence of cancer treatments" ("Look Good, Feel Better" 1998).

For women like Ellen Hobbs, Elenore Pred, and the thousands of women who joined organizations like Save Our Selves and BCA, exposing the real impact of breast cancer on women's lives would be necessary before moving toward cure and prevention. Neither make-up nor a prosthesis would change the effects of breast cancer; that would take political action. The ACS, with its focus on make-up, and on mammograms as a so-called prevention strategy for breast cancer, was seen by these activists as a barrier to change rather than as an ally in addressing the needs of women with and at risk for breast cancer.[4]

While activists were demonstrating in California's capital, women on the other side of the country were organizing political action to respond to a New York State Department of Health study linking the high rate of breast cancer on Long Island to high income levels and virtually ruling out environmental factors (New York State Department of Health 1990). When the report was released in 1990, women with breast cancer on Long Island came together to demand explanations for the high rates of the disease in their communities. Unwilling to accept their income levels as the cause of their breast cancer, these women wanted the government to examine environmental hazards that might be contributing to the incidence of breast cancer on Long Island. Having supported each other through their diagnoses and treatments, women were now supporting each other by demanding that political and scientific attention be directed toward the causes of breast cancer in their communities.

PUSHING THE POLICYMAKERS

The first demands of the politically oriented breast cancer organizations were for state legislative changes that would guarantee women access to breast cancer screening and treatment information, and for policy changes at the federal level that would assure that increased research funds would be devoted to breast cancer.

In 1991, Vermont breast cancer activists successfully lobbied the state legislature for a bill requiring insurance companies to pay for mammograms (Altman 1996:301).[5] In 1992, the Vermont legislature declared breast cancer a national health emergency at the instigation of state breast cancer activists, a step that had little impact at the state level but lent credence to what would shortly become a national political effort. The same year, California enacted laws guaranteeing that standardized written information about breast cancer treatments be provided to breast cancer patients and creating a state breast cancer research fund with monies generated through an income tax checkoff. Also in 1992, Massachusetts, responding to pressure from the Massachusetts Breast Cancer Coalition, became the first state to declare breast cancer an epidemic, announcing a three-part plan to address breast cancer education, licensing of mammography facilities, and monitoring of the incidence of breast cancer in the state.

Women active in breast cancer issues at the state level also began to focus attention on federal agencies. For example, breast cancer organizations on Long Island forced the Centers for Disease Control (CDC) to reexamine the conclusions of the state study of Long Island breast cancer rates that ignored possible environmental factors. By 1993, pressure from Long Island breast cancer organizations dissatisfied with the state's conclusion that higher breast cancer rates in the region were attributable to higher incomes in the area forced the National Institutes of Health (NIH) to begin the Long Island Breast Cancer Study Project. The project is an epidemiological study of possible environmental links to breast cancer on Long Island and includes an examination of biological markers for environmental factors. Breast cancer advocates took an active role in framing the research questions being examined by the project, results from which are expected in 2000.

In 1991, breast cancer activists confronted federal policymakers at the National Cancer Institute (NCI) and in Congress for the first time. They met with Samuel Broder, then Director of the NCI, to demand that the NCI focus more of its research attention on breast cancer. Dr. Broder acknowledged the need to involve breast cancer patient advocates in the research process and to focus more breast cancer research on premenopausal women, *but he insisted that politics and science would not mix* (Shayer 1998). Unpersuaded by Broder's concerns, the activists met with Ohio Congresswoman Mary Rose Oakar, whose sister had had breast cancer and who was sponsoring a bill authorizing $25 million for NCI to conduct research on breast cancer. At a press conference called by Congress-woman Oakar, Ellen Hobbs of Save Our Selves (Sacramento) again removed her wig, making the effects of breast cancer visible in new and dramatic ways in the corridors of federal power.

THE POWER OF NUMBERS—
COMING TOGETHER TO FIGHT BREAST CANCER

While breast cancer advocates throughout the United States were forming grass-roots organizations to address concerns at local and state levels and beginning to unite on federal issues, several national breast cancer organizations had been functioning for some time. The Dallas-based Susan G. Komen Breast Cancer Foundation's "Race for the Cure" began raising significant funds for the organization with its first five-kilometer race in 1983. The National Alliance of Breast Cancer Organizations (NABCO) began in 1986 as a network of breast cancer organizations providing information and referral for anyone with questions about breast cancer. With the growth of grass-roots activity, it made sense to see what national organizations in collaboration with the more local groups could accomplish together. The federal policy agenda—both legislative and scientific—quickly became the focus of their combined efforts.

Not long before Ellen Hobbs took off her wig in Washington, D.C., discussions had begun about the creation of a coordinated effort to fight breast cancer. At the end of 1990, three women from different backgrounds and organizations met to brainstorm about a coalition of grass-roots breast cancer organizations that would bring breast cancer patients to Washington to lobby for legislative and regulatory changes needed to address the breast cancer epidemic. The women were Susan Hester, Founder and Director of the Mary Helen Mautner Project for Lesbians with Cancer; Susan Love, surgeon and breast cancer researcher, then the Director of the Faulkner Breast Centre in Boston; and Amy Langer, Executive Director of NABCO. Though the faces and socioeconomic backgrounds of these women reflected the lack of racial and economic diversity that continues to plague much of the breast cancer movement, their different experiences and perspectives underscored the challenge of maintaining an effective coalition.

For example, breast cancer advocate Susan Hester was a lesbian who had grown up in feminism. The Mautner Project, though motivated by her deceased partner's experience of and death from breast cancer, served women with any kind of cancer. Susan Love, also a lesbian feminist, was on her way to becoming the most famous breast surgeon in the world. Amy Langer was a business woman who had used her business skills to transform NABCO into a national organization with close ties to the medical establishment. Could professionalism and grass-roots feminism unite in the battle against breast cancer? Could doctors and scientists function in coalition with lay people whose knowledge of and concerns about breast cancer derived from the deeply personal? Could small, underfunded organizations work with larger, more established entities without being swallowed up in the process? Many people believed that it was all possible, and in many ways they were right.

Calling on some of the same organizations that had helped to form NABCO, Amy Langer contacted representatives from Cancer Care (a New York social service agency for people with cancer), Komen, and Y-ME and suggested that it was time to undertake a joint advocacy effort. By spring of 1991, the National Breast Cancer Coalition (NBCC) was born, with a mission to eradicate breast cancer through action and advocacy. Of the founding organizational members, only three—NABCO, Y-ME, and the Faulkner Breast Centre—were exclusively focused on breast cancer. The others—Cancer Care, CAN ACT (Cancer Patients Action Alliance), the Mautner Project, and the Women's Community Cancer Project (WCCP)—had programs that addressed either all cancers or all women with cancer of any kind.

The Susan G. Komen Breast Cancer Foundation was conspicuously absent from the founding membership of NBCC. Describing itself as the largest private funder of research dedicated solely to breast cancer in the United States, the Komen Foundation had no significant competition in fund raising until NBCC was formed. By the time that breast cancer became a much-celebrated charity, the Komen Foundation had raised more than $65 million dollars, most of it between 1991 and 1996 (Belkin 1996). By 1997, the number had grown to $90 million.[6] It seems quite plausible that the Komen Foundation saw in the creation of NBCC a competitor for donations that might challenge the Foundation's stature.

Equally plausible—and not mutually exclusive—is the possibility that the unabashedly political agenda of the NBCC seemed incompatible with the Komen Foundation's more mainstream approach to breast cancer issues. The Komen Foundation's mission—to eradicate breast cancer as a life-threatening disease by advancing research, education, screening, and treatment—is significantly different from the action and advocacy message of NBCC. This difference in world views held by the Komen Foundation and other, more grass-roots types of organizations, is reflected in the fact that some breast cancer activists refer to the Komen Foundation as "the ladies' auxiliary of breast cancer," distinguishing the dedicated and well-meaning Komen Foundation volunteers from advocates who have taken it upon themselves to learn and challenge both the science and the politics of breast cancer.

Whatever the explanation, the Komen Foundation's absence did not deter NBCC. While the goals of NBCC were and are broad—promoting research, improving access to screening and care, and increasing the influence in the policy arena of women living with breast cancer—the coalition's initial efforts were focused on increasing the level of funding appropriated at the federal level for breast cancer research.

MORE MONEY FOR RESEARCH

The 1991 research funding campaign was a true grass-roots coalition effort. Coordinated by Y-ME, the effort generated letters to be delivered to Congress and President George Bush, urging them to support breast cancer–related research. The goal was to have 175,000 letters—one for every new breast cancer case expected in 1991—from women throughout the country, with every state sending the number of letters that corresponded to the expected number of new diagnoses in that state. Members of the organizations participating in NBCC spread the word across the country. Proving that the time was right, a total of 600,000 letters were collected by state coordinators in all states (Altman 1996:317).

As a direct result of the letter campaign, publicly funded breast cancer research in the United States increased significantly. In 1981, breast cancer research funded by the federal government through the NCI and National Institutes of Health (NIH) totaled less than $40 million (Marshall 1993). By 1993, due to the efforts of NBCC, breast cancer research funded by the NIH and the Department of Defense (DOD) stood at $407 million (Altman 1996:319). In 1998, the figure reached $595 million, and NBCC set its sights on $2.6 billion dollars by the year 2000.[7] To support their demand, NBCC in 1997 delivered to Congress 2.6 million signatures—one for every woman living with breast cancer in the United States (Altman 1996:321).

INFLUENCING THE RESEARCH AGENDA

Extending their political clout, women living with breast cancer created a role for themselves in setting the overall direction of federal policy on breast cancer. In late 1993, at the urging of NBCC, Secretary of Health and Human Services Donna Shalala convened a "Conference to Establish a National Action Plan on Breast Cancer." Participants included not only experts in screening, access, research, and treatment, but also breast cancer activists and survivors from throughout the United States.

The National Action Plan on Breast Cancer was announced in March 1994. A "public/private partnership," the Plan brought together representatives from the NIH and private citizens active on breast cancer issues to work on six priority issues that ranged from developing strategies for information dissemination to the etiology of breast cancer (Altman 1996:326ff). Since the Plan was established, its public/private working groups have done extensive work to advance the Plan's objectives, and clinicians, researchers, policymakers, and the general public rely on the Plan's analysis of a variety of breast cancer issues.[8] The working groups are now ending, in part because much of their work has been completed and in part as a result of fundamental disagreements between the initial co-chairs of the Plan. But the model set by these activists, scientists, and policymakers working together on challenging issues in breast cancer continues to be followed in the research funding arena.

TAKING A SEAT OR REDESIGNING THE TABLE

Reflecting the aim of many of its member organizations, NBCC has as one of its principal goals "increasing the influence of women living with breast cancer and other breast cancer activists in the decision making that impacts all issues surrounding breast cancer."[9] In the context of participating in the research funding process, the progress toward that goal to date has been real but limited.

The first example of a new model that brought women living with breast cancer into the research funding decision making process was the California Breast Cancer Research Program. Created in 1993 at the insistence of breast cancer advocates working with sympathetic state legislators, the program is funded with cigarette-tax dollars and makes grants for research into "the cause, cure, prevention and early detection of breast cancer" and into "the cultural barriers to accessing the health care system for early detection and treatment of breast cancer" (California Breast Cancer Research Program 1995:5,8).

Breast cancer advocates play a role in every step of the research funding process. They participate on an equal footing with scientists on the peer review panels that evaluate the scientific merit of grant applications, and funds are distributed based on research priorities set by a council which, by law, includes representatives from breast cancer survivor and advocacy groups (California Breast Cancer Research Program 1995:5). By including breast cancer advocates at every stage of the research funding process, the California program was the first to shift away from the funding model then used by the NIH, in which decisions about what research would be funded rested entirely with the scientists and clinicians.

The California program was copied at the federal level when the DOD became the repository of some of the breast cancer research funds appropriated by Congress. The DOD Breast Cancer Research Program was created in 1993 as a way of sheltering breast cancer research funds from Congressional budget cuts directed at all domestic spending except the defense budget. As in the California program, women living with breast cancer are involved in setting the research funding priorities for the DOD program and in evaluating the scientific merit of funding proposals.

In the DOD study groups, all proposals are assigned to primary and secondary scientific reviewers. However, because there are only two breast cancer advocates in each study section and many proposals to evaluate, some proposals are not reviewed by any advocate. Where a breast cancer advocate does review a proposal, the scientists in the study section hear a perspective about the potential value of research that would otherwise be missing.

Many women have educated themselves on the science of breast cancer, either through self-education or through programs like NBCC's Project LEAD (Leadership, Education and Advocacy Development) in which scientists train women in the biology and genetics of breast cancer. But even the best educated breast cancer advocates are unable to redirect the discourse in a room filled with scientists where discussions of merit are framed in a technical discourse and dominated by the assigned scientific reviewers and other study section members.

Although the breast cancer advocates each have a vote in ranking proposals, their votes are inevitably outweighed by the votes of the 15 to 18 scientists and clinicians assigned to the study section. It is perhaps telling that, in one of the stranger uses of the English language, the breast cancer activists who serve on the Department of Defense peer review and priority-setting panels are called "breast cancer consumers" and "breast cancer consumer advocates." The term consumer not only minimizes the role that women living with breast cancer play in the research funding process but also relegates them to the same position vis-à-vis breast cancer that they occupy relative to groceries and pharmaceutical products.

The numerical imbalance in the membership structure of the study groups makes it almost impossible for the views of the breast cancer advocates—whatever they are called—to carry the day. Nonetheless, the presence of their voices means that scientists and clinicians hear, often for the first time, what the decisions they are making mean to the women who are the ultimate targets of breast cancer research. Whether that voice will, in time, lead the scientific community to new perspectives on the research they are evaluating remains to be seen. It must be noted, however, that all government-funded cancer research is premised on a paradigm of scientific research that presumes that scientific merit must and can be evaluated before the research is conducted, and that it is best evaluated by scientists and clinicians who specialize in the field of the proposal. This paradigm makes it extremely difficult to change the type of breast cancer research being funded.

Impatient with both the incremental nature of scientific progress in treating breast cancer and the virtually nonexistent progress in preventing the disease, some women's cancer activists, including grass-roots breast cancer organizations, are challenging both what research is funded and the way it is funded. Organizations such as BCA and WCCP, both represented on the National Action Plan on Breast Cancer, criticize the failure of the cancer research establishment to tackle the difficult multidisciplinary challenge of studying the role of environmental toxins in the development or progress of breast cancer (Brenner 1999). They question whether an incremental research methodology is ever likely to lead to true understanding of what causes breast cancer and, therefore, how it might be prevented. These organizations and others, like Agatha's Sisters in Portland, Oregon,[10] also question the system of research funding that forces researchers to spend as much time scrambling for funding as looking for answers to pressing scientific and medical issues (Brenner 1997).

But the changing economics of cancer research may mean that the work of breast cancer activists—whether within the research process or from a policy perspective—to redirect government-funded scientific research may prove irrelevant in light of the amount of cancer research that is now being done by for-profit companies (Pharmaceutical Research Manufacturers Association 1999).[11] The relationship of many of these companies to breast cancer organizations is raising critical questions about the direction of the breast cancer movement.

PAYING THE PIPER, CALLING THE TUNE

A number of pharmaceutical and biotechnology companies that are involved in the investigation of potential new treatments for—or "chemo-prevention" approaches to—breast cancer see a natural alliance between themselves and breast cancer organizations interested in promoting research into cure and prevention. These companies increasingly express their affinity to breast cancer organizations in the form of cash grants. Questions have begun to arise within the breast cancer movement about the risks that accompany the obvious benefits of the grants: Does the self-interest of corporations working to increase their profits conflict with the work of breast cancer organizations? To what extent are corporate public relations efforts, reflected in the financial support of breast cancer organizations, defining the terms of the breast cancer discussion?

A pharmaceutical company plays a central role in National Breast Cancer Awareness Month (BCAM), the centerpiece of the largest educational effort on breast cancer. Every October since 1985, women throughout the country have been urged to get a mammogram and to help raise money for breast cancer research. BCAM was created by corporate giant Imperial Chemical Industries (ICI) in collaboration with Cancer Care. Zeneca Pharmaceuticals, formerly a subsidiary of ICI, took over the principal corporate sponsorship role for BCAM. Zeneca has many financial interests in cancer in general and in breast cancer in particular. The company manufactures and holds the patent for tamoxifen, the most commonly prescribed breast cancer drug. Zeneca controls a significant part of the market for tamoxifen and other cancer drugs through its majority stake in Salick Cancer Centers. Before 1999, Zeneca was also the fourth largest producer of pesticides in the United States, including at least one pesticide that is a known carcinogen (Brady 1997). Recently, in April of 1999, Zeneca merged with Astra Pharmaceuticals to become AstraZeneca, the third largest drug company in the world. Among other pharmaceuticals and agrochemicals, AstraZeneca has produced acetochlor, a herbicide that is a known carcinogen, although the company recently announced its plan to spin off its chemical manufacturing operation and merge it with that of Novartis, another company that also makes breast cancer drugs (Sorkin 1999).

As the principal corporate sponsor of BCAM, AstraZeneca controls the messages that are used in the campaign (Brady 1997).[12] AstraZeneca's misleading BCAM messages, promoted with the help of many cancer organizations, first advertised mammograms as preventing breast cancer and now tout the breast x-ray as protection against the illness. In fact, mammograms are a detection device that is not foolproof. The technology often can detect breast cancer— but it can neither prevent the illness nor protect a woman from getting it. Moreover, thanks to AstraZeneca, the word carcinogen never appears in BCAM promotional materials.

BCAM is now endorsed by federal health agencies, including the NCI and large nonprofit organizations, including NABCO and the Susan G. Komen Breast Cancer Foundation. The promotional materials related to Breast Cancer Awareness Month indicate that BCAM is made possible by an educational grant from AstraZeneca Pharmaceuticals, yet none of the endorsing organizations express any awareness of—let alone, any discomfort with—the fact that AstraZeneca has these conflicts of interest in promoting the breast cancer educational campaign.

In contrast, grass-roots organizations focused on breast cancer, on cancer generally, or on the links between environmental degradation and health *do* express concern over AstraZeneca's involvement in BCAM and over the failure of the major cancer organizations to focus any attention on the possible links between the environment and cancer. Renaming October National Cancer Industry Awareness Month in 1995,[13] grass-roots organizations attacked BCAM as a disinformation campaign that promoted mammography to camouflage the environmental causes of cancer (Greenpeace 1995). Since 1994, the same year that NABCO endorsed BCAM, a San Francisco coalition of cancer and environmental organizations called the Toxic Links Coalition has sponsored an October Toxic Tour of industries and organizations that pollute the environment and promote the "get your mammogram and you'll be fine" myth. Using the theme "Make the Link," the Toxic Tour encourages people to make the connections between corporate profits and the cancer epidemic (Klawiter 1999:108).

The National Cancer Industry Awareness Month analysis highlights not only the limitations of the BCAM educational campaign but also the dilemma for breast cancer organizations in accepting funds from corporations that profit from the breast cancer epidemic. While activists and corporations engaged in breast cancer are both interested in effective treatments, pharmaceutical products have much different consequences for women than they do for corporate profits. How are women to know, for example, whether the heralding by NABCO of the "success" of the tamoxifen Breast Cancer Prevention Trial was based on the merits of the results or the fact that NABCO receives significant funding from AstraZeneca, the manufacturer of tamoxifen? One can only speculate about what would have happened to NABCO's funding if it had criticized the tamoxifen trial. Breast cancer organizations that accept funding from drug companies also may find it against their organizational interests to advocate for a change in the direction of breast cancer research.

AstraZeneca is not the only drug company that supports breast cancer advocacy efforts, nor is NABCO the only breast cancer organization that receives significant financial support from pharmaceutical companies.[14] Disclaimers of any influence notwithstanding, the funding of breast cancer groups by pharmaceutical companies and other corporations whose profits are made by detecting or treating cancer inevitably leads to questions about whether the organization receiving the funds can and does fairly communicate information that is critically important to women with or at risk of developing breast cancer.[15]

Determined that their statements about women's health issues not be tainted by their funding sources, the National Women's Health Network, WCCP, and DES Action have consistently refused to accept any funding from pharmaceutical companies. However, with the exception of Breast Cancer Action, which in 1998 adopted a new policy prohibiting the acceptance of financial contributions from any company that makes its profits in the breast cancer field, breast cancer organizations have not generally followed this model.

The other side of the corporate funding issue focuses on the consequences—if any—of allowing corporate environmental polluters to prove their commitment to the public's health by giving money to breast cancer organizations. The debate focuses on two issues. The first issue is that, by accepting such gifts, cancer organizations permit corporations to use their philanthropy to deflect attention from the ways that they may be contributing to cancer. The second issue is that it is nearly impossible for breast cancer groups that accept such funding to build coalitions with grass-roots environmental health organizations working to change the conduct of corporate environmental polluters in the communities where their members live.

These concerns helped stimulate BCA's 1998 policy decision to refuse funds from corporations that produce products or use production methods that promulgate known or probable carcinogens (Roemer 1999). Larger breast cancer organizations, such as the Komen Foundation, NBCC, and NABCO, appear to be ignoring the debate, possibly because their agendas do not address the social and economic causes of breast cancer but, instead, focus on forcing the existing scientific and medical establishment to accommodate their interests. Thus, the Komen Foundation presumably saw no connection between air pollution and the cancer epidemic when it agreed to accept a dollar from BMW for every test mile driven.[16] In addition, NBCC appeared to be similarly indifferent when it agreed to be the beneficiary of a General Motors charity initiative. In contrast, the Breast Cancer Fund, a San Francisco-based fund-raising and funding organization that focuses on environmental issues, explicitly rejects the critique of its acceptance of funding from companies, such as Chevron, perceiving the challenge as "trying to turn an adversary into an ally by showing that it can be profitable to change" (Martin 1998:6).

The varying responses to issues of corporate funding reveal clear differences in both the strategies and goals of breast cancer organizations. As long as breast cancer remains an important charity, one at which people and companies are happy to throw money, these differences will not be discernible except by people closest to the various organizations. As other issues begin to rival breast cancer in philanthropic importance, it will become necessary for breast cancer organizations to distinguish themselves from each other. Whether the difference is in how funds are raised or in the agenda set for addressing breast cancer issues, or both, these differences will determine how much support an organization receives and, quite probably, how much influence it wields in the breast cancer movement.

ALL WOMEN ARE AT RISK

Breast cancer knows no boundaries of race, ethnicity, or social class. Addressing the needs of underserved women while pushing for the changes in diagnosis, treatment, and prevention that will ultimately end the breast cancer epidemic is the most daunting challenge facing the breast cancer movement (Hardisty and Leopold 1993). As American society becomes increasingly divided between the haves and the have-nots, breast cancer issues perceived and addressed by breast cancer activists differ considerably depending on where the activist resides on the continuum of access to health care.

One example of this divergence is seen in the discussions about mammograms and breast self-exam as techniques for breast cancer detection. Women with access to mammograms complain about the ineffectiveness of the technology to safely and without fail detect breast cancer at an early stage; they also debate issues of the age at which women should begin to have annual mammograms. For women who have no health insurance or only catastrophic insurance coverage, the pressing issues are providing access to the technology at all and making sure that women are trained in breast self-examination.

Another example is the controversy surrounding genetic testing for breast cancer risk, which presents a set of issues of great concern to women with access to insurance coverage for the very expensive tests, but is of little interest to those women whose family histories of the breast cancer may be as significant but who are unlikely to be able to pay for the test. Moreover, efforts to encourage greater participation by women of color in breast cancer clinical trials ignore the fundamental mistrust of medical experiments that arises out of the experience of the African American community in the United States. The Tuskeegee syphilis experiment (Jones 1981) as well as environmental racism, reflected in efforts to build a nuclear waste dump near the homes and sacred lands of native peoples in California (Michael and Wilkinson 1998), leave communities of color rightfully suspicious of the motives of policymakers who seek to include them in scientific research.

These disparities in the concerns that are addressed by activists, along with the relatively greater access of white middle-class women to agents of social change that include the media and legislative representatives, have led to a significant gap between what is generally portrayed as the experience of breast cancer and the real life experiences of many women with and at risk for the disease. Part of the response of large established breast cancer organizations has been to create program activities that provide underserved women with access to breast health education and mammograms. NABCO, for example, administered the Avon Breast Health Access Fund. The Komen Foundation funds mammography screening programs for women who have limited access. Unfortunately, programs limited to screening and detection do not address the many issues—such as the cost and impact of treatment and how to keep food on their tables—that confront women of limited means when they have received a breast cancer diagnosis.

In 1998, NBCC, noting the dilemma of funding screening but not treatment for low-income women, made funding for treatment for women diagnosed through the federal Breast and Cervical Cancer Early Detection Program one of its priority issues. A similar effort is underway to assure that Californians screened through the state's early detection program have access to treatment if they are found to have breast cancer.[17]

However, it is not enough for organizations to advocate on issues affecting underserved women. *A breast cancer movement that actually reflects the diversity of those who are affected by breast cancer must represent the entire range of issues that affect all women.* Such a movement is most likely to come into existence by making room for the voices of women whose stories are most often left out when breast cancer is discussed, and by making it possible for these women to take their rightful places at the front of the breast cancer movement.

One strategy for building diversity within the breast cancer movement is reflected in the Breast Cancer Oral History Action Project (BCOHAP), based in Berkeley, California. The project, which works to make "the invisible visible," is a participatory action research and social justice education project that trains low-income, limited literacy, limited English-speaking women to gather multilingual oral histories of medically underserved women with breast cancer. Drawing on this research, the women created a traveling mural entitled "Who Holds the Mirror? Breast Cancer, Women's Lives, and the Environment" that affirms the individual and collective power of underserved women to be leaders in creating the knowledge and tools to educate their communities and to act on this knowledge by becoming involved in health and social justice issues in their communities. BCOHAP provides tools that allow underserved women to speak and act for themselves within the movement rather than attempting to address their concerns by speaking for them or through them.

REFORM OR REVOLUTION? GLITZ OR GRASS-ROOTS?

The issues and challenges that confront the breast cancer movement go to the essence of how the movement will look and what it will accomplish in the years ahead. Will the movement be predominantly reformist, seeking to modify existing institutions so that women have a voice in decisions that continue to be framed by those scientific researchers, government agencies, and pharmaceutical companies that do not put women's interests first? Or, will breast cancer activists push for fundamental changes in the social, political, and economic structures that have brought us to where we are in the breast cancer epidemic? Will money to support the work of the movement be raised through benefit film and theater premiers[18] and car-driving experiences or through grass-roots fund-raising efforts? Will the breast cancer movement be closely allied with the medical establishment in a way that jeopardizes women's interests? Or, will the movement become part of a broader agenda of women's health activism and social change?

For many activists, the somewhat dismaying answer to all of these questions is a qualified yes. The breast cancer movement, like all social movements, is made up of many forces. Absent a common institutional threat that forces all of the people and organizations working on breast cancer to come together, the strategies and objectives of the movement will continue to be as diverse as the people and organizations who constitute it. As a result, social change—both in the movement itself and in the scope and nature of the breast cancer epidemic—will come slowly. When that change does come, the result will be that all women with breast cancer will have clear choices for treatments that cure their disease without causing another one, and all people will live in a world where they are protected from the known causes of breast cancer. The road from here to there remains unmapped, but the breast cancer movement may yet pave the way.

NOTES

AUTHOR'S NOTE: I am grateful to Maren Klawiter and Jennifer Ruth Fosket for the research assistance they provided in connection with this chapter.

1. Rose Kushner's book, *Breast Cancer: A Personal History and an Investigative Report* (1975) was the first to approach breast cancer through the lens of a woman treated for breast cancer. Other than Kushner and Lorde, it would be more than ten years before anyone would publish a book that would suggest from a feminist perspective the political dimensions of the breast cancer epidemic (see Brady 1991; Butler and Rosenblum 1991; Lorde 1988; Solla 1994; Stocker 1991).

2. The two women were Fan Rosenau of Philadelphia and Therese Lasser of New York. (Interview, 1998, with Nina Smith, granddaughter of Fan Rosenau.)

3. In 1969, all women diagnosed with breast cancer in the United States who received conventional surgical treatment were routinely treated with a Halsted radical mastectomy, in which the breast tissue as well as all axillary lymph nodes and the pectoral muscle were removed. The extensive surgery made it impossible for women to use the arm on the affected side normally and left them looking caved in on that side.

4. The pink ribbon that has come to symbolize breast cancer awareness is similarly criticized by some activists. The issue is crystalized by the National Alliance of Breast Cancer Organization's (NABCO) 1997 Breast Cancer Resource List. The document contains a section entitled "General Information About Breast Cancer" which contains a single entry entitled "Practical Advice: Pink Ribbons," under which readers can learn about different types of pink ribbons available for purchase. For a thorough analysis of how the pink ribbon came to symbolize breast cancer, see Sandy Fernandez, "Pretty in Pink," *Mamm Magazine*, June/July 1998.

5. This effort mirrored that of the Susan G. Komen Foundation in Texas in 1987 (Altman 1996:312).

6. Information on the Komen Foundation can be found at the organization's website at www.komen.org.

7. NBCC website at www.stopbreastcancer.org.

8. Information on the mission, goals, and accomplishments of the National Action Plan on Breast Cancer (NAPBC) can be found at their website, www.napbc.org.

9. As stated at the NBCC website, www.stopbreastcancer.org.

10. Agatha's Sisters, a group named for a saint who was punished for her transgressions by having her breasts cut off, originally focused on understanding and exposing where and how the billions of dollars in cancer research are spent. The name of the group has since changed to Rachel's Friends and shifted its focus to the environmental concerns first articulated by Rachel Carson.

11. Using the bellicose language that has dominated the cancer discussion since Richard Nixon's declaration of the War on Cancer in the early 1970s, the Pharmaceutical Research Manufacturers Association's advertisements feature the word cancer in large red letters on a black page, below which the following text appears: "It's a War. That's why we're developing 316 new weapons." The ad goes on to describe that the medicines being developed are "all new weapons in the high-tech, high-stakes war against cancer." The web address for the association is published as www.searchforcures.org.

12. AstraZeneca's role in Breast Cancer Awareness Month is featured on the company's website: www.astrazeneca-us.com/corp/nbcam.htm

13. The term National Cancer Industry Awareness Month was coined in 1993 by Jeannie Marshall, a founding member of the Women's Community Cancer Project. Marshall died in 1995 at the age of 36 from chordoma, cancer of the spinal cord.

14. NBCC's Project LEAD science training program for breast cancer advocates is funded by pharmaceutical companies involved in the breast cancer market, including Bristol-Myers Squibb, Genentech, Pfizer, Glaxo-Wellcome, Eli Lilly, and Rhône-Poulenc Rorer (NBCC 1998). Many of the

same companies sponsored the NBCC World Conference on Breast Cancer Advocacy (NBCC 1997).

15. For an example of a disclaimer about the influence of corporate funding, see NABCO's website at www.nabco.org. NABCO's claim to act as a voice for the interests and concerns of women with and at risk for breast cancer is questionable when, for example, it promotes educational materials on genetic testing for breast cancer susceptibility that indicate a greater risk of carrying a genetic mutation and a greater benefit from genetic testing than are scientifically supported. These educational materials—prepared by Myriad Genetics Laboratories (1996), the major marketer of genetic testing—were distributed by NABCO to breast cancer organizations at a time when NABCO received funding from Myriad. In a 1996 report funded by Bristol-Myers Squibb Oncology, NABCO's list of pharmaceutical funders—at levels of $5,000 to $25,000, $25,000 to $50,000, and $100,000-and-up—is a virtual Fortune 500 of drug companies.

16. The Komen Foundation devotes little if any of its considerable resources to addressing issues related to the environment and cancer and, in the early years of its existence, it promoted mammograms as prevention. In 1999, Komen did join a public relations campaign urging that more public research dollars be devoted to environmental links to breast cancer.

17. A Breast Cancer Treatment Act introduced in the California legislature in February 1998 was vetoed by then-Governor Pete Wilson. The veto became an issue in the gubernatorial election that was underway at the time, and a legislative solution to the problem continues to be an important issue for many California breast cancer and women's health organizations.

18. NBCC was the beneficiary of a June 1998, screening of the film *Six Days, Seven Nights* starring Anne Heche and Harrison Ford. Ticket prices started at $250 and topped out at $10,000. In January 1998, The Breast Cancer Research Foundation benefited from a production of *Ragtime* for which tickets were priced at $1,000 and $2,500.

REFERENCES

Altman, Roberta. 1996. *Waking Up, Fighting Back: The Politics of Breast Cancer.* New York: Little, Brown.

American Cancer Society. 1998. *Cancer Facts and Figures, 1998.* Atlanta: American Cancer Society.

Batt, Sharon. 1994. *Patient No More: The Politics of Breast Cancer.* Charlottetown, P. E. I., Canada: Gynergy Books.

Belkin, Lisa. 1996. "How Breast Cancer Became This Year's Hottest Charity." *New York Times Magazine* (December 22) 40.

Brady, Judy. 1997. "Public Relations and Cancer." *Center News.* Berkeley: Women's Cancer Resource Center.

Brady, Judy (ed.). 1991. *One in Three: Women with Cancer Confront an Epidemic.* Pittsburgh: Cleis Press.

Brenner, Barbara. 1997. "Cash and Cancer: An Unholy Alliance." *Breast Cancer Action Newsletter* (June/July) 1.

———. 1998/1999. "Thinking Out Loud—Toward a New Research Strategy." *Breast Cancer Action Newsletter* (December/January) 7.

Butler, Sandra, and Barbara Rosenblum. 1991. *Cancer in Two Voices*. San Francisco: Spinsters.

California Breast Cancer Research Program. 1995. "Annual Report to the State of California Legislature 1995." Oakland: University of California.

Dickersin, Kay, and Lauren Schnaper. 1996. "Reinventing Medical Research." Pp. 57-76 in *Man-Made Medicine: Women's Health, Public Policy, and Reform* ed. Kary Moss. Durham, N.C.: Duke University Press.

Fonfa, Ann. 1998. Interviewed by Maren Klawiter.

Greenpeace. 1995. "October: National Cancer Industry Awareness Month." Flier.

Hardisty, Jean, and Ellen Leopold. 1993. "Cancer and Poverty: Double Jeopardy for Women." Pp. 213 in *Confronting Cancer, Constructing Change*, ed. Midge Stocker. Chicago: Third Side Press.

Jones, James. 1981. *Bad Blood: The Tuskegee Syphilis Experiment: A Tragedy of Race and Medicine*. New York: Free Press.

Klawiter, Maren. 1999. "Racing for the Cure, Walking Women, and Toxic Touring: Mapping Cultures of Action within the Bay Area Terrain of Breast Cancer." *Social Problems* 46:104-25.

Kushner, Rose. 1975. *Breast Cancer: A Personal History and an Investigative Report*. New York: Harcourt Brace Jovanovich.

"Look Good, Feel Better." 1998. *Mamm Magazine* (February/March) 1.

Lorde, Audre. 1980. *The Cancer Journals*. Argyle, NY: Spinsters Ink.

————. 1988. *A Burst of Light*. Ithaca, NY: Firebrand Books.

Marshall, Eliot. 1993. "The Politics of Breast Cancer." *Science* 259:616-36.

Martin, Andrea. 1998. "Letter." *Women's Cancer Resource Center Newsletter*. Berkeley: Women's Cancer Resource Center.

Michael, Nancy, and Kathleen Wilkinson. 1998. "Raising the Stakes at Ward Valley." *Breast Cancer Action Newsletter* (April/May).

Myriad Genetics Laboratories. 1996. "Genetic Analysis for Risk of Breast and Ovarian Cancer: Is It Right for You?" Salt Lake City: Myriad Genetics Laboratories.

National Alliance of Breast Cancer Organizations (NABCO). 1996. "The First Ten Years." New York: National Alliance of Breast Cancer Organization.

National Breast Cancer Coalition (NBCC). 1997. "World Conference on Breast Cancer Advocacy Program Announcement." Washington, D.C.: National Breast Cancer Coalition.

————. 1998. "Project Lead Program Announcement." Washington, D.C.: National Breast Cancer Coalition.

National Cancer Institute. 1995. "Cancer Facts: Hispanic American Women Breast Cancer and Mammography Facts." Bethesda, MD: National Cancer Institute.

————. 1995. "Breast Cancer Research and Programs: An Overview." Bethesda, Md: National Cancer Institute.

New York State Department of Health. 1990. "The Long Island Breast Cancer Study, Report Number 1." Albany: New York State Department of Health.

Pharmaceutical Research Manufacturers Association. 1999. "Advertisement." *New Yorker* (Feb. 22), 61.

Roemer, Jennifer. 1999. "Thanks, But No Thanks: Breast Cancer Group Declines Funding." *Journal of the National Cancer Institute* 91:108.

Shayer, Belle. 1998. Interview. (Belle Shayer is a woman living with breast cancer and a founder of Breast Cancer Action.)

Soffa, Virginia. 1994. *The Journey Beyond Breast Cancer: From the Personal to the Political.* Rochester, VT: Healing Arts Press.

Sorkin, Andrew Ross. 1999. "AstraZeneca and Novartis Shed Agricultural Units." *New York Times* (December 3).

Spiegel, David. 1993. "Psychosocial Intervention in Cancer." *Journal of the National Cancer Institute* 85:1198-1205.

Stocker, Midge, ed. 1991. *Cancer as a Women's Issue: Scratching the Surface.* Chicago: Third Side Press.

Eliminating Breast Cancer from Our Future

Anne S. Kasper, Ph.D., and Susan J. Ferguson, Ph.D.

The chapters in this book have raised issues that are critical to advancing our understanding of breast cancer. They also provide us with a vision for ending the epidemic of breast cancer. As we have seen, breast cancer is no longer defined solely by its medical dimensions or by the narratives of individual women who have lived with the illness. The candor with which the chapters in this book were written owes much to the ever-increasing attention being paid to breast cancer. This public visibility was created by the massive efforts of thousands of breast cancer activists and by the willingness of many more women living with breast cancer to be outspoken about their illness. In addition, breast cancer's public face and force owes much to the far too many women who have suffered and died from this terrible disease.

The chapter authors have investigated breast cancer as a social problem, creating a framework to understand this illness in new ways. The authors have used a social lens to highlight the ways society and social institutions have shaped what we know about breast cancer and its impact on women and their lives. Whether examining how breast cancer research and policymaking are accomplished or how the media and social expectations influence women's breast cancer experiences, this book demonstrates that, all too frequently, the best interests of women and women with breast cancer are ignored or undermined.

CALLING FOR FUNDAMENTAL SOCIAL CHANGE

Most importantly, the chapters in this book raise a number of issues that will have to be addressed in order for the breast cancer epidemic to come to an end. Indeed, taken together, the chapters make clear the need for fundamental social change. Such change would include reframing how scientific research is conducted, making prevention rather than cure the goal of both research and clinical practice, eliminating corporate interests in making profits from the disease, and breaking the silence about environmental connections to breast cancer. Change also would include deconstructing the policymaking process so that political and economic interests are revealed, reversing the current path of the mismanaged health care delivery system, and bringing to the forefront the long-ignored needs of minority, disadvantaged, and underserved women with breast cancer. Social change also calls for exposing the misconceptions and false messages about breast cancer that women often receive, acknowledging the full range of women's breast cancer experiences, and making accurate and useful information about the disease available to women. It also calls for changing media portrayals of women with breast cancer, and strengthening the grass-roots breast cancer advocacy movement.

CHANGING THE SCIENCE OF BREAST CANCER

For example, in her chapter on breast cancer research, Sue V. Rosser argues that the ways that scientific research is conducted preclude finding answers to what women most want to know—how breast cancer can be prevented. Indeed, we may be astonished that, despite the many millions of dollars spent on basic and clinical cancer research, we still know little about the causes of breast cancer or the biological mechanisms of the disease. We do, however, have much, and often conflicting, information about the detection and treatment of the disease. Treatments for breast cancer (termed "slash, burn, and poison" by Dr. Susan Love) are still barbaric while methods of detection rely less on technology than on the simple act of an individual woman finding her own lump with her own hand. Rosser's cogent argument is that a male-defined, biomedical, scientific world not only has little interest in understanding breast cancer but also uses methods in breast cancer research that are flawed.

A different science of breast cancer would have research dollars and interested scientists probing for the causes of the disease as well as for more precise and reliable means of detecting it. Treatments would be less invasive and destructive yet assure survival and well-being. The scientific agenda would be set by, and grant applications reviewed with, the full participation of women living with breast cancer, equal to the decision-making authority of scientists. Social and behavioral studies would be at least as important as the current, overemphasized, biomedical investigations of genetic, molecular, and hormonal factors in breast cancer.

MOVING FROM CURE TO PREVENTION

It should come as no surprise that vast amounts of research money and effort are currently spent, sometimes unwisely, on treatments for breast cancer. Barron H. Lerner in his chapter on the history of breast cancer, points out that medicine was intent on transforming breast cancer from its long-time status as an incurable disease into a "curable" disease. Nineteenth-century medicine, as a social institution of increasing power, essentially saw breast cancer as an opportunity to put its newly acquired authority and technological skills to use. Surgeon William Halsted devised the radical mastectomy, an operation that removed large sections of a woman's anatomy, often leaving her with a collapsed chest wall and no greater chance of survival than with more limited surgery. Lerner makes it clear that the enduring idea of a "cure" for breast cancer was and is congruent with the social construction of medicine as a powerful, interventionist, and self-defining social institution. Then, as now, prevention was not a priority.

If history is to be instructive, it helps us to see that a search for a cure has been a fruitless quest for more than a century. The time for prevention to take center stage in breast cancer research and medical practice is long overdue. With the decline in power of traditional medical practices and the rise of complementary and alternative therapies, Americans may be more receptive to a paradigm of prevention than previously. Prevention means that disease does not occur because society and individuals have taken steps to promote the principles of public health, clean up and protect the environment, and end poverty, violence, and discrimination in all their forms. True prevention also means providing people with the resources to live in communities that support good jobs and housing, high standards of education, healthful food and health care, and strong values of civil engagement and social cooperation. However, real prevention still confronts formidable obstacles. One such obstacle might be gene therapy manipulations to insert genetic material in hopes of precluding the growth of cancer. Another prospect is of pharmaceutical companies offering the emotional appeal of prevention with a pill.

TO END PROFITING FROM BREAST CANCER

Jane S. Zones in her chapter on the political economy of breast cancer, helps explain why preventing breast cancer is still not a priority. The economics of breast cancer are such that its high visibility, the widespread fear it generates, and the tens of thousands of newly diagnosed women create new breast cancer customers each year. This disease is a growth industry in a capitalist marketplace (think of all those hospitals, doctors, radiation machines, and chemotherapy drugs ready for use). Women rightfully want answers, and they certainly need treatments when diagnosed with breast cancer. However, the proliferation of products, procedures, drugs, and devices have created a breast cancer supermarket. Yet, these offerings are not nearly as innocuous as a new brand of potato chip. Many have not been tested as rigorously as we have a right to expect given their import, long-term uses, and effects (in the case of new anticancer drugs); others (for example, genetic testing and high-dose chemotherapy) are of questionable therapeutic value; and still others (breast implants) have been sold to women as safe, and even necessary, although they are not a treatment for breast cancer. Zones argues that prevention, on the other hand, would provide profits to no one.

Preventing profit making from breast cancer will be difficult. In a hyperproductive economy predicated on marketing, selling, and profiting from increasing numbers of products and services, it is often difficult to distinguish between what is legitimately needed and what is an unnecessary or even dangerous item produced for profits. Guidelines are needed that would separate what is necessary, effective, and safe from what is solely in the interest of making money. A high-level, government-supported panel of informed women living with breast cancer, scientists concerned with the public interest, and enlightened members of industry could begin the task of discerning ways to accomplish this goal. Such a panel could be formed under the auspices of the National Action Plan on Breast Cancer, the President's National Cancer Advisory Board, or a to-be-created Citizen's Commission on Breast Cancer.

UNMASKING ENVIRONMENTAL CAUSES OF BREAST CANCER

Profits are important to the full range of industries, businesses, corporations, and the medical marketplace that are the economic engine of our society. However, as Sandra Steingraber points out, this engine is often a dirty, poisonous one that imperils the planet and may be a primary causal factor in breast cancer. In her chapter on the environment and breast cancer, Steingraber looks at the environmental evidence that most others ignore. While many breast cancer activists are increasingly calling for research into chemicals, pollutants, pesticides, and the associations between cancer clusters and industrial sites, manufacturers and others continue to ply arguments that no problem exists. Steingraber causes us to wonder if breast cancer is the canary in the mine that no one has realized has stopped breathing.

Thus, it is time to reverse the direction of the science on breast cancer and the environment. To date, few people have been willing to implicate environmental factors without scientific evidence of the certainty of cause and effect. This relationship is often difficult to prove, as scientists willingly admit. In the meantime, breast cancer and other cancers claim millions of lives. To reverse this trend, we should implement the Precautionary Principle, long articulated as both sensible and scientifically sound by public health experts. The Precautionary Principle calls for no substance to be released into the environment until it has been proven safe. In July 1999, the Second World Conference on Breast Cancer adopted a resolution calling for implementation of the Precautionary Principle, stating that "[r]elying on scientific certainty of human harm prevents action to reduce the incidence of breast cancer." In addition, we need far more research funding and attention paid to those many areas of the environment and environmental science that are promising but languish due to the lack of funds and commitment. We also must study and scrutinize environmental factors that have been hidden from public view because industries and polluters have had their public relations firms convince us that there is no link between profits and pollution.

REMAKING BREAST CANCER POLICYMAKING

In her chapter, Carol S. Weisman describes the world of breast cancer policymaking, the decisions society and its stakeholders make to allocate money, research, programs, and services to breast cancer. Weisman argues that the controversies that the salience of breast cancer has brought to public policy are evidence of the process of constructing breast cancer as a social problem. Many players, including Congress, government agencies, cancer organizations, industry, and advocacy groups, jockey for influence in the decisions that are made affecting the course of breast cancer research and treatment. These stakeholders know that breast cancer, unlike abortion, is a leading women's health issue with a broad, almost mom-and-apple pie appeal. Moreover, while everyone wants to be seen as an advocate for breast cancer, each stakeholder has its own political or economic agenda into which it hopes breast cancer will neatly fit. In fact, breast cancer does not fit neatly, as Weisman illustrates, leaving breast cancer decision making in the hands of often competing and powerful interests that may or may not coincide with the interests of women.

While we might hope that policymaking, unlike the economic interests of industry and the marketplace, would be governed by the more virtuous rules of public service, this is most often not the case. In particular, breast cancer has become fertile ground for influence peddling by various interests. Government agencies, such as the National Cancer Institute and its parent organization, the National Institutes of Health, have a vested interest in assuring the tax-paying public that we are winning the War on Cancer. Similarly, the American Cancer Society and other cancer organizations can increase contributions to their work only if people believe that progress against cancer is being made. Members of Congress want to please their constituents and appear to be doing good things for breast cancer. (When women with breast cancer were invisible and had little clout, Congress ignored the issue and allocated few dollars to research.) These and other stakeholders confound the policy-making process. What is needed is a policy agenda crafted by and in the interests of women. By reversing the status quo, the agenda would no longer be directed by Congress, government agencies, cancer organizations, medical specialties, and industry; instead, these players would be called upon as needed to support the agenda set by women.

LOOKING TOWARD A NEW HEALTH SYSTEM

One of the powerful forces with a stake in breast cancer are the industries and organizations that constitute the health care system. Whether this social institution that delivers the services we rely on to stay well and overcome illness can meet the needs of women with breast cancer is the subject of the chapter written by Ellen R. Shaffer. Shaffer provides abundant evidence that the current evolving health system is not meeting the needs of women with breast cancer. In addition, she indicts the ways this system is organized to generate profits at the expense of patients. As a result, women with breast cancer suffer the consequences of poor quality care, limited access to needed services, fragmented and disorganized care, bureaucratic miseries and mistakes, and gender, social class, race, and insurance discrimination. Shaffer argues that these frequently insurmountable obstacles are the result of the rise of corporate medicine, which is a marketplace for competition and profit making but an inappropriate structure for providing the accessible, coordinated, affordable, and appropriate services that women with breast cancer—and all patients—must have.

We can all remain witnesses to and patients in the current, unforgiving health system. Or, we can help to hasten its demise by becoming advocates for a system that serves people instead of profits. Many patients, health practitioners, policymakers, and activists have argued for a universal health care system to replace managed care. The idea of universal health care is not new and has been revisited several times this century. Some observers have argued that managed care might become so intolerable that universal health care might finally capture the political will of both patients and policymakers. At a time of economic prosperity, what better way to share the wealth than to provide the security of health services to all? Many nations, far less prosperous than the United States, have provided universal health care for a long time. Women with breast cancer would certainly benefit from such changes. Assurances that timely diagnosis, optimal and appropriate treatment and care are available would probably improve breast cancer statistics. Knowing care was assured would certainly remove the terror many women face not knowing if they are insured for or can afford breast cancer services.

MEETING THE NEEDS OF
UNDERSERVED WOMEN WITH BREAST CANCER

Poor women are one group of women who live with the terror of whether they will be treated when they find a breast lump. Anne S. Kasper, in her chapter on a group of 24 poor women with breast cancer, situates these women's lives in the larger social contexts of income inequality, poverty, and the ever-growing numbers of the uninsured. The women's difficult circumstances are indictments of a health system that fails to meet their needs and of a society that appears to deliberately ignore the lives and necessities of people who are poor. These women do not fit within the current health system not only because they are uninsured or underinsured, but because poverty has created formidable barriers and burdens the women cannot overcome when they are diagnosed with breast cancer. As a result, Kasper reports, the women faced delays of months or years before being diagnosed or treated, received treatments well below the standard of care for breast cancer, and encountered extraordinary difficulties when attempting to arrange for their own treatments and to care for themselves and their families. This picture of social inequality explains the women's high risk for more serious morbidity and mortality from breast cancer.

Poor women are but one of several groups of women who are at risk for being ill served for breast health and breast cancer care. Women of every racial and ethnic minority, medically underserved women, rural women, lesbians, geographically and socially isolated women, uninsured and underinsured women, and both older and younger women are all at risk. Breast cancer has long appeared to be an illness of white, middle- and upper-middle-class, heterosexual women because they are more likely to be insured, more likely to make health visits, and, of course, are portrayed as the stereotype of the U.S. female population. Breast cancer, however, knows no boundaries of race, social class, age, sexual orientation, or geography. Nevertheless, as some breast cancer activists have noted, the task of the breast cancer movement and, we would add, society at large, is to make visible and prominent the full diversity of women with breast cancer. It is not enough to have the faces of minority women on government reports and breast cancer brochures. Under served and ignored women with breast cancer must become full partners in activism, decision making, and the breast cancer agenda. Simultaneously, research, programs, and services to meet their breast health and breast cancer needs are urgently warranted. With representation in positions of influence of the full spectrum of women with breast cancer, the result will likely be research, programs, and services designed to meet the needs of all women with the disease.

CHANGING THE SOCIAL MESSAGES ABOUT BREAST CANCER

Women's experiences of breast cancer are affected by overt structural factors such as poverty. However, how women cope with the illness also is influenced by more subtle social factors, such as the messages women receive from the culture about their breasts, their bodies, and what it means to be a woman with breast cancer. In their chapter on women's experiences of breast cancer, Marcy E. Rosenbaum and Gun M. Roos explore the contradictions between society's expectations for women diagnosed with breast cancer and women's actual experiences with the illness. The authors illustrate these messages and discrepancies with the stories of three women diagnosed with breast cancer, and the reader vividly realizes that women with breast cancer face more than a disease, its consequences, and their potential mortality. The women also encounter and are forced to negotiate compelling and coercive messages about how they should behave and feel. The chapter clearly demonstrates how society has entered the hearts and minds of women with breast cancer, attempting to construct women's responses to their bodies and to this illness.

Difficult as it is to cope with breast cancer as a health crisis and as a life-threatening disease, women also confront the ways that society attempts to construct what it means to be a woman with breast cancer. In no other disease does a patient hear the social message that she will lose her gender identity and sexuality, suffer the loss of relationships, and be unable to renew her sense of herself. Breast cancer is unique as an illness because it continues to mirror socially sanctioned forms of discrimination against women. In spite of all the advances feminism has brought to women's lives, and the constancy of breast cancer advocates to shatter all forms of discrimination against women with breast cancer, further progress is needed. Women have begun the work of changing these social messages as individuals and in breast cancer support groups. We can be hopeful, moreover, as more women come forward to publicly recount their experiences and the power of their lives after breast cancer, and as women continue to become more empowered in all sectors of society, that these terrible psychological and emotional burdens will fall away.

ENDING MEDICAL CONTROL OF WOMEN'S BODIES

Susan J. Ferguson, in her chapter on the medicalization of women's breasts, demonstrates that society, historically, has not only sexually objectified women's breasts but viewed them as deformed or diseased. The messages women have received about breasts that do not conform to society's idealized image are that they should be treated medically—that is, shaped, reshaped, enlarged, implanted, and otherwise made to fit a socially defined breast size and shape. Women have, over time, undergone dangerous and even life-threatening procedures to have an almost unimaginable assortment of substances implanted in their breasts, ranging from small glass balls to ox cartilage to transformer coolant. This chapter delineates the historical continuum of breast augmentation in which twentieth-century silicone and saline implants are but the latest entry. Ferguson details how current breast implants are another abhorrent example in the long history of society's attempts to medicalize and control women, their bodies, and their breasts.

Controlling women and their breasts is a troubling aspect of medical practice regarding breast cancer. Women are offered breast implants and breast reconstruction after losing a breast because, their doctors tell them, these procedures are a part of breast cancer treatment. While implants and reconstruction do not treat cancer, physicians have defined them as doing so, thereby reinforcing social messages that women must have the appearance of two normal breasts in order to recover from breast cancer. At the same time, plastic and reconstructive surgeons also have created a lucrative addition to their medical practices. Before agreeing to any type of breast reconstruction, women must have more accurate information about and consider the medical risks and costs of additional surgery. They also need to know about the uncertain long-term effects of having an implanted device in their bodies, the possibilities of implant rupture and explantation (the surgical removal of the implant), and other problems associated with implants and reconstruction. With more information, women can weigh the risks and the social messages against their own best interests for health and well-being. Many women who have breast reconstruction report that replacing the breast lost to cancer did not play an important role in their recovery and their return to feeling good about themselves. While breast reconstruction and implants should remain options for all women, they should not be decreed an essential part of breast cancer treatment. The millions of dollars expended on these cosmetic procedures might be better spent on finding ways to prevent breast cancer.

REVISITING MEDIA PORTRAYALS
OF WOMEN WITH BREAST CANCER

Jennifer Fosket, Angela Karran, and Christine LaFia examined one source of the messages women receive about breast cancer. In their chapter on breast cancer in women's magazines, the authors reveal that popular women's magazines, widely thought to be reflective of women's viewpoints and concerns, are actually a powerful vehicle for transmitting society's expectations to women. The authors looked at magazine articles since 1913 and found that women were consistently told that all that they need to know about breast cancer is located within themselves. The pervasive message is that women are responsible for avoiding breast cancer through healthy behaviors and early detection, and that a positive attitude and looking attractive in the face of breast cancer are the keys to survival. The messages imply that failure to do so may explain why some women do not survive this disease. Women's magazines do not address social and environmental causes of breast cancer, nor are the articles concerned with access to care, discrimination, social class, or racial inequalities. Moreover, they rarely, if ever, tell the stories of women whose struggles with breast cancer end with suffering and death.

Women's magazines have long been a powerful purveyor of social messages to women. One of the reasons we read almost exclusively positive and uplifting magazine stories about women with breast cancer is because bad news does not sell in this form of popular literature. Magazine publishers and editors must answer to their advertisers, who want women to think of their products and services in an atmosphere of good feelings. However, there is another reason why these articles are about women's triumphs and happy endings with breast cancer. Many magazines and their advertisers are part of giant media and corporate conglomerates that may also own or have financial interests in an array of industries, chemical and manufacturing companies, as well as pharmaceutical, tobacco, insurance, medical, and other businesses. If magazine breast cancer stories moved beyond individual women's success stories and focused on the possible causes of breast cancer and its widespread destruction in the lives of women and their families, readers might begin to look for connections that owners of the media do not want them to see. Many women do triumph over breast cancer, and we enthusiastically celebrate their lives and health. However, the single-minded illusions sold in magazine form should be exposed for what they are, as well as for their connections to intersecting corporate interests, which may do as much to promote breast cancer as to pacify it.

GROWING THE GRASS-ROOTS BREAST CANCER MOVEMENT

Barbara A. Brenner, in her chapter on the breast cancer advocacy movement, traces the search of women with breast cancer to find support and answers they could not locate in a society that largely ignored them or treated them as pariahs. The women turned to each other and began to find the strength among themselves to both support one another and to challenge the medical, social, political, and economic issues constructing breast cancer. They challenged the status quo and, in so doing, became a bold movement for social change. As a result of their efforts, breast cancer has become, indisputably, the single most openly discussed women's health issue. As a result of this visibility, many activists in the breast cancer movement have recognized breast cancer as a social problem and created an opportunity to examine the social factors that influence how health and illness are socially constructed. In her chapter, Brenner also discusses how the growth of this movement has meant a divergence of views among differing organizations regarding research funding, political action, and other breast cancer agenda items, resulting in an unclear future for breast cancer advocacy.

The growth of the breast cancer movement, much like the growth of the contemporary Women's Health Movement before it, has resulted in a multiplicity of organizations, members, and interested others. A kind of mainstreaming has taken place in both movements, whereby a range of other interests have been added to the views and goals of the original founders. Some would call this democracy at work, while others would argue that the door has been open to those who would use women's health for personal, political, and profitable gain. One of the antidotes to the latter is to support the continuing grass-roots growth of the breast cancer movement, to assure that ordinary women have the strongest say in the direction of the breast cancer agenda, and to move away from self-interested corporate, government, medical, and other influences.

PROSPECTS FOR ENDING THE BREAST CANCER EPIDEMIC

What, then, does this volume tell us about breast cancer as a social problem and the prospects for bringing the epidemic of breast cancer to an end? The answer is that social changes that are necessary to eliminate breast cancer from our future will not come easily. However, this book has mapped some of the most important avenues of change to pursue. In addition, there is hope, more limited with some issues and more expansive with others, that changes are possible or already underway. For instance, there are some positive signs that breast cancer research is being modified. While we have no illusions that a major paradigm shift in the conduct of science and biomedicine is occurring, we do see some changes. The chapters in this book demonstrate that more breast cancer activists and concerned scientists are playing a role in setting the research agenda and the magnitude of funding. There have been important increases in behavioral and social sciences research in breast cancer, even at the National Institutes of Health, the home of biomedicine. In 1999, the Institute of Medicine of the National Academy of Sciences called for more research into cancer, minorities, and the underserved, and highlighted the need to address social causes of cancer.

There is also reason to be cautiously hopeful that attention will turn more toward prevention. The focus on preventive health measures, such as regular health visits, exercise, good nutrition, vitamins, and reducing stress, seems to have reached many Americans, making us health conscious in new ways. Americans have far more health information on a daily basis than ever before, and the proliferation of health magazines, brochures at drugstores and doctors' offices, and health sections in newspapers attest to the public's interest in health matters. However, messages about prevention are becoming muddled by the proliferation of pharmaceutical, nutraceutical, and other products, making it increasingly difficult for Americans to distinguish between prevention and cure. Perhaps most troubling, many individuals believe that prevention is dependent on their lifestyle choices and that it is not located in the social, economic, political, and environmental changes needed to avert disease.

One of the least promising areas for change may be eliminating financial interests in and profits made from breast cancer. As we have seen, many players, from pharmaceutical companies to cancer centers to Wall Street, have economic and political interests in breast cancer. In today's powerful, competitive, and globalized market, the creation and distribution of new products and services have taken on increasingly aggressive and persuasive practices. Much of this economic influence has been abetted by advertising and public relations firms that often exaggerate benefits, minimize risks, and make false claims, leaving the patient unsure of the accuracy of much needed, important information.

Similarly, the accuracy of reports of scientific breakthroughs may be difficult to assess when the work of some scientists is underwritten by corporations that benefit from findings in their favor. Women concerned about breast cancer may not know that some of the breast cancer or women's health organizations to which they turn for information may be supported by industries with vested interests in having their products, services, or images made visible.

Breast cancer policymaking is another challenge about which we should not be overly optimistic. As with the marketplace, we have seen that the policy process has multiple players with competing interests. Breast cancer's prominence in the health and medical worlds has yielded up many intersecting interest holders who want to influence funding, laws and regulations, policies, programs, and outcomes for breast cancer. Policymaking is inherently political and powerful, making it less likely to be in the interests of ordinary women with breast cancer.

We may have more reason to be sanguine about changes in the health care delivery system. Anger against managed care, the increasing numbers of the uninsured, and the reemergence of interest and political action on behalf of health care reform may bring changes to the health care delivery system that will be welcomed by women with breast cancer. We may also hold some cautious optimism about making the connections between breast cancer and the environment. Surveys show that more Americans care about the environment and would like to see it protected. Many citizens vote for environmental protection measures even when these same individuals vote against social and human service measures on their ballots. Whether this concern for the environment will translate into a willingness to call industries, chemical companies, and others to account for their role in causing disease remains to be seen.

There may be some reasons to be guardedly encouraged that minority and underserved women will eventually take their rightful place in the world of breast cancer. The increasing political will and clout of several minority groups (such as Latinos), as well as the proliferation of health activism and health education among groups of minority women augur well for these women. The nationwide breast and cervical cancer detection program for low-income and underserved women stands as an important model, despite its flaws, of federal efforts to reach these women with screening for both diseases. In addition, at this writing, there is some hope that medically underserved women screened in this program may find treatment services provided under a newly mandated provision in the Medicaid law.

The breast cancer advocacy movement has been at the forefront of changing some of the subtle but powerful social messages that have long discriminated against women with breast cancer. We have every reason to be encouraged by the willingness of women to expose false messages about what it means to be a woman with this illness. Women have claimed this territory, and fewer will allow themselves to be seen as defective, defeated, desexualized, and less a woman because they have breast cancer. In fact, many women now publicly, even proudly, wear the scars of their struggles. The full range of women's experiences with breast cancer also is gaining ground as women have become more vocal about their bodies, breasts, and breast cancer, even when they do not have positive outcomes. We can be hopeful that the media, and women's magazines in particular, will catch up with women's progress in these areas. Although women certainly like to hear good news, women want to see real lives portrayed. With breast cancer's conspicuousness, most women know that breast cancer is not always a triumphant story. Stories about women's unsuccessful struggles with breast cancer, including their death and dying, may be frightening, but they are also the truth telling of women's lives and are tributes to women's strength and power.

Finally, we can be optimistic that the strength of the grass-roots breast cancer movement will continue to grow. As the staggering numbers of women with breast cancer remain in the public eye and more women consider their breast cancer risks and those of their daughters and granddaughters, the acknowledgment that this epidemic can no longer be tolerated may grow. Although the public often tires of even the most outrageous occurrences if they are displayed or repeated too often, we can trust that breast cancer activists will find innovative ways to keep the focus clear on ways to end this epidemic.

Our hope, and that of the contributing authors, is that this book will have played some small part in creating workable strategies for eliminating breast cancer from all our futures.

REFERENCES

Second World Conference on Breast Cancer. 1999. "'Precautionary Principle' Resolution." Adopted by the Second World Conference on Breast Cancer, July 26-31, Ottawa, Canada. At http://www.brcancerconf.kos.net.

About the Contributors

BARBARA A. BRENNER holds an A.B. degree from Smith College (1973) and a J.D. degree from the University of California at Berkeley (Boalt Hall, 1981). Prior to her diagnosis of breast cancer for the first time at age 41, she was a partner in the San Francisco law firm of Remcho, Johansen & Purcell. Since 1995, Brenner has been Executive Director of Breast Cancer Action, a national education and advocacy organization based in San Francisco, California. She has been a "consumer" peer reviewer on the Department of Defense Breast Cancer Research Program, and now serves on the California Breast Cancer Research Council, the National Action Plan on Breast Cancer, and on numerous advisory boards for breast cancer projects.

SUSAN J. FERGUSON is an Associate Professor of Sociology at Grinnell College. She received her M.A. in sociology from Colorado State University in 1988 and her Ph.D. in sociology from the University of Massachusetts at Amherst in 1993. At Grinnell, Ferguson teaches courses on the sociology of the family, women and work, medical sociology, and research methods. Research within these areas includes the never married, racial-ethnic differences in marriage, and the intersection of gender and health, especially as it relates to the medicalization of women's health issues, such as breast cancer, breast implants, menopause, and women with HIV/AIDS. Ferguson has also edited two anthologies: *Mapping the Social Landscape: Readings in Sociology* (1996, 1999) and *Shifting the Center: Understanding Contemporary Families* (1998).

JENNIFER RUTH FOSKET is a Ph.D. candidate in sociology at the University of California, San Francisco. She is currently working on a dissertation that explores breast cancer risk and the politics of breast cancer prevention that emerge with pharmaceutical technologies such as the drugs tamoxifen and raloxifene.

ANGELA KARRAN is a sociology student, writer, and researcher. She received her B.A. from Mills College, and her work on chapter 10 in this volume reflects several years of writing and teaching in the field of media literacy, youth, and popular culture.

ANNE S. KASPER is a founding member of the contemporary U.S. Women's Health Movement. She also has been an activist, public policy expert, sociologist, and researcher in women's health for almost 30 years. As the first co-chair of the Board of Directors of the National Women's Health Network in 1976, she was instrumental in bringing national attention to women's health. From 1990 to 1994, Kasper was the Director of the Campaign for Women's Health, a national coalition of more than 100 organizations addressing health care reform. Kasper is a Senior Research Scientist with the Center for Research on Women and Gender at the University of Illinois at Chicago. She is also a partner in Finding My Way, an advocacy service for individual women with breast cancer.

CHRISTINE LAFIA received her Ph.D. in sociology from the University of Chicago after receiving an M.A. in international relations. In 1992, she joined the sociology faculty at Mills College. Her primary research interests included gender, work, mass media, and education. LaFia died in 1996 after fighting breast cancer.

BARRON H. LERNER is the Arnold P. Gold Foundation Assistant Professor of Medicine and Public Health at the Columbia University College of Physicians and Surgeons. A practicing internist, Lerner received his M.D. from Columbia in 1986 and his Ph.D. in history from the University of Washington in 1996. He is the author of *Contagion and Confinement: Controlling Tuberculosis along the Skid*

Road (1998) and is currently working on a book on the history of breast cancer screening and treatment in the twentieth century.

GUN M. ROOS is a researcher at the Finnish National Public Health Institute. Roos has an M.S. in nutritional sciences, and she received her Ph.D. in anthropology from the University of Kentucky. Roos is currently working on a qualitative exploration of health behavior and lifestyle among various occupational groups and a review of socioeconomic differences in food habits.

MARCY E. ROSENBAUM received her M.A. and Ph.D. in anthropology from the University of Kentucky. She is currently an Assistant Professor of Family Medicine at the University of Iowa College of Medicine. She has published in the areas of medical education and physician-patient communication. Her research interests include psychosocial oncology, qualitative health research, complementary and alternative medicine, and health communication.

SUE V. ROSSER received her Ph.D. in Zoology from the University of Wisconsin at Madison. She currently serves as Dean of the Ivan Allen College, the liberal arts college of the Georgia Institute of Technology in Atlanta, Georgia, where she is also Professor of History, Technology, and Society. She has published more than 80 journal articles on theoretical and applied aspects of women's health and women in science. She has authored eight books, including *Women's Health: Missing from U.S. Medicine* (1994), *Teaching the Majority* (1995), *Re-engineering Female Friendly Science* (1997), and *Women, Science, and Society: The Crucial Union* (2000).

ELLEN R. SHAFFER is Director of Policy for the Robert Wood Johnson Foundation Initiative on the Patient Provider Relationship in a Changing Health Care Environment. Shaffer was a senior staff advisor on health care in the United States Senate from 1992 to 1995 and has worked as a consultant on health system change in Washington, D.C., and San Francisco. Her publications include an article in the *New England Journal of Medicine* on the single-payer reform proposal, and she was a contributing editor for *The New Our*

Bodies, Ourselves (1998). She is completing a doctoral degree at the School of Public Health at Johns Hopkins University.

SANDRA STEINGRABER received her Ph.D. in biology from the University of Michigan. She is the author of the acclaimed *Living Downstream: An Ecologist Looks at Cancer and the Environment* (1997). The author of *Post-Diagnosis* (1995), a volume of poetry, and co-author of a report on ecology and human rights in Africa, *The Spoils of Famine* (1988), she has been called "a poet with a knife." She was recently appointed to serve on the National Action Plan on Breast Cancer. As an ecologist, she has conducted field work in northern Minnesota, East Africa, and Costa Rica. In 1997, Steingraber was named a Woman of the Year by *Ms.* magazine. Steingraber is currently a visiting faculty member at Cornell University's Center for the Environment in Ithaca, New York.

CAROL S. WEISMAN is Professor of Health Management and Policy and Director of the Interdepartmental Concentration in Reproductive and Women's Health at the University of Michigan School of Public Health in Ann Arbor, Michigan. She received her B.A. from Wellesley College and her Ph.D. in social relations from Johns Hopkins University. Her major research interests are in women's access to and use of health care services, quality assessment in women's health care, and organizational issues in health care delivery. She serves on the Board of Governors of the Jacobs Institute of Women's Health and as Associate Editor of *Women's Health Issues.* She is the author of over 70 publications, including *Women's Health Care: Activist Traditions and Institutional Change* (1998).

JANE SRAGUE ZONES is an adjunct faculty member of the Department of Social and Behavioral Sciences, School of Nursing, University of California, San Francisco. She received her Ph.D. in sociology from the University of North Carolina, Chapel Hill. A long-time women's health advocate, she currently chairs the California Women's Health Council and serves on the boards of Breast Cancer Action and the National Women's Health Network.

Index